Blueprints Notes & Cases
Pharmacology

Blueprints Notes & Cases
Series Editor: Aaron B. Caughey MD, MPP, MPH

Blueprints *Notes & Cases—Microbiology and Immunology*
Monica Gandhi, Paul Baum, C. Bradley Hare, Aaron B. Caughey

Blueprints *Notes & Cases—Biochemistry, Genetics, and Embryology*
Juan E. Vargas, Aaron B. Caughey, Annie Tan, Jonathan Z. Li

Blueprints *Notes & Cases—Pharmacology*
Katherine Y. Yang, Larissa R. Graff, Aaron B. Caughey

Blueprints *Notes & Cases—Pathophysiology: Cardiovascular, Endocrine, and Reproduction*
Gordon Leung, Susan H. Tran, Tina O. Tan, Aaron B. Caughey

Blueprints *Notes & Cases—Pathophysiology: Pulmonary, Gastrointestinal, and Rheumatology*
Michael Filbin, Lisa M. Lee, Brian L. Shaffer, Aaron B. Caughey

Blueprints *Notes & Cases—Pathophysiology: Renal, Hematology, and Oncology*
Aaron B. Caughey, Christie del Castillo, Nancy Palmer, Karen Spizer, Dana N. Tuttle

Blueprints *Notes & Cases—Neuroscience*
Robert T. Wechsler, Alexander M. Morss, Courtney J. Wusthoff, Aaron B. Caughey

Blueprints *Notes & Cases—Behavioral Science and Epidemiology*
Judith Neugroschl, Jennifer Hoblyn, Christie del Castillo, Aaron B. Caughey

Blueprints **Notes & Cases**
Pharmacology

Katherine Y. Yang, PharmD, MPH
Assistant Clinical Professor
Department of Clinical Pharmacy
School of Pharmacy
University of California, San Francisco
Infectious Diseases Clinical Pharmacist
University of California, San Francisco Medical Center
San Francisco, California

Larissa R. Graff, PharmD
Assistant Clinical Professor
Department of Clinical Pharmacy
School of Pharmacy
University of California, San Francisco
Clinical Pharmacist—Hematology/Oncology
University of California, San Francisco Medical Center
San Francisco, California

Aaron B. Caughey, MD, MPP, MPH
Clinical Instructor in Maternal-Fetal Medicine
Department of Obstetrics and Gynecology
University of California, San Francisco
San Francisco, California
Doctoral Candidate, Health Services and Policy Analysis
University of California, Berkeley
Berkeley, California

Series Editor: Aaron B. Caughey, MD, MPP, MPH

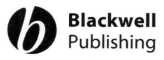
Blackwell
Publishing

© 2004 by Blackwell Publishing

Blackwell Publishing, Inc., 350 Main Street, Malden, Massachusetts 02148-5018, USA
Blackwell Publishing Ltd, 9600 Garsington Road, Oxford OX4 2DQ, UK
Blackwell Science Asia Pty Ltd, 550 Swanston Street, Carlton, Victoria 3053, Australia

03 04 05 06 5 4 3 2 1

ISBN: 1–4051-0348-5

Library of Congress Cataloging-in-Publication Data

Yang, Katherine Y.
    Blueprints notes & cases : pharmacology / Katherine Y. Yang, Larissa R. Graff, Aaron B. Caughey.
        p. ; cm. — (Blueprints notes & cases)
    Includes index.
    ISBN 1-4051-0348-5 (pbk.)
    1. Pharmacology—Case studies.
    [DNLM: 1. Drug Therapy—Case Report. 2. Drug Therapy—Problems and Exercises. 3. Pharmacology—Case Report.
  4. Pharmacology—Problems and Exercises. QV 18.2 Y219b 2004] I. Title: Pharmacology. II. Title: Blueprints notes and cases
  III. Graff, Larissa R. IV. Caughey, Aaron B. V. Title. VI. Series.
    RM301.14.Y36 2004
    615′.7—dc21   2003010569

A catalogue record for this title is available from the British Library

Acquisitions: Beverly Copland
Development: Julia Casson
Production: Debra Lally
Cover design: Hannus Design Associates
Interior design: Janet Alleyn
Typesetter: Peirce Graphic Services in Stuart, Florida
Printed and bound by Courier Companies in Westford, MA

For further information on Blackwell Publishing, visit our website: www.blackwellpublishing.com

Notice: The indications and dosages of all drugs in this book have been recommended in the
medical literature and conform to the practices of the general community. The medications
described do not necessarily have specific approval by the Food and Drug Administration for
use in the diseases and dosages for which they are recommended. The package insert for each
drug should be consulted for use and dosage as approved by the FDA. Because standards for
usage change, it is advisable to keep abreast of revised recommendations, particularly those
concerning new drugs.

Contents

Contributors

Robin L. Corelli, PharmD
Associate Clinical Professor
Department of Clinical Pharmacy
University of California, San Francisco, School of Pharmacy
San Francisco, California

Cathi Dennehy, PharmD, FCSHP
Assistant Clinical Professor
Department of Clinical Pharmacy
University of California, San Francisco, School of Pharmacy
San Francisco, California

Mai-Trang N. Dang, PharmD
Clinical Instructor
University of Washington School of Pharmacy
Clinical Pharmacist
University of Washington Medical Center
Seattle, Washington

Vicky Dudas, PharmD
Assistant Clinical Professor
Department of Clinical Pharmacy
University of California, San Francisco, School of Pharmacy
Infectious Disease Clinical Pharmacist
University of California, San Francisco Medical Center
San Francisco, California

Patrick Finley, PharmD, BCPP
Associate Clinical Professor
Department of Clinical Pharmacy
University of California, San Francisco, School of Pharmacy
Psychiatric Pharmacist
University of California, San Francisco Women's Health
Center
San Francisco, California

Jamie H. Hirata, PharmD
Clinical Pharmacist
University of California, San Francisco, Medical Center
San Francisco, California

Lisa Kroon, PharmD, CDE
Associate Clinical Professor
Department of Clinical Pharmacy
University of California, San Francisco, School of Pharmacy
Clinical Pharmacist
UCSF Diabetes Practice
The Medical Center at the University of California, San
Francisco
San Francisco, California

Kelly C. Lee, PharmD
Fellow, Clinical Pharmacy
University of California, San Francisco, School of Pharmacy
University of California, San Francisco Medical Center
San Francisco, California

Lisa M. Mitsunaga, PharmD
Assistant Clinical Professor
Department of Clinical Pharmacy
University of California, San Francisco, School of Pharmacy
Clinical Pharmacist, Neurological Surgery
Department of Pharmaceutical Services
University of California, San Francisco Medical Center
San Francisco, California

David J. Quan, PharmD
Assistant Clinical Professor
Department of Clinical Pharmacy
University of California, San Francisco, School of Pharmacy
Clinical Pharmacist
University of California, San Francisco Medical Center
San Francisco, California

Deepa Setty, PharmD
Assistant Clinical Professor
Department of Clinical Pharmacy
University of California, San Francisco, School of Pharmacy
Clinical Pharmacist, Neurosurgery
University of California, San Francisco Medical Center
San Francisco, California

Cindy H. Shih, PharmD
Clinical Specialist
MedImpact Healthcare Systems, Inc
San Diego, California

Eunice Tam, PharmD
Clinical Pharmacist
University of California, San Francisco Medical Center
San Francisco, California
Clinical Pharmacist
Veterans Affairs Hospital of Palo Alto
Palo Alto, California

Lisa M. Tong, PharmD
Assistant Clinical Professor
Department of Clinical Pharmacy
University of California, San Francisco, School of Pharmacy
Clinical Pharmacist
University of California San Francisco Medical Center
San Francisco, California

Candy Tsourounis, PharmD, FCSHP
Associate Clinical Professor
Department of Clinical Pharmacy
University of California, San Francisco, School of Pharmacy
San Francisco, California

Michael E. Winter
Professor and Vice Chair
Department of Clinical Pharmacy
University of California, San Francisco, School of Pharmacy
San Francisco, California

Sharon Youmans, PharmD
Assistant Professor of Clinical Pharmacy
Department of Clinical Pharmacy
University of California, San Francisco, School of Pharmacy
San Francisco, California

Courtney Yuen, PharmD
Assistant Clinical Professor
Department of Clinical Pharmacy
University of California, San Francisco, School of Pharmacy
Oncology Pharmacist
University of California San Francisco Medical Center
San Francisco, California

Reviewers

Celeste Chu
Class of 2004
Washington University School of Medicine
St. Louis, Missouri

Andrew N. Cohen
Class of 2004
New York College of Osteopathic Medicine
Glen Cove, New York

Minisha Kochar
Class of 2004
Temple University School of Medicine
Philadelphia, Pennsylvania

Arne Olson
Class of 2004
Medical College of Wisconsin
Milwaukee, Wisconsin

Kevin N. Sheth
Class of 2003
University of Pennsylvania Medical School
Philadelphia, Pennsylvania

Evelyn R. Vento
Class of 2004
State University of New York at Buffalo School of Medicine
and Biomedical Sciences
Buffalo, New York

Preface

The first two years of medical school are a demanding time for medical students. Whether the school follows a traditional curriculum or one that is case-based, every student is expected to learn and be able to apply basic science information in a clinical situation.

Medical schools are increasingly using clinical presentations as the background to teach the basic sciences. Case-based learning has become more common at many medical schools as it offers a way to catalogue the multitude of symptoms, syndromes, and diseases in medicine.

Blueprints **Notes & Cases is a new series by Blackwell Publishing designed to provide students a textbook to study the basic science topics combined with clinical data.** This method of learning is also the way to prepare for the clinical case format of USMLE questions. The eight books in this series will make the basic science topics not only more interesting, but also more meaningful and memorable. Students will be learning not only the why of a principle, but also how it might commonly be seen in practice.

The books in the *Blueprints* Notes & Cases series feature a comprehensive collection of cases that are designed to introduce one or more basic science topics. Through these cases, students gain an understanding of the coursework as they learn to:

- Think through the cases
- Look for classic presentations of most common diseases and syndromes
- Integrate the basic science content with clinical application
- Prepare for course exams and Step 1 USMLE
- Be prepared for clinical rotations

This series covers all the essential material needed in the basic science courses. Where possible, the books are organized in an organ-based system.

Clinical cases lead off and are the basis for discussion of the basic science content.

A list of **"thought questions"** follows the case presentation. These questions are designed to challenge the reader to begin to think about how basic science topics apply to real-life clinical situations. The **answers to these questions** are integrated within the **basic science review and discussion** that follows. This offers a clinical framework from which to understand the basic content.

The discussion section is followed by a high-yield **Thumbnail table and Key Points box,** which highlight and summarize the essential information presented in the discussion.

The cases also include two **multiple-choice questions** that allow readers to check their knowledge of that topic. Many of the answer explanations provide an opportunity for further discussion by delving into more depth in related areas. An **answer key** for these questions is at the end of the book for easy reference, and **full answer explanations** can be found at the end of the book, as well.

This new series was designed to provide comprehensive content in a concise and templated format for ease in learning. A dedicated attempt was made to include sufficient art, tables, and clinical treatment, all while keeping the books from becoming too lengthy. We know you have much to read and that what you want is high-yield, vital facts.

The authors and series editor for these eight books, as well as everyone in editorial, production, sales and marketing at Blackwell Publishing, have worked long and hard to provide new textbooks to help you learn and be able to apply what you've learned. We engaged in multiple student email surveys and many focus groups to "hear what you needed" in new basic science level textbooks to meet the current curriculums, tests, and coursework. We know that you value this "student to student" approach, and sincerely hope you like what we have put together **just for you.**

Blackwell Publishing and the authors wish you success in your studies and your future medical career. Please feel free to offer us any comments or suggestions on these new books at blue@bos.blackwellpublishing.com.

Dedication

To my parents, Warren and Sandy, for their constant encouragement and support. And to my husband, Ray, for his love, patience, and never-ending faith in me.
—Katherine Y. Yang

To my parents, Donald and Theodora, and my sister Dena. Thank you for your love, support, and encouragement. To my husband, Micheal, for all your patience, friendship, and love. And to my daughter, Riley, for inspiring me to see life in so many new and exciting ways.
—Larissa R. Graff

We would like to thank all of the staff at Blackwell, in particular Julia and Jen who kept us organized and on track. I want to thank Kathy and Larissa for organizing and revising the text and tables. I would also like to acknowledge the support I receive from my mentors at UCSF and UC Berkeley, Gene Washington, Mary Norton, Miriam Kuppermann, Hal Luft, Jamie Robinson, Matthew Rabin, and Teh-Wei Hu. I also want to thank my parents, Bill and Carol, my siblings Ethan and Samara, my closest friends Jim and Wendy and my wife, Susan, for all of the support over the years.
—Aaron B. Caughey

Abbreviations

5-FU	fluorouracil		BTB	break-through bleeding
5-HT	serotonin		BUN	blood urea nitrogen
Ab	antibody		c/o	complaints of
ABVD	Adriamycin (doxorubicin) + bleomycin + vinblastine + dacarbazine		CABG	coronary artery bypass graft
			CAD	coronary artery disease
AC	Adriamycin (doxorubicin) + cyclophosphamide		cAMP	cyclic adenosine monophosphate
ACE	angiotensin-converting enzyme		CBC	complete blood count
ACE-I	angiotensin-converting enzyme inhibitor		CBG	cortisol binding globulin
ACLS	advanced cardiac life support		CBZ	carbamazepine
ACS	acute coronary syndrome		CC	chief complaint
ADA	American Diabetic Association		CD	cluster differentiation
ADH	antidiuretic hormone		CEE	conjugated equine estrogen
ADP	adenosine diphosphate		CHD	coronary heart disease
AF	atrial fibrillation		CHF	congestive heart failure
AFI	atrial flutter		CK	creatine kinase
AIDS	acquired immunodeficiency syndrome		CML	chronic myelogenous leukemia
Alb	albumin		CMV	cytomegalovirus
AlkPhos	alkaline phosphatase		CNS	central nervous system
ALL	acute lymphocytic leukemia		COC	combined oral contraceptive
ALL	allergies		COPD	chronic obstructive pulmonary disease
ALT	alanine aminotransferase		COX	cyclooxygenase
AML	acute myelogenous leukemia		CP	chest pain
ANA	antinuclear antibody		Cr	creatinine
ANC	absolute neutrophil count		CrCl	creatinine clearance
aPTT	activated partial thromboplastin time (may be PTT)		CRP	C-reactive protein
AraC	cytarabine		CSA	cyclosporine
ARB	angiotensin receptor blocker		CSF	cerebral spinal fluid
ARV	antiretrovirals		CXR	chest x-ray
AST	aspartate aminotransferase		CYP450	cytochrome P-450
ATG	antithymocyte globulin		D_2	dopamine
AV node	atrioventricular node		DES	diethylstilbestrol
bid	twice daily		DHE	dihydroergotamine
BMD	bone mineral density		DHFR	dihydrofolate reductase
BMI	body mass index		DM	diabetes mellitus
BP	blood pressure		DMARD	disease modifying anti-rheumatic drug
BPH	benign prostatic hypertrophy		DMPA	depo-medroxyprogesterone acetate

DNA	deoxyribonucleic acid	HCTZ	hydrochlorothiazide
DPH	phenytoin	HCV	hepatitis C virus
DTR	deep tendon reflex	HDL	high density lipoprotein
DVT	deep vein thrombosis	HgbA1c	hemoglobin A1c
EBV	Epstein-Barr virus	Hgb	hemoglobin
ECG	electrocardiography	HHV	human herpes virus
ED	emergency department	HIT	heparin-induced thrombocytopenia
EE	ethinyl estradiol	HIV	human immunodeficiency virus
EF	ejection fraction	HR	heart rate
EGD	esophagogastroduodenoscopy	HRT	hormone replacement therapy
EIB	exercise-induced bronchospasm	HSV	herpes simplex virus
EPS	extrapyramidal symptoms	HTN	hypertension
ER	estrogen receptor	IBD	inflammatory bowel disease
ESR	erythrocyte sedimentation rate	ICD	implantable automatic cardioverter defibrillation
FAC	fluorouracil + Adriamycin (doxorubicin) + cyclophosphamide	ICU	intensive care unit
FBG	fasting blood glucose	IFG	impaired fasting glucose
FDA	Food and Drug Administration	IL-2	interleukin 2
FEV1	forced expiratory volume in the first second	IM	intramuscular
FH	family history	IN	intranasal
FNA	fine needle aspirate	INR	international normalized ratio
FSH	follicle stimulating hormone	IOP	intraocular pressure
FVC	forced vital capacity	ISDN	isosorbide dinitrate
G6PD	glucose-6-phosphate dehydrogenase	ISA	intrinsic sympathomimetic
GABA	gamma aminobutyric acid	ISH	isolated systolic hypertension
GAD	generalized anxiety disorder	ISMO	isosorbide mononitrate
GERD	gastroesophageal reflux disease	IV	intravenous
GFR	glomerular filtration rate	kg	kilogram
GI	gastrointestinal	LDH	lactate dehydrogenase
GIST	gastrointestinal stromal tumor	LDL	low density lipoprotein
GMP	guanosine monophosphate	LES	lower esophageal sphincter
GpIIb/IIIa	glycoprotein IIb/IIIa	LFTs	liver function tests
GT	gastric tube	LH	luteinizing hormone
GX	glycinexylidide	LHRH	luteinizing hormone releasing hormone
GxPy	gravidy (x = # pregnancy) parody (y = # deliveries)	LLE	left lower extremity
HAART	highly active antiretroviral therapy	LMWH	low molecular weight heparin
HCT	hematocrit	LNG	levonorgestrel
		LP	lumbar puncture

Lytes	electrolytes	PCP	*Pneumocystis carinii* pneumonia
MAO	monoamine oxidase	PE	physical exam
MEGX	monoethylglycinexylidide	PE	pulmonary embolism
mg	milligram	PFT	pulmonary function tests
MI	myocardial infarction	PGT	per gastric tube
mL	milliliter	Ph+	Philadelphia chromosome
MOA	mechanism of action	PI	protease inhibitor
MoAb	monoclonal antibody	PICC	peripherally inserted central catheter
MPA	medroxyprogesterone acetate	Plt	platelets
MRSA	methicillin-resistant *Staphylococcus aureus*	PMH	past medical history
MRSE	methicillin-resistant *Staphylococcus epidermidis*	PMN	polymorphonuclear
msec	millisecond	PO	per oral
MTB	*Mycobacterium tuberculosis*	POAG	primary open angle glaucoma
N/V	nausea/vomiting	PPI	proton pump inhibitor
NAPA	*N*-acetylprocainamide	PR	per rectum
NE	norepinephrine	PSVT	paroxysmal supraventricular tachycardia
NGU	nongonococcal urethritis	PT	prothrombin time
NHL	non-Hodgkin's lymphoma	PTSD	posttraumatic stress disorder
NK	natural killer	PTU	propylthiouracil
NKDA	no known drug allergies	PUD	peptic ulcer disease
NMS	neuroleptic malignant syndrome	PVC	premature ventricular contraction
NNRTI	non-nucleoside reverse transcriptase inhibitor	PVD	peripheral vascular disease
NPO	nothing per oral	RA	rheumatoid arthritis
NRTI	nucleoside reverse transcriptase inhibitor	RAI	radioactive iodine
NS	normal saline	RBC	red blood cells
NSAID	nonsteroidal anti-inflammatory drug	RNA	ribonucleic acid
NSR	normal sinus rhythm	RR	respiratory rate
NtRTI	nucleotide reverse transcriptase inhibitor	RSV	respiratory syncytial virus
OA	osteoarthritis	RT	reverse transcriptase
OCD	obsessive compulsive disorder	RUQ	right upper quadrant
OD	right eye	s/p	status post
OS	left eye	Sao$_2$	oxygen saturation
PACU	postanesthesia care unit	SC	subcutaneous
PB	phenobarbital	SCD	sequential compression device
PBP	penicillin binding protein	SCLC	small cell lung cancer
PCA	patient controlled analgesia	SCr	serum creatinine
PCI	percutaneous coronary intervention	SE	status epilepticus

SERMs	selective estrogen receptor modulators		TMP	trimethoprim
SH	social history		TMP-SMX	trimethoprim-sulfamethoxazole
SHBG	sex-hormone binding globulin		topo	topoisomerase
SIADH	syndrome of inappropriate secretion of ADH		TSH	thyroid-stimulating hormone
SL	sublingual		TXA2	thromboxane A2
SLE	systemic lupus erythematosus		UA	urinalysis
SOB	shortness of breath		UC	ulcerative colitis
SPS	sodium polystyrene sulfonate		UFH	unfractionated heparin
SSRI	selective serotonin reuptake inhibitor		ULN	upper limit of normal
STD	sexually transmitted disease		UTI	urinary tract infection
SuVT	sustained ventricular tachycardia		VAD	vincristine + Adriamycin (doxorubicin) + dexamethasone
T_3	triiodothyronine		VF	ventricular fibrillation
T_4	thyroxine (aka levothyroxine)		VLDL	very low density lipoprotein
$T^{1/2}$	half-life		VP16	etoposide
TB	tuberculosis		VPA	valproic acid
TBG	thyroid binding globulin		VS	vital signs
Tbili	total bilirubin		VT	ventricular tachycardia
TCA	tricyclic antidepressant		VZV	varicella zoster virus
TD	tardive dyskinesia		WBC	white blood cell
TED	thromboembolic deterrent		wnl	within normal limits
Temp or T	temperature		Wt	weight
TG	triglycerides			

Normal Ranges of Laboratory Values

BLOOD, PLASMA, SERUM

Alanine aminotransferase (ALT, GPT at 30 C)	8–20 U/L
Amylase, serum	25–125 U/L
Aspartate aminotransferase (AST, GOT at 30 C)	8–20 U/L
Bilirubin, serum (adult) Total // Direct	0.1–1.0 mg/dL // 0.0–0.3 mg/dL
Calcium, serum (Ca^{2+})	8.4–10.2 mg/dL
Cholesterol, serum	Rec: < 200 mg/dL
Cortisol, serum	0800 h: 5–23 μg/dL // 1600 h: 3–15 μg/dL
	2000 h: $\leq$ 50% of 0800 h
Creatine kinase, serum	Male: 25–90 U/L
	Female: 10–70 U/L
Creatinine, serum	0.6–1.2 mg/dL
Electrolytes, serum	
Sodium (Na^+)	136–145 mEq/L
Chloride (Cl^-)	95–105 mEq/L
Potassium (K^+)	3.5–5.0 mEq/L
Bicarbonate (HCO_3^-)	22–28 mEq/L
Magnesium (Mg^{2+})	1.5–2.0 mEq/L
Ferritin, serum	Male: 15–200 ng/mL
	Female: 12–150 ng/mL
Follicle-stimulating hormone, serum/plasma	Male: 4–25 mIU/mL
	Female: premenopause 4–30 mIU/mL
	midcycle peak 10–90 mIU/mL
	postmenopause 40–250 mIU/mL
Gases, arterial blood (room air)	
pH	7.35–7.45
P_{CO_2}	33–45 mm Hg
PO_2	75–105 mm Hg
Glucose, serum	Fasting: 70–110 mg/dL
	2-h postprandial: < 120 mg/dL
Growth hormone—arginine stimulation	Fasting: < 5 ng/mL
	provocative stimuli: > 7 ng/mL
Iron	50–70 μg/dL
Lactate dehydrogenase, serum	45–90 U/L
Luteinizing hormone, serum/plasma	Male: 6–23 mIU/mL
	Female: follicular phase 5–30 mIU/mL
	midcycle 75–150 mIU/mL
	postmenopause 30–200 mIU/mL
Osmolality, serum	275–295 mOsmol/kg
Parathyroid hormone, serum, N-terminal	230–630 pg/mL
Phosphate (alkaline), serum (p-NPP at 30 C)	20–70 U/L
Phosphorus (inorganic), serum	3.0–4.5 mg/dL
Prolactin, serum (hPRL)	< 20 ng/mL
Proteins, serum	
Total (recumbent)	6.0–7.8 g/dL
Albumin	3.5–5.5 g/dL
Globulin	2.3–3.5 g/dL
Thyroid-stimulating hormone, serum or plasma	0.5–5.0 μU/mL
Thyroidal iodine (^{123}I) uptake	8–30% of administered dose/24 h
Thyroxine (T_4), serum	5–12 μg/dL
Transferrin	221–300 μg/dL
Triglycerides, serum	35–160 mg/dL
Triiodothyronine (T_3), serum (RIA)	115–190 ng/dL
Triiodothyronine (T_3), resin uptake	25–35%
Urea nitrogen, serum (BUN)	7–18 mg/dL
Uric acid, serum	3.0–8.2 mg/dL

CEREBROSPINAL FLUID

Cell count	0–5 cells/mm^3
Chloride	118–132 mEq/L
Gamma globulin	3–12% total proteins
Glucose	40–70 mg/dL
Pressure	70–180 mm H$_2$O
Proteins, total	< 40 mg/dL

HEMATOLOGIC

Bleeding time (template)	2–7 minutes
Erythrocyte count	Male: 4.3–5.9 million/mm^3
	Female: 3.5–5.5 million/mm^3
Erythrocyte sedimentation rate (Westergren)	Male: 0–15 mm/h
	Female: 0–20 mm/h
Hematocrit	Male: 41–53%
	Female: 36–46%
Hemoglobin A$_{1C}$	≤ 6%
Hemoglobin, blood	Male: 13.5–17.5 g/dL
	Female: 12.0–16.0 g/dL
Leukocyte count and differential	
Leukocyte count	4500–11,000/mm^3
Segmented neutrophils	54–62%
Bands	3–5%
Eosinophils	1–3%
Basophils	0–0.75%
Lymphocytes	25–33%
Monocytes	3–7%
Mean corpuscular hemoglobin	25.4–34.6 pg/cell
Mean corpuscular hemoglobin concentration	31–36% Hb/cell
Mean corpuscular volume	80–100 μm^3
Partial thromboplastin time (activated)	25–40 seconds
Platelet count	150,000–400,000/mm^3
Prothrombin time	11–15 seconds
Reticulocyte count	0.5–1.5% of red cells
Thrombin time	< 2 seconds deviation from control
Volume	
Plasma	Male: 25–43 mL/kg
	Female: 28–45 mL/kg
Red cell	Male: 20–36 mL/kg
	Female: 19–31 mL/kg

SWEAT

Chloride	0–35 mmol/L

URINE

Calcium	100–300 mg/24 h
Chloride	Varies with intake
Creatine clearance	Male: 97–137 mL/min
	Female: 88–128 mL/min
Osmolality	50–1400 mOsmol/kg
Oxalate	8–40 μg/mL
Potassium	Varies with diet
Proteins, total	< 150 mg/24 h
Sodium	Varies with diet
Uric acid	Varies with diet

Presentation 1 HPI: BK is a 72-year-old 60-kg man who is admitted to the hospital for treatment of sepsis. He has a long history of diabetes mellitus for which he has been receiving glipizide. He has a leg wound that is erythematous and tender. Blood cultures and a needle aspirate of the leg ulcer were taken and sent to the laboratory for culture and sensitivity.

Labs: His labs include serum creatinine (Cr) level 2.4 mg/dL, blood urea nitrogen (BUN) 44 mg/dL, fasting blood glucose (FBG) 85 mg/dL, white blood cell (WBC) count 18,000/mL. He is currently febrile at 38.5°C. He has an allergy to penicillin (rash and shortness of breath).

As empiric therapy for sepsis and the leg ulcer, BK is started on vancomycin 1 g intravenously (IV) every 12 hours and tobramycin 100 mg IV every 8 hours.

Thought Questions

- What is BK's renal function?

- Should vancomycin or tobramycin therapy be initiated with a "loading" dose?

- Is the initial maintenance dose appropriate?

- If a decrease in the "dose" is required, would it be more appropriate to decrease the dose and maintain the same interval or to keep the same dose and extend the interval?

Presentation 2 HPI: TE is a 62-year-old 75-kg man who is admitted to the hospital for shortness of breath (SOB) and "palpitations." He has experienced in the past short episodes of "chest pounding," but previously it always spontaneously resolved. TE has essentially normal laboratory values. Electrocardiography indicates he is in atrial fibrillation. His previous medical history (PMH) is significant for hypertension treated with hydrochlorothiazide only. He has no known drug allergies (NKDA).

For initial treatment, TE is to be given a 1-mg loading dose of digoxin IV and then started on a maintenance dose of 0.25 mg every morning orally (PO). Following rate control, TE is to be started on amiodarone 400 mg a day PO for 1 month and then the maintenance dose will be reduced to 200 mg each morning PO. He was instructed to continue on the hydrochlorothiazide.

Thought Questions

- Is the loading dose of digoxin appropriate for TE?

- Is TE's maintenance dose appropriate?

Basic Pharmacokinetic Principles

Absorption (Bioavailability) It is assumed that when a drug is given parenterally (IV) that the entire dose is available for pharmacologic effect. Following oral administration not all drugs are completely or even well absorbed (i.e., have a limited or poor oral bioavailability). Absorption following oral administration is a complex process, and any number of factors can limit absorption, including water versus lipid solubility, stability of the drug in the gastrointestinal (GI) tract, and metabolism by enzymes in the gut wall or liver.

Volume of Distribution Volume of distribution is the space in which the drug appears to distribute. Volume of distribution is a complex relationship between water and lipid solubility, drug binding to plasma and tissue proteins, and active transport systems.

Volume of distribution can be used to estimate a loading dose in order to rapidly achieve effective drug concentrations and therapeutic effects. In clinical practice the use of a loading dose is not always necessary. The three most common reasons for not administering a loading dose are (a) the first maintenance achieves a therapeutic effect, (b) the nonacute clinical setting dictates that immediate effect is not necessary or desirable, and (c) the pharmacologic effect is delayed due to a sequence of biologic processes.

Volume of Distribution, Two Compartment Model Following rapid intravenous administration, most drugs have an initial distribution phase where drug is distributing from plasma to the more slowly equilibrating tissues (Figure 1-1).

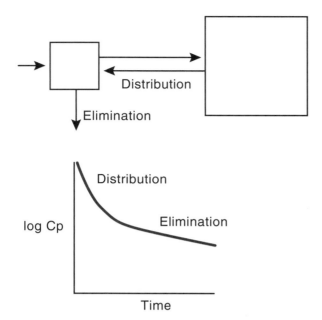

Figure 1-1 Plasma drug concentrations.

The above graph depicts plasma drug concentrations following rapid input into the plasma compartment. The initial rapid decline represents a distribution phase where drug is moving into the more slowly equilibrating tissues. The elimination phase represents equilibrium between the rapidly and slowly equilibrating tissues and drug elimination from the body.

Because of the potential for an intense and rapid onset of drug effect when the initial drug concentrations are high, the rate at which many drugs are infused into the body must be carefully controlled.

Clearance   Clearance is the term describing how the body eliminates solute from the body. Clearance is the key pharmacokinetic parameter to consider when determining maintenance doses of drugs.

For most drugs the two primary routes of clearance or elimination are hepatic, renal, or a combination of these two pathways. As a general rule the maintenance dose of a drug would be reduced in proportion to the patient's decrease in clearance.

Hepatic Clearance   Patients with significant hepatic dysfunction would be expected to have a decreased ability to metabolize or clear drugs. An increase in liver enzymes (aspartate aminotransferase [AST], alanine aminotransferase [ALT], and alkaline phosphatase [AlkPhos]) or an increase in bilirubin, prothrombin time and a decrease in serum albumin usually indicates hepatic dysfunction.

Renal Clearance   Serum creatinine and **creatinine clearance** (CrCl) rate are the most common measurements of renal

function. In adult patients the normal value for serum Cr is 1 mg/dL (range 0.7 to 1.4) and in the average 70-kg young individual (approximately 20 to 30 years of age) this serum Cr corresponds to a CrCl rate of approximately 100 mL/min. As a general rule every doubling of the serum Cr represents a halving of a patient's renal function.

The following equation by Cockcroft and Gault, which considers age, weight, sex, and serum Cr at steady state, is commonly used to estimate CrCl rate.

Creatinine clearance (mL/min) =
$$\frac{(140 - \text{age in years})(\text{weight in kg})}{(72)(\text{Cr in mg/dL})} (0.85 \text{ if female})$$

Capacity-Limited Metabolism   For some drugs clearance changes with the drug concentration. Increases in maintenance doses will result in a disproportionate increase in the steady-state drug concentration. Phenytoin is the classic capacity-limited drug.

Half-Life   The drug half-life ($T\frac{1}{2}$) is defined as the time required for the drug to decline by half (Figure 1-2).

The $T\frac{1}{2}$ is determined by the drug's volume of distribution and clearance or elimination from the body. $T\frac{1}{2}$ can be used to determine the rate at which the drug will accumulate once a maintenance regimen is started. In one half-life a drug will achieve 50% of the final steady state plateau value, in two half-lives 75%, in three 87.5%, and in 3.3 half-lives 90% of steady state (Figure 1-3).

Most clinicians use between 3.3 and 5 half-lives as the time required to achieve steady state.

Half-life is also useful in determining the dosing interval. For some drugs the goal is to maintain a relatively constant drug concentration. In these cases the drug should be either given as a constant IV infusion, a sustained oral dosage form, or with a dosing interval that is short compared with the drug $T\frac{1}{2}$. In other cases, it is clinically acceptable to have wide swings in the drug concentration within the dosing interval (drugs with a wide therapeutic window or a

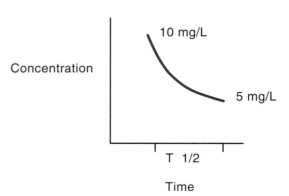

Figure 1-2 Drug half-life.

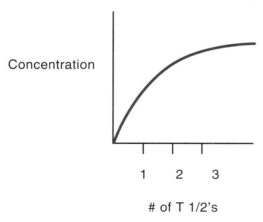

Figure 1-3 Drug half-life.

pharmacologic reason for having the peak concentration much higher than the trough concentration (e.g., aminoglycoside antibiotics, which exhibit a concentration-dependent antibacterial effect). In these cases it would be acceptable to intermittently administer the drug with a dosing interval that is longer than the drug T½ .

Plasma Samples for Therapeutic Monitoring   In most cases it is recommended that routine drug plasma samples for therapeutic monitoring be obtained after steady state has been achieved (i.e., 3.3 to 5 half-lives after starting on a maintenance regimen). In addition, most drug samples are obtained at a specific time within the dosing interval, usually at the drug trough or just before the next scheduled dose. Care should be taken to avoid obtaining drug samples during the distribution phase (i.e., soon after drug administration).

Presentation 1 Conclusion   Both vancomycin and tobramycin are administered with dosing intervals that are longer than the drugs T½ . Under these conditions there is little accumulation, and loading doses are not usually administered. Both vancomycin and tobramycin are eliminated from the body primarily by the renal route. BK is a 72-year-old man with a serum Cr level of 2.4 mg/dL. As a first estimate, his renal function would appear to be approximately half of the normal value. Using the equation that accounts for age, body size, sex, and serum Cr, his estimated CrCl rate is expected to be approximately 25 mL/min.

$$\text{CrCl for males (mL/min)} = \frac{(140 - \text{age})(\text{weight})}{(72)(\text{Cr})}$$

$$= \frac{(140 - 72 \text{ yrs})(60 \text{ kg})}{(72)(2.4 \text{ mg/dL})}$$

$$= 23.6 \text{ mL/min} \approx 25 \text{ mL/min}$$

Assuming 100 mL/min to be the "normal" value, BK's renal function is only about one fourth of normal. Clearly some type of dose adjustment seems warranted for both vancomycin and tobramycin. The question is whether to decrease the dose and maintain the same interval or to keep the same dose and increase the interval. In any case, we would expect to administer the two drugs at about one fourth the usual rate.

Vancomycin exhibits **time-dependent** antibacterial activity; thus, the primary goal is to keep the minimum drug concentration above the minimum inhibitory concentration. Therefore, decreasing the dose would be the proper approach. Administering 250 mg (one fourth the usual dose) every 12 hours (the usual interval) might be appropriate. An alternative might be to administer 500 mg (half the usual dose) every 24 hours (twice the usual interval). These two regimens represent the same rate but the second has the convenience of once daily dosing.

Tobramycin exhibits **concentration-dependent** antibacterial activity. The higher the drug level, the better the bacterial killing. Achieving high peak concentrations is an important therapeutic goal. Therefore, the most logical approach would be to keep the same dose of 100 mg and extend the interval by a factor of 4. Unfortunately this produces an interval of 32 hours, which would result in an inconsistent time of administration each day and increase the possibility of missing a dose or administering the dose at the wrong time. Most clinicians would probably compromise and give the tobramycin every 24 hours.

Presentation 2 Conclusion   Because digoxin has a usual T½ of approximately 2 days, it would take approximately 7 to 10 days (3.3 to 5 half-lives) for digoxin to accumulate to the final steady-state concentration. In order to shorten the time required to achieve therapeutic concentrations, it is common to administer a digoxin loading dose. However, this process of loading digoxin is usually restricted to the acute care setting, where the patient can be closely monitored for adverse events. Digoxin is approximately 80% eliminated by the renal route. Although TE has a "normal" serum Cr level (assumed to be approximately 1 mg/dL), he is 62 years of age and would have an expected CrCl rate of approximately 80 mL/min based on the equation of Cockcroft and Gault. Although 80 mL/min is slightly below the usually accepted normal of approximately 100 mL/min, TE's renal function would not be considered to be "compromised." At first inspection the initial loading and maintenance dose of digoxin would appear to be reasonable. However, with the addition of amiodarone the digoxin level would be expected to increase. This is because there is a drug-drug interaction such that amiodarone inhibits the body's ability to metabolize and renally eliminate digoxin by a factor of 0.5 (i.e., clearance is half of normal). In order to prevent the undesired increase in the digoxin concentration, TE should have his digoxin maintenance reduced to about half of the prescribed amount. This could be accomplished by either doubling the interval to 2 days or decreasing the dose to 0.125 mg/day. Because daily dosing is probably more convenient and most likely to result in adherence, the previous regimen would be discontinued and a new digoxin regimen of 0.125 mg each day would be prescribed.

Thumbnail: Pharmacokinetics

Absorption/bioavailability: The percentage or fraction of a drug that reaches the systemic circulation. Drugs administered by the parenteral route (IV, IM, or SC) are assumed to have 100% absorption. Some drugs administered orally have very good (> 80%) and some very poor (< 20%) absorption. The percent absorption must be taken into account when changing from the parenteral to the oral route. Some drugs have such a low bioavailability that to achieve systemic effects they must be administered parenterally.

Volume of distribution: The space into which the drug appears to distribute. Most important when administering a loading dose.

Loading dose = (volume of distribution) × (plasma concentration)

and

$$\text{Plasma concentration} = \frac{(\text{loading dose})}{(\text{volume of distribution})}$$

All drugs when administered by the IV route display two compartment pharmacokinetics. Therefore, many drugs must have the rate of IV drug input controlled in order to avoid acute toxicities.

Clearance: Clearance of drugs is almost always either hepatic or renal. Hepatic and renal function as well as the route by which a drug is eliminated must be assessed when determining maintenance doses.

Maintenance dose = (clearance) × (steady-state plasma concentration)

and

$$\text{Steady-state plasma concentration} = \frac{(\text{maintenance dose})}{(\text{clearance})}$$

Creatinine clearance: The normal CrCl rate for an adult is approximately 100 mL/min. The most common equation for estimating renal function is:

$$\text{CrCl (mL/min)} = \frac{(140 - \text{age in yrs})(\text{weight in kg})}{(72)(\text{Cr in mg/dL})} \ (\times\ 0.85 \text{ if female})$$

Half-life: The time required for a drug to decline to half its value. (Assumes no drug input and volume of distribution and clearance are constant or "first order" elimination)

$$\text{T½} = \frac{(0.693)(\text{volume of distribution})}{\text{clearance}}$$

Time to decay: With each half-life a drug concentration will decline by half. After 3.3 half-lives, 90% of the drug will have been eliminated.

Time to steady state: When on a consistent maintenance regimen, 90% of steady state is achieve in 3.3 half-lives. Steady state is assumed after 3.3 to 5 half-lives.

Dosing interval: The time between doses. Usually determined by the T½ of the drug and the desire to maintain a relative constant drug concentration (dosing interval less than the drug T½) or a drug concentration that swings widely within the interval (dosing interval longer than the drug T½).

Time to obtain plasma sample: Most drug samples are obtained as trough concentrations at steady state. If a peak sample is to be obtained, the absorption/distribution phase should be avoided. Recording the time of sampling is important.

Questions

1. A 55-year-old woman is admitted for treatment of her heart failure. She is experiencing frequent premature ventricular contractions (PVC) and chest pain. In addition she has had a recent weight gain of 11 pounds. Her medications include benazepril, digoxin, furosemide, and amiodarone. Her labs are significant for the following: potassium 2.8 mEq/L, digoxin 3.6 µg/L, Cr 2.2 mg/dL. You may assume that the patient has been taking all medications as directed and the T½ of digoxin in this patient is approximately 4 days. Which of the following is/are true statement(s):

   A. The potassium value of 2.8 mEq/L is in part responsible for the elevated digoxin level.
   B. The amiodarone is in part responsible for the elevated digoxin level.
   C. The digoxin should be held for 4 days in order for the digoxin level to decline to approximately 1 µg/L.
   D. Digoxin is primarily eliminated by the liver.
   E. Benazepril reduces the elimination of digoxin and is in part responsible for the elevated digoxin level.

2. HS is an 80-year-old man with a postoperative infection. You are asked to write an order for cefepime. HS weighs 72 kg and has a serum Cr level of 3 mg/dL. The hospital dosing guidelines for cefepime are given in Table 1-1.

Table 1-1 Dosing guidelines for cefepime based on renal function

	Creatinine Clearance			
	> 60 mL/min	30–60 mL/min	10–30 mL/min	< 10 mL/min
Cefepime dose	1–2 g	1–2 g	0.5–1 g	0.25–0.5 g
Dosing interval	Every 12 hr	Every 24 hr	Every 24 hr	Every 24 hr

Which of the following dosing regimens is/are appropriate based on the hospital's dosing guidelines?
   A. 1 g IV Q 12 hr
   B. 2 g IV Q 12 hr
   C. 1 g IV Q 24 hr
   D. 2 g IV Q 24 hr
   E. 0.5 g IV Q 24 hr
   F. 0.25 g IV Q 24 hr
   G. C and E

HPI: DD is a 67-year-old woman who presents to the clinic complaining of headache, dizziness, and "buzzing in her ears." She states that her symptoms have been present for about 4 days. One week prior, the patient was discharged from the hospital for atrial fibrillation (AF). Rate control was achieved and she was converted to normal sinus rhythm (NSR). She was placed on a new antiarrhythmic medication to prevent further episodes of AF. PMH: Episodic AF, cirrhosis.

PE: Vitals within normal limits (WNL). ECG is normal.

Labs: Normal, except for elevated LFTs and an elevated serum level of her new antiarrhythmic medication.

Thought Questions

- How do antiarrhythmic drugs act?

- What are the major toxicities of class IA and IC antiarrhythmics?

- Which drug do you suspect is causing this patient's side effects?

Basic Science Review and Discussion

Arrhythmias are caused by abnormal pacemaker activity or abnormal impulse propagation. Antiarrhythmic drugs are often classified according to the Vaughan-William scheme, which organizes agents based on channel or receptor involved (Table 2-1). Class I agents block sodium channels and are sometimes referred to as "local anesthetics." The

Table 2-1 Vaughan-William classification of antiarrhythmics

Class I: Na⁺ channel blockers		
Class IA	*Class IB*	*Class IC*
• Disopyramide	• Lidocaine	• Flecainide
• Procainamide	• Tocainide	• Moricizine
• Quinidine	• Mexiletine	• Propafenone

Class II: Beta-blockers
• Propranolol
• Metoprolol

Class III: K⁺ channel blockers
• Amiodarone
• Dofetilide
• Ibutilide
• Sotalol

Class IV: Ca²⁺ channel blockers
• Verapamil
• Diltiazem

class I drugs are further subdivided according to their effects on action potential duration. Class IA agents prolong the action potential, class IB agents shorten it, and class IC agents have no effect on action potential duration.

All class I antiarrhythmics slow or block conduction (especially in depolarized cells) and slow or eliminate abnormal pacemakers. These drugs affect abnormal tissue more readily than normal channels because the ion channels in arrhythmic tissue spend more time in open or inactivated states and the drugs bind to the receptors more avidly under these conditions.

Class IA agents (quinidine, procainamide, disopyramide) affect both atrial and ventricular arrhythmias. These drugs block both sodium channels and reduce potassium current. They increase action potential duration and effective refractory period, which results in slowed conduction velocity and inhibition of ectopic pacemakers. They may **prolong the QT$_c$ interval** as a result of increased action potential duration. This may precipitate torsade de pointes.

Quinidine may be associated with a syndrome called **cinchonism,** which is characterized by headache, vertigo, and tinnitus. Procainamide may result in hypotension or a reversible syndrome similar to **lupus erythematosus.** Patients may develop positive antinuclear antibody (ANA) titers and complain of rash, arthralgia, and arthritis. Disopyramide is poorly tolerated due to its **anticholinergic** effects (urinary retention, dry mouth, blurred vision), and its use should be avoided in patients with congestive heart failure (CHF) due to negative inotropic effects.

Class IC drugs (flecainide, moricizine, propafenone) block sodium channels but do not affect potassium current. Therefore, they do not prolong the ventricular action potential or increase the QT interval. However, this class of drugs is quite proarrhythmic, and its use should be reserved for patients who have arrhythmias refractory to other treatments. Additionally, these drugs should not be used in patients with underlying heart disease.

Case Conclusion Further work-up yielded negative results, and the patient's complaints were attributed to her quinidine. She is at a somewhat higher risk for cinchonism due to her age and decreased hepatic function (cirrhosis). Her dose was reduced and her symptoms resolved.

Thumbnail: Class IA and IC Antiarrhythmics

Drug class	Class IA	Class IC
Prototypic agents	Quinidine Procainamide Disopyramide	Flecainide Moricizine Propafenone
Clinical uses	PVC, paroxysmal atrial tachycardia, AF, VT	Documented life-threatening ventricular arrhythmias. Flecainide also may be used for AF and supraventricular tachycardias in patients **without** structural heart disease. Propafenone is also indicated for paroxysmal AF.
MOA	For both class IA and IC—Decrease influx of sodium during repolarization → reduces conduction velocity Also prolong duration of action potential and increase effective refractory period	No effect or variable effect on refractory period
Pharmacokinetics		
Absorption/distribution	All have good oral absorption.	Absorption: Flecainaide: very good Moricizine: good Propafenone: poor
Metabolism/elimination	Procainamide is hepatically acetylated to *N*-acetylprocainamide (NAPA), an active metabolite that is renally cleared. Adjust doses in renal impairment. Quinidine is hepatically eliminated; levels may be increased in patients with CHF, liver cirrhosis, and in the elderly. Disopyramide is both hepatically and renally cleared.	Both propafenone and moricizine are mainly hepatically eliminated, while flecainide is 75% liver and 25% renally cleared.
Adverse effects	All may prolong QT_c interval and increase risk for torsade de pointes. Disopyramide: anticholinergic effects, hypotension, and heart failure. Procainamide and quinidine commonly cause GI upset (nausea, vomiting, diarrhea) and hypotension. Less commonly, procainamide is associated with agranulocytosis and lupus-like syndrome. Additional side effects of quinidine include thrombocytopenia and cinchonism.	All may cause dizziness and nausea. Moricizine also may cause perioral numbness and euphoria. All antiarrhythmics can be proarrhythmic.

Questions

1. A 62-year-old woman currently taking an antiarrhythmic to maintain normal sinus rhythm has a sudden onset of malaise and develops a "butterfly rash." Vitals: T 38.4°C, BP 140/95 mm Hg, HR 90 beats/min, RR 16 breaths/min. Stat labs: ANA positive. Which of the following drugs is the most likely cause of these findings?

   A. Amiodarone
   B. Ibutilide
   C. Lidocaine
   D. Procainamide
   E. None of the above

2. KM is a 71-year-old man with CHF, benign prostatic hypertrophy (BPH), renal dysfunction, and paroxysmal AF. Which of the following agents should be avoided in this patient?

   A. Disopyramide
   B. Flecainide
   C. Procainamide
   D. A and C
   E. All of the above

HPI: BB is a 72-year-old man who presents to the ED with complaints of palpitations. PMH includes anterior myocardial infarction (MI), hypertension (HTN), and depression.

PE: Vital signs: BP 105/75 mm Hg, HR 160 beats/min, RR 14 breaths/min. ECG showed sustained ventricular tachycardia (SuVT).

Thought Questions

- What are the acute treatment options for SuVT?

- What is the primary pharmacology and side effects of lidocaine?

- What factors may reduce the clearance of lidocaine?

- What medications can be given orally for long-term maintenance of normal sinus rhythm in patients who have had ventricular tachycardia?

Basic Science Review and Discussion

Sustained ventricular tachycardia is defined as consecutive premature ventricular contractions lasting more than 30 seconds. Nonsustained ventricular tachycardia (VT) usually self-terminates and lasts for less than 30 seconds. The acute treatment of SuVT depends on the hemodynamic stability and symptoms of the patient. Unstable patients should receive immediate **cardioversion.** If patients are stable with mild symptoms, they can be treated with IV antiarrhythmics.

The antiarrhythmic of choice for SuVT is lidocaine because of its fast onset and ease of administration. Lidocaine is a class IB antiarrhythmic that inhibits sodium ion channels, decreasing the action potential duration and effective refractory period. Lidocaine raises the electrical stimulation threshold and suppresses spontaneous depolarization of the ventricle. It is given as a bolus dose, but an additional bolus may be required 8 to 10 minutes after the first one due to the short distribution half-life. Once converted to normal sinus rhythm (NSR), the patient can be placed on a continuous infusion of lidocaine.

Side effects should be monitored after the initiation of lidocaine. The most common adverse reactions are drowsiness, dizziness, paresthesia, and euphoria. Patients also may experience serious **central nervous system** (CNS) side effects such as confusion, agitation, psychosis, seizures, and coma, but usually only at supratherapeutic levels. The active metabolites of lidocaine are responsible for most of the CNS toxicities. Cardiovascular side effects, including atrioventricular block, hypotension, and circulatory collapse, are not as well correlated to lidocaine levels.

Lidocaine is mostly cleared by hepatic metabolism. Any condition that impairs **liver function** or compromises liver blood flow may increase lidocaine levels. Lower infusion rates should be administered in patients with CHF, shock, advanced age, and liver cirrhosis.

Alternative intravenous antiarrhythmics that may be used for SuVT include procainamide and amiodarone. For maintenance, oral antiarrhythmics such as sotalol, procainamide, amiodarone, and quinidine are possible options.

Case Conclusion Two lidocaine boluses were given 10 minutes apart, followed by a continuous infusion. BB's VT resolved with lidocaine therapy. Upon careful review of the ECG, it was noted that he had experienced a new lateral MI. The cardiac catherization revealed triple-vessel disease, and he underwent a coronary artery bypass graft.

Thumbnail: Class IB Antiarrhythmics

Prototypical agent: Lidocaine.

Other agents: Tocainide and mexiletine are analogues of lidocaine with improved oral bioavailability.

Clinical use: Only for ventricular arrhythmias. Lidocaine is also used as a local anesthetic.

Mechanism of action: Class IB antiarrhythmics inhibit sodium ion channels and decrease the action potential duration and effective refractory period.

Pharmacokinetics

Absorption: Lidocaine is ineffective orally; 60% to 70% of an oral dose is metabolized by the liver before reaching the systemic circulation. It is only administered IV for arrhythmias. Both mexiletine and tocainide are well absorbed orally.

Distribution and elimination: Lidocaine is extensively biotransformed in the liver to at least two active metabolites: monoethylglycinexylidide and glycinexylidide. The distribution phase (T½ = 10 minutes) accounts for the short duration of action following IV bolus administration, and continuous infusion of lidocaine is necessary to maintain antiarrhythmic effects. The elimination half-life is 1.5 to 2 hours, and 3 hours following infusions of more than 24 hours. Less than 10% of the parent drug is excreted unchanged in the urine, but renal elimination is important in the elimination of the active metabolites. Mexiletine has a large volume of distribution and is mainly hepatically eliminated. Tocainide is eliminated via conjugation and 40% unchanged in the urine.

Therapeutic range: Lidocaine = 1.5–5 μg/mL.

Adverse reactions: Minor side effects of lidocaine are drowsiness, dizziness, paresthesia, and euphoria. More serious side effects include CNS and cardiovascular effects. Tocainide and mexiletine both have a high incidence of **GI** side effects (nausea and vomiting) and CNS side effects (dizziness, numbness, and paresthesias). Additionally, tocainide has a 15% incidence of rash and may cause agranulocytosis.

Precautions: For lidocaine, use caution with repeated or prolonged administration in patients with liver or renal disease because toxic accumulation of lidocaine or its metabolites may occur.

Questions

1. A 55-year-old man is admitted to the ED for VT. Vital signs: BP 105/86 mm Hg, HR 138 beats/min, and RR 20 breaths/min. PMH: diabetes, CHF, atrial flutter, mitral valve regurgitation, and HTN. Labs are within normal limits except for a slightly low serum sodium. What is a reason for starting lidocaine at a lower dose in this patient?

   A. Diabetes
   B. Atrial flutter
   C. Increased heart rate
   D. Low serum sodium
   E. Congestive heart failure

2. SA is a 63-year-old woman who recently had an MI and an episode of ventricular arrhythmia. Lidocaine was started 10 hours previously and now she is exhibiting drowsiness, dizziness, severe agitation, and psychosis. Labs are within normal limits except for an elevated serum Cr (1.8 mg/dL). Which following reactions are adverse effects associated with lidocaine?

   A. Drowsiness
   B. Dizziness
   C. Agitation
   D. Psychosis
   E. All of the above

> **HPI:** CS is a 58-year-old man admitted for an anterior MI. Three days after admission, the patient's nurse found him unresponsive. His vital signs included no detectable blood pressure or pulse. ECG showed VT that progressed to ventricular fibrillation (VF). Immediate electrical defibrillation was applied. Other treatments instituted include airway management, chest compression, and establishment of IV access. After three shocks, 1 mg epinephrine was given and patient was shocked again. However, he was still in VF and amiodarone was administered.

Thought Questions

- When should drug treatment be initiated during cardiopulmonary resuscitation?

- What are the antiarrhythmic agents used for VF?

- Describe the pharmacology and side effects of amiodarone.

- What are the other class III antiarrhythmics and how do they differ from amiodarone?

Basic Science Review and Discussion

The treatment of cardiac arrest should follow the American Heart Association guidelines for Advance Cardiac Life Support. After three shocks, epinephrine or vasopression are administered. If this fails, then **antiarrhythmics** are given to facilitate the conversion and maintenance of NSR.

Amiodarone, lidocaine, and procainamide are commonly used antiarrhythmics for conversion in VF. Of these, amiodarone is the antiarrhythmic agent recommended first. In the Amiodarone versus Lidocaine in Ventricular Emergency (ALIVE) trial, patients administered amiodarone had a better rate of survival to hospital admission than those given lidocaine. Amiodarone contains sodium channel, potassium channel, β-adrenergic, and calcium channel blocking effects. It may be used for both **atrial and ventricular arrhythmias.** Amiodarone has a large volume of distribution because it is extensively bound to tissue and highly lipophilic. Its half-life is about 50 days after chronic administration. Amiodarone is metabolized to an active metabolite, desethylamiodarone, but its contribution to amiodarone's antiarrhythmic effect is not well delineated.

Amiodarone has many adverse effects involving a number of organ systems. The most common side effects include nausea, constipation, and bradycardia. Other possible side effects are hypo- or hyperthyroidism, bilateral corneal microdeposits, hepatoxicity, dermatologic (photosensitivity and gray-blue discoloration of the skin), anorexia, tremor, and ataxia. **Pulmonary fibrosis** is the most serious adverse effect. This occurs in 5% to 10% of the population and is dose dependent. A baseline chest radiograph and pulmonary function tests are recommended. Patient education regarding symptoms such as dyspnea, nonproductive cough, and weight loss should be given to assist in early detection. Other baseline and follow-up labs, including LFTs, thyroid function tests, and slit-lamp eye examination, are recommended.

Other class III antiarrhythmics include sotalol, ibutilide, and dofetilide. These agents do not have a role in the acute treatment of ventricular fibrillation.

Case Conclusion Once the patient is resuscitated, antiarrhythmics should be continued until the patient is more stable. The requirement for long-term treatment with antiarrhythmics and/or implantable automatic cardioverter defibrillation should be evaluated.

Thumbnail: Class III Antiarrhythmics

	Amiodarone	Sotalol	Ibutilide	Dofetilide
Clinical uses	Conversion and maintenance of AF to NSR; ventricular arrhythmias	Ventricular arrhythmias; maintenance of NSR after conversion from AF	Rapid conversion of AF or atrial flutter (AFl) of recent onset to NSR	Conversion of AF/AFl to NSR
MOA	All class III antiarrhythmics inhibit outward potassium channels (prolongs action potential duration and repolarization)			
	Also blocks sodium and calcium channels; blocks β-adrenergic receptors; impedes atrioventricular (AV) node conduction and slows heart rate	Also has nonselective beta-blocking activity	Relies on activation of slow inward sodium current to prolong action potential and effective refractory period	
Pharmacokinetics				
Absorption/ distribution	Fair oral absorption (40% to 60%); available IV and PO; high concentration in adipose tissue	Great oral absorption (90% to 100%), PO only	IV only	Great oral absorption (90% to 100%); PO only
Metabolism/ elimination	Hepatic; long half-life (50 days)	Renal	Mostly hepatic	Mostly renal (some metabolism by CYP450)
Adverse reactions	All class III antiarrhythmics can cause QT_c prolongation and increase risk of torsade de pointes			
	Hypo- or hyperthryroidism, bradycardia, corneal microdeposits, hepatotoxicity, GI upset, tremor, ataxia, pulmonary fibrosis, dermatologic reactions	Fatigue, dyspnea, bradycardia, headache. May cause bronchospasm in patients with asthma or COPD	Arrhythmias (VT, supraventricular tachycardia), AV block, headache, hypotension, bradycardia	Headache, dizziness, insomnia, rash, nausea, diarrhea, dyspnea, arrhythmias (VT and torsade de pointes)
Drug interactions	May increase levels of digoxin (two-fold), procainamide, warfarin, quinidine			Contraindicated in combination with medications that may increase its level (verapamil, cimetidine, ketoconazole, megestrol, trimethoprim, prochlorperazine). Avoid use with drugs that may prolong QT (cisapride, phenothiazines, fluoroquinolones, bepridil, class I or III antiarrhythmic)
Warnings/ precautions		Contraindicated in patients with renal impairment (CrCl rate of < 40 mL/min) or prolonged QT interval (> 450 msec).	Administer in setting of continuous ECG monitoring (to identify acute ventricular arrhythmias)	Administer in setting with continuous ECG monitoring for at least 3 days (high risk for arrhythmia); contraindicated in patients with renal impairment (CrCl < 30 mL/min)

Questions

1. A 57-year-old woman recently started on an antiarrhythmic for her ventricular tachycardia returns 2 days later complaining of shortness of breath. PMH: VT, s/p MI, hyperlipidemia, asthma, and osteoporosis. Which of the following antiarrhythmic drugs was probably prescribed for this patient?
   A. Sotalol
   B. Amiodarone
   C. Procainamide
   D. Lidocaine
   E. Quinidine

2. TA is a 61-year-old man converted from VF to NSR on lidocaine. Now he is able to take oral medications and the team would like to switch him over to an oral antiarrhythmic that is safe in systolic heart failure. Which of the following would you recommend?
   A. Disopyramide
   B. Quinidine
   C. Sotalol
   D. Amiodarone
   E. Lidocaine

HPI: MD, a 28-year-old woman, presents to the ED diaphoretic and complaining of palpitations. She reports experiencing occasional episodes of palpitations over the past few years, usually after exercise. MD is not in acute distress.

PE: Vitals: T 37.2°C, BP 105/86 mm Hg, HR 185 beats/min, and RR 22 breaths/min. ECG: HR 180 beats/min, regular rhythm, no P waves, and narrow QRS complexes.

Thought Questions

- When should drug treatment be initiated in patients with **paroxysmal supraventricular tachycardia (PSVT)?**

- What are the pharmacologic action and side effects of adenosine?

- What are the other drug options for acute treatment of PSVT?

Basic Science Review and Discussion

When a patient presents with PSVT, hemodynamics should be assessed first. If a patient is hemodynamically unstable, shock is required. If the patient is hemodynamically stable, then **vagal maneuvers** should be considered. The success rate of vagal maneuvers is over 85%. However, patients with PSVT who present to the ED usually have more refractory PSVT and have already failed vagal maneuvers. Pharmacologic treatment should then be attempted.

Adenosine is the treatment of choice for PSVT. It slows the conduction and interrupts the re-entry pathways through the **atrioventricular node,** restoring dysrhythmia to NSR. Adenosine is not effective in treating other atrial arrhythmias such as atrial flutter or atrial fibrillation or in treating ventricular arrhythmias. Adenosine is rapidly degraded enzymatically or cleared from the circulation by vascular endothelial cells. The half-life is approximately 6–10 seconds; therefore, a flush of the IV line is required after each bolus dose and this drug should be administered through a large IV catheter. **Flushing, chest pain,** and dyspnea often occur after adenosine administration, but these discomforts are brief.

The nondihydropyridine calcium channel blockers, such as **verapamil** and **diltiazem,** have efficacy rates similar to that of adenosine, but are considered second line. Intravenous calcium channel blockers have a few disadvantages. In contrast to adenosine, caution should be taken in hypotensive patients. Adenosine may cause hypotension, but appears to be safe in patients who present with hypotension due to the short half-life. In addition, calcium channel blockers also should be used with caution in patients with systolic heart failure, patients receiving concurrent beta-blocker therapy, and in those with accessory pathways.

Intravenous **beta-blockers** also may be used for PSVT. However, they are less effective than adenosine and calcium channel blockers. Furthermore, they may cause bronchoconstriction, hypotension, or cardiac dysfunction. Intravenous **digoxin** is another option, but it has a delayed onset and is dangerous in the presence of accessory pathways.

Case Conclusion The patient was diagnosed with PSVT and vagal maneuvers were tried and failed. Adenosine was administered with rapid conversion to normal sinus rhythm. MD experienced transient flushing and dyspnea but she was reassured that these were common effects of the adenosine. She was discharged from the ED in good condition.

Thumbnail: Adenosine

Clinical use: Adenosine is used to convert PSVT to NSR. Adenosine may also be used in conjunction with thallium to assess patients with suspected coronary artery disease.

MOA: Adenosine slows the conduction and interrupts the re-entry pathways through the AV node, restoring dysrhythmia to NSR.

Pharmacokinetics

Absorption: Adenosine is only given IV.

Distribution and elimination: Adenosine is rapidly taken up by most types of cells and rapidly degraded by deamination or phosphorylation.

Adverse reactions: Flushing, chest pain, and dyspnea often occur after adenosine administration, but these discomforts are brief. Similarly, if hypotension occurs, it lasts only a few seconds.

Warning: Adenosine may provoke **bronchospasm**; therefore, use adenosine with caution in patients with obstructive lung disease (e.g., emphysema and bronchitis) and avoid use in patients with asthma. Also, administration of adenosine may result in brief periods of bradycardia or asystole and should be used cautiously in patients with sinus node dysfunction.

Drug interactions: Methylxanthines (e.g., theophylline) and dipyridamole are adenosine antagonists.

Questions

1. A 35-year-old woman presents with sudden onset of palpitations. The ECG showed that she has PSVT. She failed vagal maneuvers, and was given adenosine. After two doses of adenosine, the patient still did not convert to normal sinus rhythm. Which of the following concurrent medications may have affected the efficacy of adenosine?

   A. Doxycycline
   B. Furosemide
   C. Theophylline
   D. Pantoprazole
   E. Hydrochlorothiazide

2. A 48-year-old man presents to the clinic with another recurrent episode of PSVT. He has shortness of breath and is requesting assistance. He has a PMH of asthma, and wheezing is noted on the lung examination. Which drug (or drug class) would be the best option for his recurrent PSVT?

   A. Beta-blocker
   B. Calcium channel blocker
   C. Digoxin
   D. Adenosine
   E. Amiodarone

HPI: MM is a 67-year-old woman brought into the ED complaining of loss of appetite and nausea for the preceding 2 days. She also reports hazy vision with "halos" but thinks it is due to her tiredness. PMH: CHF, HTN. Medications: Digoxin. She recently started taking an angiotensin-converting enzyme inhibitor (ACE-I).

Labs: Digoxin level pending. Potassium pending.

Thought Questions

- What is digoxin's mechanism of action?
- What is the importance of monitoring digoxin levels?
- What are some important drug interactions associated with digoxin?
- What are common signs of digoxin toxicity?

Basic Science Review and Discussion

Congestive heart failure is a clinical syndrome that occurs when the heart is unable to supply blood and oxygen to meet the metabolic needs of the body. Impaired ventricular function leads to decreased **cardiac output,** and hypoperfusion occurs leading to inadequate oxygen delivery to the tissues. The result is pulmonary and systemic congestion. Patients typically present with symptoms of **dyspnea, fatigue,** and **fluid retention.** Pharmacotherapy is aimed at correcting hemodynamic abnormalities to preserve quality of life and to slow down the progression of the disease. **Beta-blockers, ACE inhibitors, spironolactone,** and **digoxin** have been shown to decrease the rate of mortality in CHF patients.

Digoxin increases contractility of the heart muscle by inhibiting the **Na^+/K^+ ATPase pump.** In a normally functioning heart, intracellular calcium stored in the sarcoplasmic reticulum is released and activates the contractility of the muscle. The Na^+/Ca^{2+} exchanger located in the cell membrane controls normal intracellular calcium levels. Exchangers use the Na^+ ion gradient, maintained by the Na^+/K^+ ATPase, to move calcium ions out of the cell. When digoxin inhibits the Na^+/K^+ ATPase, intracellular sodium levels increase. This increase in sodium shifts the balance of the Na^+/Ca^{2+} exchanger, leading to increased stores of intracellular calcium available in the sarcoplasmic reticulum and stronger contraction of the heart muscle.

When starting digoxin therapy, it is important to obtain baseline electrolyte levels and renal function. Electrolyte imbalances (**hypokalemia, hypomagnesemia,** or **hypercalcemia**) predispose patients to digoxin toxicity. When serum potassium is low, digoxin uptake increases because digoxin and potassium compete for the same site on the Na^+/K^+ ATPase. Increases in serum calcium can facilitate digitalis toxicity by causing overloading of intracellular calcium stores that can induce arrhythmias. Low magnesium also can contribute to toxicity. In addition, digoxin is cleared by the kidney; therefore, it is important to obtain baseline renal function values to determine if dose adjustments are necessary.

Serum levels of digoxin are recommended when toxicity is suspected, especially when compliance, efficacy, or renal function changes are a concern. Digoxin has a narrow therapeutic range of 0.5–2 µg/L. However, levels should only be used as a guide because overlap can occur between the therapeutic and toxic ranges. Levels should be obtained at least 4 hours after an IV dose or 6 hours after oral dose to allow the distribution of digoxin to equilibrate between the plasma and the heart muscle. Monitoring of digoxin levels should be done 5 to 7 days after a dosage change.

Because of digoxin's narrow therapeutic range, toxicity can often occur, especially in those who have predisposing factors, such as hypokalemia, concurrent therapy with potassium wasting diuretics, age (elderly and pediatrics), small body size, and drug interactions. Common signs of toxicity include GI complaints (nausea, vomiting, and anorexia), arrhythmias, and CNS effects (i.e., confusion, hallucinations, and visual disturbances).

In most cases of mild digoxin toxicity, stopping digoxin as well as correcting hypokalemia (if present) usually is the only treatment required. In severe overdose, the Na^+/K^+ ATPase is blocked in all cells, leading to a large leak of potassium from skeletal muscle. Hyperkalemia is treated with sodium polystyrene sulfonate or sodium bicarbonate and glucose with insulin. Patients who have severe hyperkalemia and life-threatening arrhythmias may receive digoxin immune Fab (digoxin antibodies that bind digoxin molecules).

Case Conclusion MM's presentation was consistent with digoxin toxicity. Labs returned with a normal potassium value (3.9 mEq/L) and a supratherapeutic digoxin level (2.6 μg/L). Her digoxin and ACE-I were immediately discontinued. Within 2 days, MM was starting to feel like herself again. The ACE-I and oral digoxin were restarted (at lower doses).

Thumbnail: Digoxin

Clinical use: Used to improve cardiac output in CHF. Also used in atrial arrhythmias for rate control.

MOA: Digoxin (cardiac glycoside) is a **positive inotropic** agent that inhibits the Na^+/K^+ ATPase pump. Inhibition of the pump causes an increase in intracellular sodium that allows the Na^+/Ca^{2+} exchanger to increase intracellular calcium. The heart is then able to use the increased intracellular calcium to increase contractility.

Pharmacokinetics

Absorption: Available intravenously and orally. Oral absorption depends on formulation (soft gelatin capsules > elixir > tablets).

Elimination: Renally cleared. $T\frac{1}{2}$ 2 days ($T\frac{1}{2}$ 4 days in renal impairment). May also undergo enterohepatic recycling.

Therapeutic plasma range: 0.5 to 2 μg/L.

Adverse reactions: Arrhythmias, visual disturbances (blurred vision, yellow or green tinting, "halos," red-green color blindness), GI complaints (abdominal discomfort, nausea, vomiting, anorexia).

Drug interactions: Amphotericin B or potassium-wasting diuretics may contribute to digoxin toxicity; ACE-I, amiodarone, bepridil, diltiazem, quinidine, and verapamil may increase digoxin levels.

Questions

1. DM is a 55-year-old man who has been on chronic digoxin therapy for CHF for 3 years. He is currently undergoing treatment with amphotericin B for a fungal pneumonia. Today he complains of dizziness and nausea. Cr 0.8 mg/dL, weight 70 kg. What is the most likely reason for his digoxin toxicity?

   A. Hyperkalemia
   B. Hypokalemia
   C. Decreased renal clearance
   D. Hypermagnesemia
   E. Hypocalcemia

2. AH is a 70-year-old depressed woman who took suicidal doses of digoxin. When brought into the ED, she had a potassium level of 5.1 mEq/L and electrocardiography showed a bradycardic arrhythmia unresponsive to atropine. Which of the following drugs would be the most appropriate therapy?

   A. Atropine
   B. Glucose with insulin
   C. Sodium polystyrene sulfonate
   D. Lidocaine
   E. Digoxin-immune Fab

HPI: TT is a 48-year-old man who presents to the general medicine clinic complaining of recent onset of chest pain (CP) on exertion. He says that he was feeling fine until about a week ago when he started experiencing intermittent CP while mowing the lawn. He also states that the CP subsides after sitting down in the shade and resting for about 5 minutes. FH: Father who died at age 46 secondary to coronary artery disease (CAD). Smoking History: One pack of cigarettes per week for 20 years.

Thought Questions

- What are the different types of angina?
- What is the drug of choice for acute chest pain?
- What is nitrate tolerance? How do you minimize tolerance?

Basic Science Review and Discussion

Angina pectoris is a symptom of **ischemic heart disease** that is frequently characterized by chest pain. There are three basic categories of angina: stable (exertional) angina, unstable angina, and vasospastic angina. Both stable and unstable angina reflect underlying **atherosclerotic** narrowing of coronary arteries. Vasospastic angina, or Prinzmetal's variant angina, is usually not associated with CAD and is due to coronary spasms that result in decreased myocardial blood flow.

Angina occurs when atherosclerotic plaques obstruct coronary blood flow, therefore decreasing the oxygen supply to myocardial tissues. Atherosclerotic plaques are composed of cholesterol and foam cells (derivatives of macrophages) enclosed within a fibrous capsule. Thrombus formation occurs within the plaque, and as erosion of the endothelium occurs, the thrombus extends into the arterial lumen. Coronary blood flow may become occluded depending on the size of the atherosclerotic plaque and therefore produce symptoms of angina.

Nitrates are the drugs of choice for relieving angina because they decrease preload and myocardial oxygen demand by **venous dilatation.** In addition, nitrates dilate coronary arteries even in the setting of atherosclerosis. The two proposed mechanisms by which nitrates promote venodilatation are stimulation of cyclic guanosine monophosphate (GMP) production and inhibition of thromboxane synthetase.

Short-acting nitrates, such as sublingual (SL) tablets or translingual sprays, are the preparation of choice for quick relief, especially in the setting of exertional angina. Long-acting nitrates (e.g., isosorbide dinitrate [ISDN] and isosorbide mononitrate [ISMO]) become useful when the number, severity, and duration of anginal attacks increase.

When using long-acting nitrates, it is important to schedule a 10- to 12-hour nitrate-free interval to minimize **tolerance.** With continuous exposure to nitrates, tolerance or the loss of antianginal and hemodynamic effects occurs. When exposure is discontinued, symptoms of withdrawal (severe headache, chest pain, or sudden cardiac death) can occur. Short-acting nitrates are not likely to lead to tolerance due to their rapid onset of action and short duration.

Case Conclusion After the cardiac work-up for TT, it was concluded that he had a diagnosis of unstable angina. He was prescribed nitroglycerin sublingual tablets for chest pain and a beta-blocker to help decrease the workload of the heart and decrease myocardial oxygen demand. His lipid panel revealed elevated cholesterol (250 mg/dL with low-density lipoprotein [LDL] 140 mg/dL and high-density lipoprotein [HDL] 40 mg/dL) and triglycerides (296 mg/dL). He was started on atorvastatin to help lower his cholesterol because it is a component of atherosclerotic plaques. Smoking cessation counseling was given, and the patient was advised to start on nicotine patches.

Thumbnail: Nitrates

Prototypical agent: Nitroglycerin

Clinical use: Primarily for the management of anginal symptoms of CAD.

MOA: Nitrates cause venous and arterial dilatation. However, venous dilatation is more evident because it increases venous pooling, therefore decreasing preload and reducing myocardial oxygen demand. In addition, nitrates dilate epicardial coronary arteries, consequently decreasing coronary vasospasm.

Adverse reactions: Headache, postural hypotension, and syncope are common. After several days of therapy, tolerance develops and headache and hypotension should resolve. Patients with nitrate-induced syncope should have their doses reduced. Dizziness, facial flushing, nausea, and tachycardia also occur. Methemoglobinemia may develop with large doses of IV nitroglycerin.

Drug interactions: The concurrent use of sildenafil (used for erectile dysfunction) is contraindicated due to potentiation of hypotensive effects of nitrates. Ergot alkaloids (used for migraine headaches) may cause increased blood pressure and decreased antianginal effects of nitrates—avoid concurrent use.

Questions

1. KB is a 59-year-old man who presents to the clinic with unresolved mild chest pain after taking numerous SL nitroglycerin tablets (one every 5 minutes over a total of 30 minutes). He reports that he hasn't used these pills for over a year, but still keeps them by his bedside. He also adds, "Now that I need these pills, they don't work!" Which is the most logical reason for the ineffective SL tablets?

   A. Nitrate tolerance
   B. Expired sublingual tablets
   C. Took too many tablets
   D. Took the wrong medication
   E. Nitrate intolerance

2. JK is a 70-year-old woman who has had angina for 5 years. She was well controlled on SL nitroglycerin until 3 weeks ago, when she started to note an increase in anginal episodes, ranging from three to five times per week. The attacks usually occurred on the fairways of the local golf course, where she meets and plays golf with friends three times a week. Today's vital signs are BP 119/69 mm Hg, HR 68 beats/min, RR 14 breaths/min. What is the most reasonable therapeutic option?

   A. Isosorbide dinitrate tablets
   B. Atenolol
   C. Verapamil
   D. Nitroglycerin ointment plus SL nitroglycerin
   E. SL isosorbide dinitrate

HPI: AV is a 62-year-old white man with a 6-year history of HTN. His current antihypertensive therapy consists of enalapril and hydrochlorothiazide, but AV's BP is still elevated at 165/94 mm Hg. PMH: COPD, peptic ulcer disease (PUD), HTN, and chronic back pain.

PE: Vitals: HR 85 beats/min, RR 14 breaths/min. Medications: Omeprazole, enalapril, hydrochlorothiazide, acetaminophen. Metoprolol was initiated.

Labs: Serum Cr 1.5 mg/dL, K^+ 5.0 mEq/L.

Thought Questions

- What is the primary pharmacology of beta-blockers?

- Which of the beta-blockers are α_1 selective?

- Which beta-blockers provide alpha blockade as well?

- Which beta-blocker is the most lipid soluble?

- What are the advantages and disadvantages of having intrinsic sympathomimetic properties?

- When might a beta-blocker be chosen over some of the other antihypertensives?

- Which beta-blocker is the shortest acting?

Basic Science Review and Discussion

Beta-blockers are one of the antihypertensive agents useful in patients with CAD because they have been shown to reduce morbidity and mortality. Beta-blockers competitively block both β_1 and β_2, but with different selectivity. Blocking β_1 receptors, which are found primarily on cardiac muscle, will lead to negative chronotropic and inotropic effects. In hypertensive patients, this will lower their blood pressure. β_2 receptors are found predominantly on the outer membrane of the smooth muscle cells of the vasculature, bronchioles, and myometrium and regulate the relaxation of these cells. Blockage of this receptor can lead to vasoconstriction and bronchoconstriction.

Some beta-blockers demonstrate β_1 selectivity. At low doses, metoprolol and atenolol predominantly antagonize the receptors on cardiac tissues with less activity on β_2-receptors. Therefore, they are less likely to cause bronchospasm in patients with COPD or asthma. The nonselective beta-blockers also have the disadvantage of masking hypoglycemic symptoms, especially in insulin-dependent diabetics. Blocking β_2-receptors also leaves the alpha-mediated vasoconstriction unopposed and, as a result, may worsen Raynaud's disease or peripheral vascular disease. Some beta-blockers, such as labetolol and carvedilol, also possess alpha-blocking properties.

Another important difference among the beta-blockers is their relative lipophilicity. Propranolol is the most lipophilic agent. It undergoes a more extensive first-pass hepatic metabolism than other less lipophilic beta-blockers. Hence, propranolol has more interpatient variability in serum concentrations. Less lipophilic beta-blockers are excreted more by the kidney and may require dosage adjustments in renal impairment. More lipophilic beta-blockers also have an extensive volume of distribution, even crossing the blood–brain barrier. Consequently, these agents may have more CNS adverse effects such as drowsiness, nightmares, confusion, and depression. On the other hand, because propranolol penetrates the CNS, it is useful in treating migraines and anxiety.

Beta-blockers with intrinsic sympathomimetic (ISA) properties are not pure antagonists. These agents partially stimulate the beta-receptors as well. Theoretically, these agents are less likely to cause bradycardia and bronchospasm, increase lipids, decrease cardiac output, and cause peripheral vasoconstriction. However, these agents can still cause bronchospasm or exacerbate heart failure. ISA beta-blockers may have a role in patients who experiences severe bradycardia with non-ISA agents. When these agents are given to someone with a slow heart rate at rest, they may increase the heart rate. Conversely, ISA agents in someone with exercise-induced tachycardia may decrease the heart rate because the beta-blocking activity predominates. Avoid these agents in patients who are s/p MI because the agonistic properties may be detrimental.

In addition to their use as antihypertensive agents, beta-blockers are useful in treating many other conditions. Beta-blockers are considered first-line therapy in the management of chronic stable angina because they decrease the cardiac workload. Patients with a history of MI should receive beta-blockers if they do not have contraindications. Furthermore, they are used as antiarrhythmic agents in supraventricular and ventricular arrhythmias. Propranolol is used in the setting of hyperthyroidism to reduce symptoms and heart rate as well as decrease the conversion of thyroxine (T_4) to triiodothyronine (T_3), migraines, headaches, anxiety, and essential tremors. The nonselective beta-blockers are also used for hepatic portal hypertension in patients with liver cirrhosis. Topical beta-blockers are used in glaucoma to reduce intraocular pressures.

Table 8-1 Beta-blockers: Selectivity, activity, and metabolism

Agent	Selectivity	Lipid solubility	Metabolism	T½	Notes
Acebutolol	β_1	Moderate	Hepatic/renal	3–4 h	Partial agonist
Atenolol	β_1	Low	Renal	6–7 h	
Betaxolol	β_1	Low	Hepatic/renal	14–22 h	Used in glaucoma
Bisoprolol	β_1	Low	Hepatic/renal	9–12 h	
Carteolol	β_1 and β_2	Low	Hepatic/renal	6 h	Partial agonist. Used in glaucoma
Carvedilol	β_1, β_2, and α_1	High	Hepatic	6–10 h	Used mostly for CHF
Esmolol	β_1	Low	RBCs	10 min	Used IV, short-acting
Labetolol	β_1, β_2, and α_1	Moderate	Hepatic/renal	6–8 h	β blockade
Metoprolol	β_1	Moderate-high	Hepatic/renal	3–7 h	
Nadolol	β_1 and β_2	Low	Renal	20–24 h	Long-acting
Penbutolol	β_1 and β_2	High	Hepatic/renal	5 h	Partial agonist
Pindolol	β_1 and β_2	Moderate	Hepatic/renal	3–4 h	Partial agonist
Propranolol	β_1 and β_2	High	Hepatic	4–6 h	
Timolol	β_1 and β_2	Low-moderate	Hepatic/renal	4–5 h	Used in glaucoma

Case Conclusion   Although this patient has a history of COPD, a β_1-selective agent may still be used, especially at low doses. In addition, the patient has renal impairment; thus, metoprolol was selected because it is hepatically metabolized.

Thumbnail: Beta-Blockers

Prototypical agent: Propranolol has no beta-receptor selectivity. Metoprolol and atenolol were developed with more β_1 selectivity.

Clinical use: Primarily as an antihypertensive agent. Also used for controlling ventricular rate in AF, post-MI, CHF, angina, and hyperthyroidism. Additionally, propranolol may be used for migraine headaches, essential tremors, and anxiety. The nonselective beta-blockers are useful in the treatment of hepatic portal hypertension in patients with liver cirrhosis. Topical agents are used to lower intraocular pressures in patients with glaucoma.

MOA: Beta-blockers competitively antagonize beta-receptors, leading to decreased calcium influx into myocardial cells, which in turn leads to both decreased heart rate (chronotropic effect) and cardiac contractility (inotropic effect).

Pharmacokinetics

Absorption: Most are well absorbed orally; however, propranolol undergoes a large first-pass effect by the liver. Increasing the dose may compensate for this effect.

Distribution: Large volumes of distribution. Propranolol crosses the blood-brain barrier.

Elimination: Most are hepatically metabolized. The exceptions are atenolol and nadolol, which are renally excreted unchanged.

Adverse reactions: The most important adverse reactions are seen in asthmatics. In asthmatics, beta-blockers may lead to constriction of the airways via smooth muscle contraction. Although α_1-selective agents may have less of an effect, they should still be used cautiously. The most common adverse effects are fatigue, bradycardia, hypotension, dizziness, nausea, diarrhea, and exercise intolerance. They are also associated with increased triglycerides and hyperglycemia. Additionally, beta-blockers can block some of the symptoms normally induced by hypoglycemia, particularly in insulin-dependent diabetics. Other side effects seen are depression, sleep disturbance, and impotence. The more lipophilic agents have more CNS adverse effects, such as drowsiness, nightmares, confusion, and depression. Beta-blockers with β_1-antagonist activity may produce more vasodilation activity and have a higher incidence of postural dizziness, lightheadedness, and fatigue.

Warning: If beta-blockers are stopped abruptly, they can cause rebound hypertension.

Drug interactions: An interaction at the level of cardiac activity may be seen, particularly with the calcium-channel blocker verapamil. This can lead to bradycardia and severely diminished cardiac output.

Questions

1. A 66-year-old man who has been taking furosemide, atenolol, and loratadine for 5 months, ran out of his medication for 1 week. The patient's blood pressure is 173/96 mm Hg compared with 155/90 mm Hg 5 months ago before drug therapy. PMH includes HTN, asthma, and diabetes. What is the most likely reason for the increased BP?

   A. Antihypertensive medication not adequate
   B. Rebound hypertension
   C. Loratadine
   D. Hyperglycemia
   E. Asthma

2. An 82-year-old patient presents to the clinic with untreated HTN. PMH includes CAD, MI, COPD, and renal impairment. There is a strong indication for initiating a beta-blocker in this patient. Which one would you select?

   A. Atenolol
   B. Nadolol
   C. Metoprolol
   D. Propranolol
   E. Labetolol

HPI: A 60-year-old woman presents to the clinic for a 6-month follow-up examination for newly diagnosed HTN, which has not been adequately controlled by dietary and lifestyle changes. PMH: Angina and asthma.

PE: Vital signs: BP 160/99 mm Hg, HR 55 beats/min. Allergies: Sulfa-based drugs. Medications: Albuterol inhaler, fluticasone inhaler, and nitroglycerin sublingual tablets.

Thought Questions

- What are the different mechanisms of actions for calcium channel blockers?

- How do the four types of calcium channel blockers differ?

- What are some indications for calcium channel blocker use?

- What are the common side effects of calcium channel blockers?

Basic Science Review and Discussion

There are 10 calcium channel blockers available today in the United States. As a diverse class of drugs, they have many roles in the treatment of cardiovascular diseases. One calcium channel blocker, **nimodipine,** also has a specific role in treating subarachnoid hemorrhages.

Calcium channel blockers inhibit L-type calcium channels in cardiac and smooth muscle. As a result, inhibition of calcium influx into cells occurs, causing a **decrease in myocardial contractility** and rate, resulting in reduced oxygen demand. **Cardiac rate** is slowed by the ability of calcium channel blockers to block electrical conduction through the **atrioventricular (AV) node.** In addition, calcium channel blockers can reduce systemic arterial pressure by relaxing arterial smooth muscle and **decreasing systemic vascular resistance.**

Four categories of calcium channel blockers can be defined based on their chemical structures and actions: diphenylalkylamines, benzothiazepines, dihydropyridines, and bepridil. Both diphenylalkylamines (verapamil) and benzothiazepines (diltiazem) exhibit effects on both cardiac and vascular tissue. With specificity for the heart tissue, these two types of calcium channel blockers can slow conduction through the AV node and are useful in treating arrhythmias. The dihydropyridines (nifedipine is the prototypical agent) are more potent peripheral and coronary artery **vasodilators.** They do not affect cardiac conduction, but can dilate coronary arteries. They are particularly useful as antianginal agents. Bepridil is unique in that it blocks both fast sodium channels and calcium channels in the heart. All calcium channel blockers, except nimodipine and bepridil, are effective in treating HTN.

Most side effects of the calcium channel blockers are related to their mechanism of action. Verapamil and diltiazem can both cause **sinus bradycardia** and may worsen CHF. **Constipation** has been associated with verapamil use. The dihydropyridines often cause symptoms associated with vasodilatation, such as facial flushing, peripheral edema, hypotension, and headache. Because dihydropyridines are potent vasodilators, they can cause reflex tachycardia, which may precipitate palpitations, worsening angina, or MI. Lastly, all calcium channel blockers can cause GI complaints and fatigue.

Case Conclusion Diuretics and beta-blockers are first-line agents for treating HTN. Because this patient has asthma, beta-blockers should be avoided. Calcium channel blockers are favorable therapeutic options in patients with both angina and HTN. Because her heart rate is low, diltiazem and verapamil are not optimal choices because they can slow down AV nodal conduction. A long-acting dihydropyridine, amlodipine, was started.

Thumbnail: Calcium Channel Blockers

Agent	Verapamil	Diltiazem	Nifedipine	Bepridil
Clinical use	Angina (vasospastic, chronic stable and unstable), HTN, arrhythmias, migraine prophylaxis	Angina (vasospastic, chronic stable and unstable), HTN, arrhythmias	Vasospastic angina, HTN, nimodipine is used for subarachnoid hemorrhage	Chronic stable angina
MOA	Calcium channel antagonists bind to L-type channels in cardiac and smooth muscle, and inhibit influx of calcium into cardiac muscle, which decreases contractility and rate.			
Hemodynamic properties				
AV node conduction	↓↓↓	↓↓	0	↓
Myocardial contractility	↓↓	↓	↓	↓
Peripheral vascular resistance	↓↓	↓	↓↓↓	↓
Pharmacokinetics				
Route of administration	PO, IV	PO, IV	PO	PO
Metabolism	Liver (T½ 3–7 hours)	Liver (T½ 3–7 hours)	Liver (T½ 2–5 hours)	Liver (T½ 24 hours)
Adverse reactions	Sinus bradycardia, constipation, gingival hyperplasia	Sinus bradycardia	Facial flushing, peripheral edema, hypotension, headache, gingival hyperplasia, reflex tachycardia (palpitations, angina, myocardial infarct)	Agranulocytosis, arrhythmias (torsade de pointes)
Drug interactions	Increased levels of digoxin, carbamazepine, cyclosporine, theophylline; additive AV nodal block with concurrent beta-blockers		Grapefruit juice may increase levels of some dihydropyridine agents	

Questions

1. A 55-year-old man is hospitalized for observation after an anginal attack. He suddenly develops shortness of breath and fatigue and tells his nurse that his heart feels like its ready to "jump out" of his chest. His ECG monitor shows AF with a ventricular rate of 160 beats/min. PMH: COPD and diabetes. Which of the following medications is best to control his ventricular rate?

   A. Quinidine
   B. Metoprolol
   C. Diltiazem
   D. Amlodipine
   E. Nimodipine

2. A 25-year-old woman with a history of migraine headaches was started on a calcium channel blocker 6 months ago for prophylaxis therapy. She now reveals that she has been having problems with constipation since starting therapy. In addition, she says that her gums are "overgrowing." PMH: Depression and diabetes. Which calcium channel blocker is the most likely cause of her side effects?

   A. Diltiazem
   B. Amlodipine
   C. Bepridil
   D. Verapamil
   E. Nifedipine

HPI:	MS is a 64-year-old woman newly diagnosed with HTN.

PMH: Osteoporosis. Her current medications include calcium carbonate, estrogen, and medroxyprogesterone acetate.

PE: Vitals: T 37.3°C, BP 162/70 mm Hg, HR 65 beats/min, RR 18 breaths/min.

Labs: K+ 3.7 mEq/L, BUN 18 mg/dL, Cr 1.0 mg/dL. Hydrochlorothiazide was started to lower her blood pressure.

Thought Questions

- What are the three main classes of diuretics?

- Why choose thiazide diuretics over other diuretics for the treatment of hypertension?

- Discuss the differences in pharmacology between the classes.

Basic Science Review and Discussion

The three main diuretic classes are **thiazide, loop,** and **potassium-sparing diuretics** (Table 10-1). Thiazide diuretics are considered one of the first-line agents for the treatment of HTN. Acutely, thiazide diuretics lower blood pressure by inhibiting sodium chloride cotransporters in the ascending loop of Henle and distal tubule, increasing sodium excretion and causing diuresis. The reduction in plasma volume decreases cardiac output and consequently reduces blood pressure. However, with continued therapy, the plasma volume returns to pretreatment level and there is a decrease in peripheral vascular resistance, which is responsible for the long-term antihypertensive effects. The most common indication for thiazide diuretics is HTN.

The loop diuretics, including furosemide, bumetanide, torsemide, and ethacrynic acid, are the most potent diuretics available. They inhibit sodium and chloride channels in the thick ascending limb of the loop of Henle and prevent sodium reabsorption leading to diuresis. In general, they do not reduce peripheral vasodilatation to the same extent as thiazide diuretics; therefore, they do not consistently and are not as effective at lowering blood pressure. Loop diuretics are more potent than thiazides for diuresis and are most commonly used in patients with fluid overload.

Spironolactone, triamterene, and amiloride are potassium-sparing diuretics. They inhibit sodium reabsorption in the distal and collecting tubules and decrease potassium excretion through different modes. Spironolactone is a competitive aldosterone antagonist in the distal tubule and prevents the formation of protein important in sodium transport. It is indicated in the management of CHF for its mortality benefits and in patients with hyperaldosteronism (e.g., patients with hepatic cirrhosis and ascites). Triamterene and amiloride reduce the passage of sodium ions by directly acting on the sodium and potassium transporters in the distal and collecting tubule. The naturetic activity of potassium-sparing diuretics is limited compared with thiazide and loop diuretics. For this reason, they are usually given in combination with thiazide or loop diuretics in HTN to reduce the potassium loss.

Table 10-1 Comparison of currently available diuretics

Diuretic class	Tubular site of action	Onset (hr) PO (IV)	Duration of effect (hr) PO (IV)	T½ (hr)
Thiazide or related	Loop of Henle and early distal tubule			
Chlorthalidone		2–3	24–72	40
Chlorothiazide		2 (15 min)	12–16	¾–2
Hydrochlorothiazide		2	12–16	5½–15
Metolazone		1	12–24	No data
Loop	Loop of Henle			
Furosemide		1 (5 min)	6–8 (2)	2
Bumetanide		½ (2 min)	4–6 (½–1)	1–1½
Torsemide		1 (10 min)	6–8	3½
Potassium-sparing	Distal and collecting tubule			
Spironolactone		24–48	48–72	20
Triamterene		2–4	12–16	3
Amiloride		2	24	6–9

Case Conclusion According to the Sixth Report of the Joint National Committee on Prevention, Detection, Evaluation, and Treatment of High Blood Pressure (JNC VI)[1] diuretics are the preferred first-line agents in patients with isolated systolic hypertension (ISH). Studies have shown significant reduction in strokes, heart attacks, and mortality with diuretics and dihydropyridine calcium channel blockers in the treatment of ISH. Because this patient has ISH and adequate renal function, a thiazide diuretic is appropriate as initial treatment.

Thumbnail: Diuretics

	Thiazide	Loop	Potassium-sparing
Clinical use	HTN, adjunct to loop diuretics for edema.	Edema HTN in patients with CrCl < 30–50 mL/min	HTN Spironolactone: systolic heart failure & hepatic cirrhosis.
MOA	Inhibits reabsorption of NaCl in the ascending loop of Henle and the early distal tubules	Inhibits reabsorption of NaCl in the ascending loop of Henle and distal tubule	Spironolactone blocks aldosterone receptors in the distal renal tubules. Triamterene & amiloride interfere with K^+/Na^+ exchange in the distal and collecting tubule.
Pharmacokinetics			
Absorption	Good absorption, except for chlorothiazide (mostly given IV)	Well absorbed. In heart failure patients with edematous bowels, IV diuretics may be required.	Well absorbed
Distribution	Protein binding varies among different agents, but most have large volumes of distribution.	Highly protein bound and small volumes of distribution	Spironolactone is highly protein bound. Triamterene has moderate protein binding. Amiloride has insignificant protein binding and a very large volume of distribution.
Elimination	Renally excreted unchanged	Hepatically, except for furosemide	Spironolactone is metabolized by the liver to an active metabolite, carenone. Triamterene is hepatically cleared. Amiloride is renally excreted.
Adverse reactions	Electrolyte imbalances; ↓K^+, ↓Mg^{2+}, ↓Na^+, ↓Cl^-, ↑uric acid reabsorption in the proximal tubules can precipitate gouty attacks. Other side effects include rash, ↑glucose, dizziness, photosensitivity, ↓BP, headache, ↑lipids.	Similar to thiazide diuretics, except may also cause hypocalcemia.	↓BP, ↑K^+, constipation, and nausea. Gynecomastia can occur with spironolactone.
Comments	Electrolytes, blood glucose, and lipids need to be monitored periodically.	Ototoxicity may occur with furosemide at high infusion rates.	↑K^+ most often occurs in patients with renal impairment or in combination with ACE-I.

Questions

1. SL is an 82-year-old man admitted to the hospital 3 days ago for pulmonary edema. He received nitroglycerin and a diuretic. Now he complains of decreased hearing. Which diuretic most likely caused the ototoxicity?

   A. Hydrochlorothiazide
   B. Furosemide
   C. Bumetanide
   D. Torsemide
   E. None of the above

2. LC is a 56-year-old woman with HTN and renal insufficiency (CrCl 20 mL/min) who presents to the clinic. Her BP is elevated at 150/92 mm Hg. Which diuretic is probably not effective in this patient?

   A. Furosemide
   B. Hydrochlorothiazide
   C. Bumetanide
   D. Torsemide
   E. A, C, and D

Reference

[1]Joint National Committee on Detection, Evaluation, and Treatment of High Blood Pressure. The Sixth Report of the Joint National Committee on Detection, Evaluation and Treatment of High Blood Pressure. Arch Intern Med 1997;157:2413–2446.

HPI: MM is 64-year-old Asian man who presents to the clinic for an HTN follow-up examination after starting hydro-chlorothiazide 6 months ago. He denies chest pain, shortness of breath, dizziness, or headache. His past medical history is significant for diabetes and HTN. He is currently only receiving hydrochlorothiazide.

PE: Vital signs are T 37.5°C, BP 154/92 mm Hg, HR 82 beats/min, and RR 16 breaths/min. His BP remains elevated above goal (130/85 mm Hg), and an ACE inhibitor is begun.

Labs: K^+ 4.3 mEq/L, BUN 26 mg/dL, Cr 1.4 mg/dL. Urinalysis (UA): 3+ protein.

Thought Questions

- What is the pharmacology of ACE inhibitors (ACE-I)?
- When would an ACE inhibitor be preferred over other antihypertensive medications?
- Which ACE inhibitor has the shortest half-life?

Basic Science Review and Discussion

ACE-I block the conversion of angiotensin I to angiotensin II, which causes vasoconstriction and stimulates the production of aldosterone synthesis. Thus, ACE-I promote vasodilatation and decrease sodium retention, consequently lowering blood pressure. The inhibition of angiotensin-converting enzymes also blocks the breakdown of bradykinins. The increase in bradykinin level leads to additional vasodilatation effects. However, the increase in bradykinin is also responsible for adverse effects such as cough and angioedema.

In addition, ACE-I are particularly useful in treating patients with **diabetic nephropathy**. In these patients, ACE-I can decrease proteinuria and stabilize renal function independent of their antihypertensive effects. The benefits are attributed to their effects on renal hemodynamics. Angiotension II may adversely affect the kidney by increasing the glomerular efferent arteriole resistance. Hence, the decrease in production of angiotensin II results in vasodilatation of the efferent arteriole and lowering intra-glomerular capillary pressure. These agents also have favorable effects in patients with CHF and post-MI. ACE-I have been shown to reduce mortality and to preserve left ventricular function by reducing remodeling of the myocardium in these patients.

Captopril is the shortest and fastest acting oral ACE-I (Table 11-1). Because of these properties, it is used to titrate patients to the desired response and often converted to a longer-acting ACE-I.

Table 11-1 Comparison of currently available ACE inhibitors

Agent	Onset (min)	Duration (hr)	T½ (hr)	Elimination
Captopril	15–30	10–12	2	Renal
Enalapril	60	24	11	Renal
Lisinopril	60	24	12	Renal
Ramipril	60–120	24	13–17	Renal
Benazepril	30–60	24	10–11	Renal
Fosinopril	60	24	12	Renal + hepatic
Quinapril	60	24	2	Renal
Moexipril	90	24	2–9	Renal + hepatic
Trandolapril	240	24	10	Renal

Case Conclusion A 24-hour urine collection is performed, which reveals 780 mg of protein and a CrCl rate of 58 mL/min. Thus, this patient has chronic renal disease, most likely diabetic nephropathy. Therefore, an ACE-I would be a good choice for this patient.

Thumbnail: ACE Inhibitors

Prototypical agent: Captopril, shortest-acting ACE inhibitor. Additional agents have been developed with longer durations of action, allowing for once-daily dosing.

Clinical use: ACE-I are most commonly used for hypertension, diabetic nephropathy, CHF, and post-MI.

MOA: ACE-I block the conversion of angiotensin I to angiotensin II, promoting vasodilatation and decreasing sodium retention.

Pharmacokinetics

Absorption: Most are well absorbed, but food may reduce the absorption of captopril, moexipril, quinapril, and trandolapril.

Distribution: The distribution greatly varies depending on the protein binding of the agent: Moexipril > lisinopril > captopril > trandolapril > benazepril, fosinopril.

Elimination: Most ACE-I are renally eliminated.

Adverse reactions: The most common adverse effects are hypotension, headache, fatigue, dizziness, **hyperkalemia,** and **cough.** The incidence of ACE inhibitor-induced cough ranges from 1% to 10%. The onset may occur within a couple of weeks to months after initiation. The cough is dry, nonproductive, and not responsive to cough suppressants. It should resolve 1 to 4 days after discontinuing the ACE-I. Less common side effects are dygeusia, rash, **agranulocytosis,** and **angioedema.** The incidence of angioedema is less than 1% and may occur anytime during therapy. The swelling is usually confined to the face, lips, tongue, glottis, and larynx. Patients should not be rechallenged with an ACE-I if they have a history of angioedema.

Warning: The use of ACE-I during the second and third trimesters of pregnancy can cause injury or death to the developing fetus.

Questions

1. A 63-year-old man presents to the clinic complaining of dizziness and lightheadedness. The patient's BP is 95/62 mm Hg and HR 110 beats/min. He was recently started on benazepril 10 days ago. His PMH is notable for HTN and osteoarthritis. He is currently taking furosemide and ibuprofen. Stat labs include Na^+ < 128 mEq/L, K^+ 4.6 mEq/L, and Cr 1.1 mg/dL. What is (are) the risk factor(s) for ACE inhibitor-induced hypotension?

   A. Hyponatremia (serum sodium < 130 mEq/L)
   B. Concurrent diuretic use
   C. Concurrent NSAID use
   D. Tachycardia
   E. A and B

2. A 72-year-old woman with an anterior MI was admitted to the hospital 7 days ago and has developed swelling of her lips and tongue, and bradycardia. She also complains of flushing and hallucinations. During the hospital course, the patient was started on metoprolol, captopril, isosorbide dinitrate, aspirin, and morphine. Which of the following adverse drug reactions is mostly likely caused by captopril?

   A. Bradycardia
   B. Swelling of lips and tongue
   C. Flushing
   D. Hallucinations
   E. None of the above

> **HPI:** Six weeks after starting lisinopril for HTN, MM develops a dry nonproductive cough. After ruling out other causes of the cough, he was switched to losartan.
>
> **PE:** Vitals: T 36.8°C, BP 145/85 mm Hg, HR 80 beats/min, RR 16 breaths/min. Lungs clear to auscultation. Medications: Hydrochlorothiazide and lisinopril.
>
> **Labs:** K^+ 4.7 mEq/L, BUN 24 mg/dL, Cr 1.2 mg/dL. UA: Positive protein.

Thought Questions

- What is the primary pharmacology of angiotensin receptor blockers (ARBs)?

- When are ARBs indicated?

- What are the advantages of ARBs over ACE-I?

Basic Science Review and Discussion

Angiotensin receptor blockers are selective and competitive **angiotensin II receptor antagonists** (Table 12-1). They block vasoconstriction and aldosterone-secreting effects similar to ACE-I. However, because ARBs do not block the metabolism or increase the levels of bradykinin, they are less likely to be associated with nonrenin-angiotensin effects such as cough and angioedema.

Angiotensin II antagonists share the hemodynamic effects of ACE-I, and therefore have similar indications such as HTN, CHF, and diabetic nephropathy. However, ARBs have not been shown to be superior to ACE-I and are more expensive. In addition, there is an absence of data documenting comparable long-term cardiovascular benefits. Therefore, ARBs should be reserved principally for patients in whom ACE-I are indicated but who are unable to tolerate the medication.

Table 12-1 Comparison of currently available angiotensin receptor blockers

Agent	Onset (min)	Duration (hr)	T½ (hr)	Elimination
Losartan	60–90	24	2–9	Hepatic + renal
Valsartan	120	24	6	Hepatic
Irbesartan	60–120	24	11–15	Hepatic
Candesartan	120–240	24	9	Hepatic + renal
Telmisartan	60–180	24	24	Hepatic

Case Conclusion The patient was switched to an ARB because he was experiencing cough, a possible side effect of ACE-I. It is important to rule out other causes of cough before discontinuing ACE-I. The incidence of ACE inhibitor-induced cough may vary, ranging from 1% to 10%, and occurs less frequently with ARBs because it does not inhibit the breakdown of bradykinins. ACE inhibitor-induced cough may occur within a couple of weeks to months after initiation of therapy. After discontinuing the ACE-I, the cough should resolve within 1 to 4 days.

Thumbnail: Angiotensin Receptor Blockers

Prototypical agent: Losartan.

Clinical use: ARBs have indications similar to those for ACE inhibitors, but they are mainly used in patients who are unable to tolerate ACE inhibitors.

MOA: Angiotensin II receptor antagonist, which prevents vasoconstriction and aldosterone-secreting effects of angiotensin II.

Pharmacokinetics

Absorption: The absorption greatly varies depending on the agent: irbesartan > telmisartan > losartan, valsartan > candesartan.

Distribution: Variable depending on the protein binding of the agent.

Elimination: ARBs are predominantly eliminated through hepatic metabolism.

Adverse reactions: Similar to ACE inhibitors. The most common side effects are **cough,** hypotension, headache, fatigue, dizziness, and **hyperkalemia.** The less common adverse reactions include dygeusia, rash, diarrhea, **agranulocytosis,** and **angioedema.** Cough and angioedema occur less frequently than in ACE inhibitors, but precautions should be taken when initiating ARBs in someone who experienced angioedema with an ACE inhibitor because there is some cross-reactivity.

Warning: Use during the second and third trimesters can cause injury or death to the developing fetus.

Questions

1. A 57-year-old woman is admitted to the hospital for CHF. Losartan was started, and 2 days later her renal function began declining rapidly over the ensuing few days. PMH: Asthma, AV block, CHF, diabetes, and bilateral renal stenosis. Why are ARBs contraindicated in this patient?

    A. Bilateral renal stenosis
    B. Congestive heart failure
    C. Asthma
    D. AV block
    E. None of the above

2. A 63-year-old man recently started on valsartan for HTN. What should be monitored upon initiation of ARBs?

    A. Serum creatinine
    B. Blood pressure
    C. Serum potassium
    D. Blood urea nitrogen
    E. All of the above

> **HPI:** AF is a 55-year-old woman who is scheduled to undergo left hip replacement surgery. While in the operating room and postanesthesia care unit (PACU), she has on thromboembolic deterrent (TED) stockings and sequential compression devices (SCDs). On postoperative day 1, the SCDs are discontinued, and she is started on enoxaparin for deep vein thrombosis (DVT) prophylaxis. On postoperative day 7, as AF is getting ready for discharge, she becomes acutely short of breath and develops a painful and swollen left leg.
>
> **Labs:** Cr 1.2 mg/dL, international normalized ratio (INR) 1.1, activated partial thromboplastin time (aPTT) 35 seconds, hematocrit (Hct) 38%, platelets 247,000/mm³. Doppler ultrasound: Partial noncompressibility of the left popliteal vein, nonocclusive clot. Ventilation-perfusion scintigraphy: High probability for acute pulmonary embolism. Unmatched ventilation perfusion defect is seen in the left lower lobe.

Thought Questions

- What are some of the risk factors for venous thromboembolism?

- How does factor X contribute to clotting?

- What are the contraindications for low-molecular-weight heparins (LMWH)?

- What are some of the disadvantages of warfarin-based therapy?

Basic Science Review and Discussion

Patients with a high risk for clotting require thromboprophylaxis. Some risk factors for venous thromboembolism include age greater than 40 years, prolonged immobility, history of prior venous thromboembolism (DVT, pulmonary embolism [PE]), cancer, major surgery (abdominal, pelvic, or lower extremity), fracture (pelvis, hip, or leg), CHF, MI, stroke, obesity, and high-dose estrogen use.

The coagulation pathway can be activated by one of two pathways: the **extrinsic** (tissue factor) pathway or the **intrinsic** (contact activation) pathway (Figure 13-1). The main coagulation pathway in vivo is the tissue factor pathway. Tissue factor is exposed by damaged endothelium. This exposed tissue factor binds and activates factor VII, which, in turn, activates factor X. Factor Xa results in the generation of a thrombin (factor IIa) burst. Thrombin, in turn activates factors XI, VIII, and V, leading to the further generation of thrombin and clottable fibrin. Additionally, the tissue factor VIIa complex activates factor IX, which further contributes to the activation of factor X.

Heparins inhibit factors Xa and IIa through their interaction with antithrombin, a naturally occurring anticoagulant. **Unfractionated heparin** (UFH) is a parenteral agent that requires monitoring of the aPTT. Complications with UFH include osteoporosis, heparin-induced thrombocytopenia (HIT), and mineralocorticoid deficiency. HIT type II is observed in 1% to 5% of patients and characteristically occurs after 5 to 10 days of heparin exposure. It is characterized by a significant reduction in platelet count, often falling to the 30,000 to 80,000 cells/mm³ range or to a level less than 50% of baseline. The pathogenesis of HIT type II is immune mediated, resulting from antibodies that activate platelets in the presence of heparin.

Low-molecular-weight heparins, such as enoxaparin, dalteparin, and tinzaparin, were introduced in 1982. These are parenteral agents that have fixed or weight-adjusted dosing, involve less monitoring, and are easier to administer. The half-lives of LMWHs are longer than that of UFH. Because LMWHs are metabolized renally and due to a 90% cross-reactivity to HIT antibodies, they are contraindicated in patients with poor renal function and patients with HIT. In rare instances, antifactor Xa levels are measured. This peak level is drawn 4 hours after the third dose (prophylaxis 0.2–0.4 units/mL; treatment 0.5–1.0 units/mL).

Vitamin K antagonists, such as **warfarin,** interfere with gamma-carboxylation of vitamin K-dependent clotting proteins: factors II, VII, IX, and X and proteins C and S. Because warfarin affects the natural anticoagulants, protein C and S, and takes 4 to 5 days to become fully established, it should be overlapped with heparin. Although factor VII is quickly depleted and an initial prolongation of the prothrombin time is seen in 8 to 12 hours, maximum anticoagulation is not approached for about 4 days as the other factors are depleted and the drug achieves steady state. Its therapeutic index is narrow, so INRs need to be monitored closely. There are also many food and drug interactions with warfarin, and it is contraindicated in pregnant patients. Warfarin is metabolized by cytochrome P450 (CYP450) enzymes in the liver. Medications that are potent inhibitors (amiodarone, fluconazole, metronidazole, trimethoprim-sulfamethoxazole,

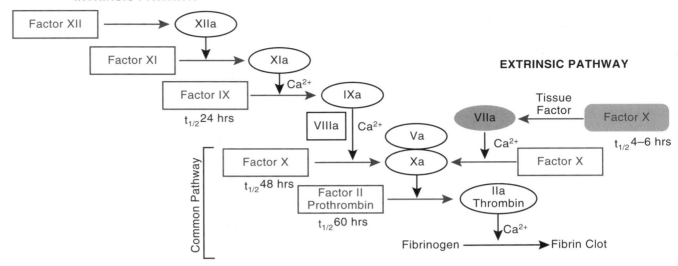

Figure 13-1 Extrinsic and intrinsic pathway.

etc.) or potent inducers (carbamazepine, rifampin, pheno-barbital, etc.) of the CYP450 system can dramatically increase or decrease warfarin effect, respectively. Concomitant illnesses, such as liver disease and hyper-thyroidism, can affect the patient's response to warfarin therapy as well. This is dependent on the synthesis of the vitamin K-dependent coagulation factors and the rate of decay.

Case Conclusion AF was started on enoxaparin 60 mg subcutaneously (SC) every 12 hours, followed by warfarin 5 mg PO at bedtime. The patient's goal INR was 2 to 3. She was discharged with warfarin and enoxaparin after being clini-cally stable, follow-up appointments were obtained, and the patient was taught how to give subcutaneous injections to herself. Once the warfarin dosing was therapeutic, the enoxaparin was discontinued and the patient was continued on warfarin, with monthly monitoring, for 6 months.

Thumbnail: Anticoagulant Agents

Drug	Unfractionated heparin	LMWHs (dalteparin, enoxaparin, tinzaparin)	Warfarin
Clinical indications	Prophylaxis and treatment mitral of venous thrombosis; PE; peripheral arterial embolism; AF	Prevention of DVT and other thromboembolic complications; treatment of acute DVT with or without PE	Prophylaxis and treatment of venous thrombosis and its extension; PE and thromboembolic complications associated with AF
Mechanism of action	Potentiates the action of antithrombin III and thereby inactivates thrombin (as well as factors IXa, Xa, XIa, XIIa, and plasmin); prevents the conversion of fibrinogen to fibrin. Molecular weights of heparin vary from 300 to 30,000 daltons.	Enhances the inhibition of factor Xa and thrombin by binding to and accelerating antithrombin III activity. Molecular weights vary from 2000 to 9000 daltons.	Interfere with the hepatic synthesis of vitamin K-dependent clotting (factors VII, IX, X and II). Anticoagulant effects are dependent on the T½ of these clotting factors.
Absorption/distribution	Must be given IV or SC (not absorbed PO); IV bolus results in immediate anticoagulant effects; peak plasma levels of heparin are achieved in 2 to 4 h following SC use; once absorbed, heparin is distributed in plasma and is extensively and nonspecifically protein bound.	Bioavailability of SC injection is about 90%. The onset of anticoagulant effect is approximately 4 h.	Rapidly and completely absorbed. Highly bound to plasma proteins, primarily albumin.
Metabolism/elimination	Rapidly cleared from plasma with an average T½ of 30–180 min. The T½ is dose dependent and nonlinear (may be prolonged at higher doses). Heparin is partially metabolized by liver heparinase and the reticuloendothelial system.	Metabolized by the kidneys.	Metabolized by hepatic microsomal enzymes and is excreted primarily in the urine as inactive metabolites.
Adverse reactions	Hemorrhage. Other side effects include thrombocytopenia, osteoporosis, cutaneous necrosis.	Similar to UFH. Incidences of HIT may occur but are rare.	Hemorrhage. Some complications may present as paralysis, headache, chest or joint pain, shortness of breath, and difficulty breathing or swallowing.
Drug interactions			Co-trimoxazole Erythromycin Metronidazole Rifampin Amiodarone
Contraindications	Allergy to heparin; uncontrolled bleeding	Allergy to heparin. Avoid in patients with CrCl of < 30 mL/min. Use in caution in patients with low body weights.	Pregnancy; hemorrhagic tendencies

Questions

1. A patient with a mechanical prosthetic mitral valve is seen in the clinic. He has been stable on 5 mg of warfarin taken every evening. His INRs have been ranging from 2.5 to 2.7 for the past 6 months. He was started on amiodarone 2 weeks ago for an arrhythmia. Today his INR is 5.1 and thyroid-stimulating hormone (TSH) level is 2.1 mIU/L. How does amiodarone play a part in this patient's anticoagulation therapy?

   A. Decreases warfarin absorption
   B. Increases metabolism of vitamin K-dependent clotting factors
   C. Additive or synergistic anticoagulant effects
   D. Decreases warfarin metabolism

2. An 80-year-old woman is admitted to the hospital with pneumonia. She has AF and takes warfarin 2.5 mg PO every morning. She reports a slight nosebleed last night. Her appetite has been poor this past week, and she has had a fever for the past 2 days. Her INR is 9.1. How would you manage this patient?

   A. Give one dose of vitamin K 2.5 mg PO, hold warfarin, and recheck INR tomorrow.
   B. Give vitamin K 10 mg SC for three doses, hold warfarin, and recheck INR tomorrow.
   C. Give vitamin K 5 mg IV, hold warfarin, and recheck INR tomorrow.
   D. Hold patient's warfarin dosage and recheck INR tomorrow.

HPI: PB is a 70-year-old man who was brought to the ED with "crushing" chest pain radiating down his left arm. He was found on the couch looking pale, diaphoretic, and clutching his chest, and was given a total of three sublingual nitroglycerin tablets, with recurrent pain in between. En route to the ED, the patient was told to chew an aspirin.

PE: His initial vital signs were significant for BP 210/120 mm Hg, HR 80 beats/min, RR 18 breaths/min, and O_2 saturation 98% on 6 liters oxygen by nasal cannula. In the ED, PB was started on IV infusions of nitroglycerin, metoprolol, and heparin. The patient was ruled in for acute MI, with first creatine kinase (CK) of 137 IU/L, then peaking to 467 IU/L. Troponin was elevated at 0.95. ECG showed an ST segment elevation with no Q wave.

Thought Questions

- What is the role of platelet aggregation in acute coronary syndromes?

- What are the different pathways of platelet activation?

- What is the final common pathway in platelet aggregation?

- What are drug interactions with aspirin?

- What is the mechanism of action for glycoprotein IIb/IIIa inhibitors?

Basic Science Review and Discussion

Platelet aggregation plays an important role in the pathogenesis of acute coronary syndromes (ACS). **Myocardial infarction** is an ACS that occurs when atherosclerotic plaques embedded in artery walls rupture, leading to thrombus formation and coronary occlusion. Patients with high-risk coronary stenosis may need **percutaneous coronary interventions** (PCI) with or without stent placement to revascularize the arteries.

Atherosclerotic plaques contain a lipid core that is highly thrombogenic. The lipid core contains lipids, collagen, macrophages, tissue factor, and von Willebrand factor that can further accelerate coagulation. When the plaque ruptures, platelets adhere to exposed collagen and von Willebrand factor, which leads to additional platelet activation and recruitment.

Once platelets are activated, the **glycoprotein IIb/IIIa (GpIIb/IIIa) receptors** located on the platelet surface undergo a conformational change, causing fibrinogen to cross-link platelets. Release of thrombin, thromboxane-2 (TXA_2), epinephrine, and adenosine diphosphate (ADP) leads to increased expression of GpIIb/IIIa receptors on the platelet surface.

Antiplatelet therapy plays a key role in the treatment of ACS, such as MI. **Aspirin** has been shown to decrease overall mortality and reinfarction and is recommended for all patients in this setting unless contraindicated. Aspirin should be given at the lowest effective dose, to ensure efficacy and to limit adverse reactions. If aspirin is contraindicated or not tolerated, **thienopyridines (clopidogrel** or **ticlopidine)** may be used. Comparisons of oral antiplatelet agents are summarized in Thumbnail.

Concomitant use of heparin and oral anticoagulants can increase the risk for bleeding due to the antiplatelet effect of aspirin. In addition, use with alcohol can increase the risk of GI bleeding. Aspirin displaces a number of drugs (e.g., tolbutamide, nonsteroidal anti-inflammatory drugs [NSAIDs], methotrexate, phenytoin, and probenecid) from protein binding sites in the blood. Corticosteroid use can reduce serum salicylate levels by increasing the clearance of aspirin.

Patients undergoing PCIs to revascularize arteries are also subject to arterial injury, new plaque rupture, and thrombus formation. GpIIb/IIIa inhibitors are used in conjunction with heparin and aspirin to treat patients with ACS that will undergo PCI. GpIIb/IIIa inhibitors have been shown to reduce mortality, reinfarction, and revascularization in this patient population. The use of GpIIb/IIIa inhibitors decreases the ischemic events and angioplasty complications and improves outcomes of coronary stenting.

Case Conclusion Despite treatment with nitroglycerin, metoprolol, and heparin drips in the ED, PB continued to have chest pain. He was scheduled for an emergent coronary catheterization to improve symptoms and prevent further ischemia. He was started on an eptifibatide IV drip for 24 hours and oral clopidogrel for 4 weeks.

Thumbnail: Antiplatelet Agents

A. Oral Antiplatelet Agents

Agent	Aspirin	Ticlopidine	Clopidogrel
Clinical use	MI, unstable angina, cerebrovascular disease	MI, unstable angina, coronary artery stenting, cerebrovascular disease	MI, unstable angina, coronary artery stenting, cerebrovascular disease
MOA	Nonselective cyclooxygenase (COX) inhibitor. Inhibits TXA_2 platelet aggregation.	Inhibits ADP platelet receptor.	Inhibits ADP platelet receptor.
Absorption	Rapid absorption	80% absorbed	Rapid absorption
Antiplatelet effect	Can be detected within 60 min, lasts ~ 10 days	3–5 days	3–5 days
Metabolism	Hydrolyzed by esterases; salicylate hepatically metabolized	CYP450 activation	CYP450 activation
Adverse effects	GI upset, ulceration, or bleeding, tinnitis in high doses, renal dysfunction. Patients with preexisting asthmatic disease or intolerance to aspirin may develop bronchoconstriction, rhinitis, or urticaria.	Diarrhea, nausea, vomiting, skin rash, neutropenia, bone marrow aplasia, thrombocytopenic purpura, cholestatic jaundice	Diarrhea, nausea, vomiting
Comments	Antiplatelet activity lasts the duration of the life of the platelet, since platelets cannot generate new COX enzyme.		

B. Intravenous GpIIb/IIIa Inhibitors

Agent	Abciximab	Eptifibatide	Tirofiban
Structure	Monoclonal antibody	Cyclic heptapeptide	Nonpeptide
MOA	Blocks GpIIb/IIIa receptors by steric hindrance and conformation effect	Reversible GpIIb/IIIa inhibitor	Reversible GpIIb/IIIa inhibitor
Receptor specificity	Nonspecific	Specific	Specific
Platelet inhibition	> 80% inhibition	40%–50% inhibition	> 90% inhibition
Return of platelet function	Slow	Fast	Fast
Pharmacokinetics	$T\frac{1}{2}$ = 10–30 min	$T\frac{1}{2}$ = 2.5 h	$T\frac{1}{2}$ = 2 h
Elimination	Senescent platelets	About 50% renal	Mostly renal
Comments	Active bleeding is an absolute contraindication. Relative contraindications include major surgery within the past 3 months, stroke within the past 6 months, or recent trauma.		

Questions

1. JG is a 61-year-old woman who was recently hospitalized for an MI. Her PMH includes hyperlipidemia, hypertension, and asthma. Which antiplatelet medication should have been initiated for JG's acute coronary disease?
   - A. Aspirin
   - B. Ticlopidine
   - C. Clopidogrel
   - D. Abciximab
   - E. Eptifibatide

2. LM is a 50-year-old man who underwent PCI to revascularize a 100% occluded left anterior descending coronary artery. For the procedure he will receive heparin, abciximab, and aspirin. Baseline platelet count is 150,000/mm³. Two hours after the bolus dose of abciximab is given, platelet count is 1,000/mm³. What clinical intervention(s) should occur?
   - A. Continue abciximab until the procedure is over.
   - B. Continue abciximab, aspirin, and heparin but give a platelet transfusion.
   - C. Discontinue aspirin and heparin.
   - D. Discontinue abciximab, aspirin, and heparin.
   - E. Discontinue abciximab, aspirin, and heparin and give a platelet infusion.

> **HPI:** LG is a 28-year-old man brought into the ED by ambulance after a motor vehicle accident.
>
> **PE:** On physical examination, his vital signs were T 38.2°C, BP 140/80 mm Hg, HR 87 beats/min, and RR 22 breaths/min; lungs are clear. LG has sustained extensive contusions and superficial lacerations to the left lower extremity. The left leg is edematous, and radiography reveals a tibial fracture. The leg is initially placed in a splint while the swelling subsides. LG is complaining of severe, unremitting pain, described as sharp and throbbing. He rates the pain as an 8 on a scale of 10.

Thought Questions

- How can LG's pain be classified?

- What is the pharmacology of opioids?

- What are the differences between the various opioid agents?

- What are common adverse effects of opioid treatment?

Basic Science Review and Discussion

Pain is defined as an unpleasant sensory and emotional experience associated with actual or potential tissue damage. The nerves that transmit pain are of two types, the A-delta and C. The **A-delta** fibers are myelinated, rapidly conducting fibers that are primarily responsible for well-localized, sharp, stabbing pain, otherwise know as "first pain." **C fibers** are unmyelinated fibers that respond to noxious mechanical, thermal, and chemical stimuli at a much slower rate and mediate "second pain." Acute pain is attributable to direct injury of the tissues due to physical trauma or invasive procedures. It is generally self-limiting, but inadequate relief can impair the healing process. Acute pain is treated aggressively with opioids and non-narcotic analgesics. Chronic malignant and nonmalignant pain have musculoskeletal and neurologic origins. Chronic nonmalignant pain is associated with a traumatic event or a chronic disease.

Opioids are both natural and synthetic compounds that target endogenous opioid receptors: mu, kappa, and delta. These receptors are further subdivided into mu_1, mu_2, $kappa_1$, $kappa_2$, $kappa_3$, and $delta_1$ and $delta_2$. Endogenous opioid peptides—endorphins, enkephalins, and dynorphins—act on these receptors to mediate analgesia. Opioids mimic the activity of endogenous peptides at these receptors and act on excitatory neurotransmitters such as N-methyl-D-aspartate (NMDA) and substance P to modulate pain perception.

Severity of pain, route of administration, and patient history of opioid use should guide the selection of an appropriate opioid. Morphine is the prototypical pure agonist to which other agents are compared. Pure agonists do not exhibit a ceiling to the analgesic effects. Hence, as the dose of a pure agonist is increased, a corresponding log-linear increase in analgesia is seen. The dose may be increased until adequate analgesia is achieved or until dose-limiting adverse effects occur. Codeine, hydrocodone, and propoxyphene are less potent agents. These agents are formulated with adjunctive agents such as acetaminophen or aspirin and are used primarily for mild to moderate pain. Morphine, methadone, hydromorphone, meperidine, and fentanyl are used for moderate to severe pain. With the exception of methadone, all have short durations of action, permitting frequent titration of dose (Table 15-1). The transdermal form of fentanyl has a long onset time and lasts for 72 hours, making titration with the patch difficult. Hence, it is reserved for chronic, stable pain.

Opioid use can be limited by intolerable side effects. CNS effects include **somnolence,** cognitive impairment, and mood alterations. Opioid receptors throughout the GI system mediate the slowing of gut peristalsis, causing **constipation.** Use of stool softeners and stimulant laxatives may provide prophylaxis for constipation. Nausea and vomiting, affecting 10% to 40% of patients, are produced through direct stimulation of the medullary chemoreceptor trigger zone, enhanced vestibular sensitivity, and increased gastric antral tone. **Myoclonus** is a dose-related effect that can occur with high doses of any opioid, but the incidence is higher with meperidine. Normeperidine, the active metabolite of meperidine, has twice the seizure potential of the parent compound. **Respiratory depression,** through direct effects on the chemoreceptors of the respiratory centers in the brainstem, is the most dangerous adverse effect of opioids. The threshold for respiratory depression is above the threshold for sedation, which itself is above that for analgesia. Opioids also cause **pruritis** due to histamine release, hypotension, addiction, and miosis. **Tolerance** can develop to all side effects with the exception of constipation and miosis. Excess sedation or respiratory depression can be reversed with the opioid antagonist **naloxone,** given IV. Orally administered naloxone, which is 3% absorbed, may be given for refractory constipation without reversing systemic analgesic effects.

Table 15-1 Comparison of opioid analgesics

	Metabolites	Duration of action	Adverse effects	Comments
Morphine	Morphine–6-glucuronide is more potent than morphine sulfate; renally cleared	3–4 h	Sedation, nausea, decreased BP, constipation, pruritis	Gold standard starting agent
Codeine	10% is converted to morphine sulfate	3–4 h	Frequent nausea	Similar to morphine, less potent
Hydrocodone	Metabolized to hydromorphone	3–4 h	Less nausea/constipation than codeine	Similar to morphine
Oxycodone	Metabolized to oxymorphone	3–4 h	Less nausea/constipation than codeine	Rapid CNS dysphoria or euphoria
Hydromorphone	No active metabolites	3–4 h	Less emesis and fewer CNS effects than morphine	3–6 times more potent than morphine
Fentanyl	No active metabolites	1–2 h (IV); 3 days (transdermal patch)	Fewer effects on BP, no histamine release	Patch has slow onset; prolonged drug absorption after patch removal
Meperidine	Normeperidine has half the analgesic activity but twice the seizure potential; renally cleared	3–4 h; normeperidine T½ 15–30 h	Most potent CNS irritant	Active metabolite may accumulate
Methadone	No active metabolite	6–8 h; increases with chronic dosing secondary to accumulation	Less sedation than morphine	No cross-reactivity with morphine or meperidine
Propoxyphene	Norpropoxyphene has greater CNS depressant effects	3–4 h		Less potent than other opioids; no antitussive activity

Case Conclusion   In the ED, the patient was given IV morphine with adequate pain control. After an overnight hospital stay for observation and casting of the left leg, LG was discharged to home with a prescription for hydrocodone/acetaminophen tablets, to be taken as needed for pain.

Thumbnail: Opioids

Prototypical agent: Morphine, a naturally occurring opioid, is derived from the poppy plant. Other natural, semisynthetic and synthetic opioids include codeine, hydrocodone, oxycodone, methadone, fentanyl, and hydromorphone, among others.

Clinical usage: Primarily used as an analgesic for relief of moderate to severe acute and chronic pain. Morphine is used in MI for analgesia, venodilation, and reduction in preload and oxygen requirements. Fentanyl and sufentanil are used as general anesthesia due to their short duration and minimal effects on the cardiovascular system. Codeine is used as an antitussive and in cough associated with pulmonary edema. Diarrhea may be alleviated with diphenoxylate. Methadone is used in maintenance programs for addiction.

MOA: Binds primarily to endogenous mu, kappa, and delta receptors in the central and peripheral nervous system, altering pain perception.

Pharmacokinetics

Absorption: Oral bioavailability is variable depending on drug and formulation (morphine < hydrocodone and oxycodone < methadone). The exception is fentanyl, which is very poorly absorbed and hence is only available in IV, transdermal, and transmucosal formulations.

Distribution: Opioids are widely distributed in tissue and particularly in highly perfused organs, such as the liver, lungs, kidney, and spleen. Opioids also distribute into and accumulate in fatty tissue.

Elimination: Opioids are hepatically metabolized via the CYP2D6 enzyme into metabolites that are renally eliminated. The exception is methadone, which is metabolized via the CYP3A4 enzyme.

Adverse reactions: Sedation, respiratory depression, constipation, myoclonus, nausea, vomiting, flushing, itching, miosis, hypotension, and hallucinations. Tolerance develops to all side effects with the exception of constipation and miosis. **Physical dependence** may develop within 5 days of opioid use.

Drug interactions: Drugs utilizing the CYP2D6 (i.e., fluoxetine, cimetidine) or the CYP3A4 (i.e., macrolides, antiretrovirals) pathways may inhibit opioid metabolism and potentiate side effects. Drugs such as benzodiazepines and barbiturates should be used cautiously in combination with opioids, as they may potentiate respiratory depression or sedative effects.

Questions

1. A 76-year-old man is admitted to the hospital with severe abdominal pain and a progressive inability to swallow solid foods. He can tolerate a soft diet of pureed foods and liquid. Further work-up reveals a large, inoperable, esophageal tumor obstructing the fundus. A gastric tube (GT) is placed for medication administration and feeding. The patient continues to have severe pain, requiring opioid analgesics. Which of the following would not be a good choice for treatment of this patient's pain?

   A. Hydrocodone/acetaminophen extra-strength tablets per GT (PGT)
   B. Sustained-release oxycodone PGT
   C. Morphine sulfate elixer PGT
   D. IV hydromorphone
   E. Acetaminophen with codeine tablets PGT

2. A 62-year-old man with a history of diabetes and severe osteoarthritis of the knees undergoes a right knee replacement. He has been placed on a hydromorphone PCA (patient-controlled analgesia) and must be transitioned to an oral regimen in preparation for discharge. Labs are normal with the exception of increased BUN 32 mg/dL and serum Cr 2.4 mg/dL. Which of the following would be an appropriate pain medication to treat this patient?

   A. Morphine tablets
   B. Morphine elixir
   C. Fentanyl patch
   D. Meperidine tablets
   E. Oxycodone/acetaminophen tablets

> **HPI:** DM is a 43-year-old woman with metastatic cancer in the hospice care unit. She has long-standing uncontrolled pain from metastases to the chest wall and abdomen and reports sharp, shooting pain that travels anteriorly to posteriorly. She also reports constant, throbbing pain localized to the chest. PMH: Lymphoma for 7 years, chronic constipation.
>
> **PE:** On physical examination, her vital signs are T 37.6°C, BP 128/82 mm Hg, HR 84 beats/min, and RR 18 breaths/min. The pain is described as a chronic 9/10. Her current pain regimen includes oxycodone 10–20 mg every 4 to 6 hours as needed (prn) for pain (about 100 mg/day) and hydromorphone 0.8–1.2 mg IV every 1 to 2 hours prn for breakthrough pain (about 8 mg/day). Allergies (ALL): Morphine (itching, flushing), codeine (nausea, vomiting), meperidine (involuntary leg movements, and facial tics).

Thought Questions

- How does chronic pain present?

- What treatment options are effective for neuropathic pain?

- What factors should be taken into consideration when selecting an opioid for chronic pain?

Basic Science Review and Discussion

Chronic malignant and **chronic nonmalignant** pain has musculoskeletal and neurologic origins. Chronic malignant pain, associated with metastases or tumor lysis syndrome, increases with disease progression. Chronic nonmalignant pain is associated with a traumatic event or a chronic disease. The neuropathic component of pain occurs with physical or chemical destruction of normal neuronal pathways and does not typically respond to opioid treatment. Neurogenic pains are unpleasant sensations or pain characterized as tingling, stabbing, shocking, shooting, and traveling in quality. Temperature descriptors—such as hot, cold, or burning—are commonly used.

Neuropathic pain is treated with **membrane-stabilizing agents,** including anticonvulsants (phenytoin, carbamazepine, gabapentin, lamotrigine) and antiarrhythmics (lidocaine, mexilitine). **Tricyclic antidepressants** (TCAs) are also effective at treating neuropathic pain. Membrane stabilizers prolong the depolarization of nerves, resulting in depressed neuronal membrane excitability and a reduced rate of neural pain firing. These agents work by sodium channel blockade or by enhancing the inhibitory neurotransmitter gamma aminobutyric acid (GABA). TCAs act in the CNS brainstem dorsal horn pain modulating system, which alters or ameliorates ascending pain signals to pain perception centers in the brain. The TCAs inhibit reuptake of norepinephrine and serotonin, which in turn reduce the trafficking of pain signals along the spinal cord.

Chronic pain is often managed with short-acting or immediate-release opioids. This type of management, however, is labor intensive and not optimal in treating chronic pain. Longer-acting opioids and around-the-clock dosing should be implemented in chronic pain management. The longer-acting opioids include methadone, sustained-released formulations of oxycodone and morphine, and transdermal fentanyl. Patients with chronic pain should be converted to long-acting formulations of opioids with rescue dosing with short-acting agents available for breakthrough pain. When using methadone, it is important to titrate carefully because the drug will accumulate with chronic dosing, increasing the duration of action. Fentanyl patches are often used in patients with disabling adverse effects from morphine. Improved sleep quality, reduced constipation and emesis, and long-term pain relief are some benefits of transdermal fentanyl over morphine. Transdermal patches have a long onset time, with a peak onset of 8 hours. Additionally, there is prolonged drug absorption for 8 to 12 hours after a patch is removed.

Case Conclusion DM is converted to sustained-release oxycodone 40 mg three times daily (TID) with oxycodone 5–10 mg every 4 to 6 hours as needed for breakthrough pain. Over the next day, DM uses 7 doses of oxycodone for breakthrough pain. The dose of sustained-release oxycodone is titrated up to 60 mg TID for better pain control and to reduce the need for breakthrough pain dosing.

Thumbnail: Agents for Chronic Pain

Long-acting opioid	Onset of action			Duration of action
Methadone	0.5–1 h			Up to 12 h with chronic dosing
Fentanyl, transdermal	6–8 h			72 h
Morphine, SA	1 h			Up to 12 h
Oxycodone, SA	Biphasic absorption of drug; drug absorbed at 0.6 h and 6 h			Up to 8 h

Agents Used for Neuropathic Pain				
	MOA	Metabolism	Adverse reactions	Comments
Anticonvulsants				
Carbamazepine	Sodium channel blockade	Hepatic, may induce own metabolism	Dizziness, ataxia	Drug-drug interactions due to ability to induce and inhibit metabolism of other drugs
Gabapentin	Unknown	Unchanged drug renally eliminated	Ataxia, dizziness, nystagmus	May accumulate in patients with renal dysfunction
Antiarrhythmics				
Lidocaine	Sodium channel blockade	Hepatic	Local irritation, infusion effects	Topical or single IV doses for local nerve block
Antidepressants				
Prototypical agent: amitriptyline	Inhibits norepinephrine and serotonin reuptake	Hepatic metabolism with renal elimination	High anticholinergic and antihistamine effects; imipramine has high orthostasis profile	2nd degree amines (nortriptyline, desipramine) and doxepin have moderate anticholinergic effects

Questions

1. A 59-year-old man who is s/p thalamic stroke 3 months ago is seen in the clinic and reports continual pain in the contralateral jaw and leg. The pain is burning and marked by tingling, particularly in the knee. He also reports a hypersensitivity of the leg when long pants are worn. He tried gabapentin 100 mg TID for 2 weeks but did not feel improvement and is now asking to try another medication. Which of the following options is most appropriate.

   A. Stop gabapentin. Imipramine has less anticholinergic effects and should be the next agent tried.
   B. Stop gabapentin. Start carbamazepine and titrate to a therapeutic serum level.
   C. Continue gabapentin and add a tricyclic antidepressant.
   D. Continue gabapentin and titrate up the dose.
   E. Attempt a lidocaine nerve blockade.

2. A 72-year-old woman has chronic back pain secondary to scoliosis. She also has some neuropathic pain due to sciatica. She has been using immediate-release morphine every 3 to 4 hours as needed throughout the day. Which of the following would be the most appropriate long-acting regimen to convert this patient?

   A. Immediate-release morphine on an around-the-clock schedule.
   B. Sustained-release morphine scheduled every 8 hours.
   C. Once-daily dosing of methadone.
   D. Sustained-release morphine scheduled every 4 hours.
   E. First convert dosing to immediate-release oxycodone, then convert to sustained release oxycodone every 8 hours.

> **HPI:** KO is a 57-year-old man with a history of migraine headaches and HTN who just completed a course of antibiotics for an upper respiratory infection. He had a severe migraine headache for which he took 10 tablets of ergotamine over 6 hours. He is presenting to the ambulatory care clinic with complaints of muscle cramps and numbness in his extremities. Medications: Ergotamine 2 mg at onset of headache, then 1 mg every 30 minutes until headache resolution; metoprolol; and erythromycin for 10 days. KO has NKDA.

Thought Questions

- What agents are available for treatment of headaches?

- How does treatment of migraine headaches differ from treatment of tension and cluster headaches?

- What are some contraindications to using the serotonin agonists?

Basic Science Review and Discussion

The International Headache Society classifies **headaches** into one of 13 categories, ranging from migraine, tension-type, and cluster headaches, to headaches that are not classifiable. Effective headache treatment is thus guided by an accurate diagnosis of the headache type.

Tension headaches are initially treated with analgesics such as **aspirin, acetaminophen,** or **nonsteroidal anti-inflammatory agents** such as ibuprofen or naproxen. If these agents are ineffective, combination products such as those composed of acetaminophen/caffeine/butalbital may be effective. **Amitriptyline** is the agent most commonly used for headache prophylaxis in patients with recurrent symptoms.

The etiology of **migraine** headaches is currently attributed to the neurovascular hypothesis, with the release of vasoactive neuropeptides and subsequent vasodilation of blood vessels. Serotonin plays an important role in migraine pathophysiology, and **serotonin agonists** have an important role in migraine treatment.

Migraine headache treatment will vary according to the symptoms and severity of headache presentation. Headaches may be triggered by a variety of factors such as food (monosodium glutamate, tyramine, caffeine), exertion, stress, menses, medication, or alcohol. Individual patient triggers should be identified, and patients instructed on their minimization or avoidance. For initial pharmacologic abortive therapy, over-the-counter agents such as acetaminophen, ibuprofen, or aspirin may be used. When over-the-counter agents are not sufficient, a number of combination analgesics containing acetaminophen, butalbital, and caffeine are available. Ergotamine and dihydroergotamine are also prescription agents that can be used for moderate to severe migraines. Because migraine headaches are often accompanied by nausea and gastric stasis, **antiemetics** such as metoclopramide or prochlorperazine can be useful in these situations.

Treatment of migraine headaches changed dramatically upon the introduction of **serotonin agonists** such as sumatriptan in the 1990s. Other agents in this class are zolmitriptan, naratriptan, rizatriptan, almotriptan, and most recently frovatriptan. Sumatriptan causes vasoconstriction, affecting cranial blood vessels, and also may have effects on neuropeptide release. All of the agents in this class are available orally. Rizatriptan and zolmitriptan are also available as orally disintegrating tablets, which are particularly useful in patients with nausea. Sumatriptan is also available as a nasal spray and SC injection. This class of agents is generally more expensive than other treatments, but minimizing losses due to missed work or school days may offset this cost.

Case Conclusion KO is experiencing peripheral vasospasm from an interaction between his ergotamine and the erythromycin. It is also recommended that KO not exceed 6 tablets of ergotamine per migraine attack or 10 tablets per week. Acute **ergotism** can be manifested when these agents are used concurrently, manifesting as peripheral ischemia. Nitroprusside IV may be required in more severe cases.

Thumbnail: Agents for Headache Treatment

Drug class	Ergot alkaloids	Combination analgesics	Serotonin agonists
Prototype drug	Ergotamine	Butalbital, caffeine, and acetaminophen (Fioricet®)	Sumatriptan
Other agents in class	Dihydroergotamine (DHE), methysergide maleate	Butalbital, caffeine, aspirin (Fiorinal®)	Almotriptan, frovatriptan, naratriptan, rizatriptan, zomitriptan
Routes of administration	Ergotamine (oral, IV), methysergide (oral), DHE (intranasal [IN], IM, IV)	Oral	All available orally; orally disintegrating tablets (rizatriptan, zolmitriptan); IN and SC injection (sumatriptan)
MOA	Acts at alpha-adrenergic, dopaminergic, and tryptaminergic receptors (partial agonist or antagonist activity). Methysergide: does not affect norepinephrine reuptake.	Barbiturate (CNS depressant), vasoconstrictor, analgesic	Act as $5HT_1$ agonists
Metabolism	Hepatic	Hepatic, renal elimination	Hepatic, renal elimination. Dose adjustment required: renal or hepatic impairment (almotriptan, naratriptan).
Adverse reactions	Primarily nausea/vomiting (N/V), but also diarrhea, angina, transient bradycardia/ tachycardia, BP elevation, peripheral numbness, tingling, gangrene. Methysergide: also fibrotic disorders (retroperitoneal, endocardial, pleural), abdominal pain.	N/V, drowsiness, dizziness, sedation	N/V, dizziness, injection site pain. Cardiovascular: coronary vasospasm, chest pain, ischemic MI.
Contraindications	CAD, peripheral vascular disease (PVD), renal/liver dysfunction, pregnancy, hypersensitivity to ergot alkaloids. Methysergide: pulmonary disease.	Hypersensitivity to components, porphyria. Midrin®: CAD, CHF, PVD, renal/liver dysfunction, pregnancy, uncontrolled HTN, glaucoma; monoamine oxidase (MAO) inhibitor therapy.	CAD, CHF, uncontrolled HTN; ergot or 5HT agonist use within 24 hr; hemiplegic/basilar migraine. Specific contraindications: Wolff-Parkinson-White syndrome (zolmitriptan); PVD (frovatriptan); MAO-A inhibitor use within 2 weeks (sumatriptan, rizatriptan, zolmitriptan, frovatriptan).
Comments	Beta-blockers and macrolides: increased risk for acute ergotism. Antiemetics may increase tolerability. DHE: less emetogenic than ergotamine. Methysergide: drug holidays to minimize fibrotic complications (medication-free interval of 4 weeks following each 6 month period of treatment).	Fiorinal® is a controlled substance; also available with codeine. Isometheptene, dichloralphenazone. acetaminophen (Midrin®).	Expensive; improved bioavailability with the newer agents vs. sumatriptan. Almotriptan MAO-A, CYP2D6, and 3A4 enzyme substrate. Sumatriptan, rizatriptan, zolmitriptan: MAO-A metabolism. Frovatriptan has longest T½.

Questions

1. A 27-year-old woman with a history of migraine headaches presents to the outpatient clinic with complaints of daily headaches that have become progressively worse over the past month. The headaches are unrelieved with prescription medication, which she has been using daily for the past 3 months. She is diagnosed with headaches from overuse of analgesics. Upon withdrawal of all her medications, her headaches slowly improve over several weeks. Which medication is associated with a lower incidence of analgesic overuse headaches?

   A. Acetaminophen with codeine
   B. Combination of acetaminophen, isometheptene, and dichloralphenazone
   C. Combination of aspirin, butalbital, and caffeine
   D. Ergotamine
   E. Naratriptan

2. BA is a 37-year-old man with newly diagnosed cluster headaches. The headaches have been lasting 1 to 2 hours per attack, and come on suddenly. He has no other comorbid conditions, and lives a very active lifestyle. Which treatment would be most appropriate for abortive treatment of his headache syndrome?

   A. Ergotamine sublingual tablets
   B. Ibuprofen tablets
   C. Oxygen therapy
   D. Combination of acetaminophen, isometheptene, and dichloralphenazone tablets
   E. Sumatriptan tablets

HPI: JJ is a 50-year-old woman with metastatic lung cancer, s/p frontal-temporal craniotomy for resection of a metastatic brain lesion 2 days ago. JJ is complaining of a pruritic, erythematous rash on her back and arms that she denies having prior to admission. PMH: Metastatic lung cancer s/p chemotherapy and radiation therapy 6 months prior. Presented 3 weeks prior to admission with a new onset generalized tonic-clonic **seizure.**

PE: Vitals: T 37.8°C, BP 124/74 mm Hg, HR 80 beats/min, RR 18 breaths/min. Medications: Phenytoin (started 3 weeks ago), dexamethasone, famotidine. Patient has NKDA.

Labs: Slightly elevated transaminases (AST 78 IU/L, ALT 201 IU/L, AlkPhos 176 IU/L, Total bilirubin [Tbili] 0.9 mg/dL).

Thought Questions

- Which **antiepileptics** are indicated for which types of seizures?

- What are the most common signs of **anticonvulsant hypersensitivity**?

- What other antiepileptics can be used in a patient who is thought to have a hypersensitivity reaction to phenytoin?

Basic Science Review and Discussion

Choosing an antiepileptic agent for treatment of seizures depends on the diagnosis and classification of the seizure type. One of the first antiepileptics discovered was phenobarbital, which is used for **generalized tonic-clonic seizures** and **status epilepticus.** Phenytoin (also known as diphenylhydantoin, or DPH) is used in the treatment of partial, focal, and generalized seizures and status epilepticus. Carbamazepine and valproic acid were found to be effective in partial and generalized tonic-clonic seizures. There are also a dozen other agents that are now being used as adjunctive treatment for generalized seizures, and as adjunctive and monotherapy for **absence** and **partial seizures.** Treatment should generally start with one agent to minimize adverse effects and enhance compliance.

Many of the anticonvulsants can cause **rash,** which can range in severity from benign (resolving with dose reduction or discontinuation of therapy) to severe hypersensitivity reactions necessitating a change in therapy. Phenytoin is known to cause **hypersensitivity** reactions, most often presenting as a rash that generally occurs 2 weeks to 2 months after initiation of therapy. The rash is often described as morbilliform, although it can present in a variety of forms (scarlatiniform, maculopapular, urticarial). The rash is often pruritic and distributed on the trunk, arms, and chest. Facial edema also has been observed. Reactions are often accompanied by fever, lymphadenopathy, elevated transaminases, leukocytosis, and eosinophilia. These rashes can progress to more severe, potentially fatal reactions, such as erythema multiforme, exfoliative dermatitis, or toxic epidermal necrolysis. Thus, if phenytoin is suspected as the etiology of the reaction, it should be discontinued immediately and an alternative anticonvulsant started if necessary. Corticosteroid therapy may mask some of the signs and symptoms of a hypersensitivity reaction, and patients on concomitant corticosteroids should be evaluated carefully for any symptoms resembling a hypersensitivity reaction.

True hypersensitivity reactions to phenytoin are related to the "aromatic" anticonvulsants. Thus, in patients in whom a reaction is suspected, other arene anticonvulsants such as carbamazepine, oxcarbazepine, phenobarbital, or primidone should be avoided, as there is a high rate of cross-reactivity (estimated as high as 80%). Valproic acid is an agent that can be safely used as an alternative anticonvulsant in such patients.

Case Conclusion   Phenytoin was discontinued and JJ was started on valproic acid. She received an initial IV dose, followed by oral maintenance therapy of divalproex sodium. She was monitored closely for resolution of her reaction, which took several weeks.

Thumbnail: Anticonvulsants

Drug	Phenytoin (DPH)	Carbamazepine (CBZ)	Valproic acid (VPA) and divalproex sodium	Phenobarbital (PB)
Clinical indications	Status epilepticus, generalized tonic-clonic, complex partial, focal motor seizures. Not effective for absence seizures.	Partial, generalized tonic-clonic seizures. Pain associated with trigeminal neuralgia.	Complex partial, absence, generalized tonic-clonic, myoclonic seizures. Migraine headache prophylaxis, mania associated with bipolar disorder.	Status epilepticus, partial, generalized tonic-clonic seizures. Sedative hypnotic.
MOA	Appears to block posttetanic potentiation of synaptic transmission; with effects on sodium channels.	Thought to be similar to phenytoin, and reduces polysynaptic responses.	Not established. May be related to increased brain concentrations of gamma-aminobutyric acid (GABA).	Sodium effects similar to phenytoin, with effects on calcium and GABA.
Absorption/ distribution	Absorption: very good. Use only extended-release capsules for once-daily dosing. IM not recommended. Enteral feedings bind phenytoin.	Absorption: good. No parenteral form available. Distribution: CSF, 15%–22% of serum concentration.	Absorption: excellent. Conversion between the oral and parenteral dosage forms are equivalent. Distribution: plasma and extracellular water; CSF, 10% of serum concentrations.	Absorption: excellent. Distribution: all tissues, high concentrations in the brain.
Metabolism/ elimination	Primarily hepatic metabolism. Saturable metabolism (small dosage increases can result in large serum level fluctuations).	Hepatic metabolism (CYP450). Initially induces own metabolism, monitor closely, dose adjust when initiating therapy.	Primarily hepatic metabolism. Saturable protein binding; serum concentrations not proportional to dosage changes.	Primarily hepatic metabolism. 25%–50% of dose eliminated unchanged.
Adverse reactions	Infusion related (hypotension, cardio-vascular collapse, CNS depression). Dose related (nystagmus, ataxia, slurred speech). Diplopia, N/V, gingival hyperplasia, hepatotoxicity, hyper-sensitivity reactions, hematologic abnormalities.	Idiosyncratic aplastic anemia and agranulo-cytosis (can be fatal). Leukopenia (usually mild, monitor closely). Dose related: GI upset, ataxia, diplopia, dizziness, drowsiness. Hyper-sensitivity reactions.	Hepatic failure (monitor LFTs prior to initiation and frequently thereafter), pancreatitis. Dose related: N/V, abdominal pain. Tremor, somnolence, dizziness, asthenia, weight gain, alopecia, thrombocytopenia, and hyperammonemia.	Infusion related: hypotension (administer slowly), somnolence, CNS depression, ataxia. Hyper-sensitivity reactions. Paradoxic excitation.
Contraindications	Allergy to phenytoin or other hydantoins.	History of bone marrow suppression, hypersen-sitivity to CBZ or tricyclic antidepressants (chemically related).	Hepatic disease; hypersensitivity to drug; known urea cycle disorders.	Hypersensitivity to barbiturates, hepatic dysfunction, porphyria, severe respiratory disease.
Drug interactions	Decreased levels with CBZ, rifampin, chronic alcohol ingestion. Increased levels with amiodarone, sulfonamides, isoniazid, fluconazole. Unpredictable effects with VPA and PB. Decreased effectiveness of: warfarin, CBZ, doxycycline, estrogens.	Decreased levels with CYP450 enzyme inducers: DPH, PB. Increased levels with erythromycin, itraconazole, propoxyphene, VPA. Decreased effective-ness of DPH, VPA, warfarin, oral contraceptives.	Decreased levels with enzyme inducers: DPH, CBZ, PB. CYP450 enzyme inhibitors (i.e., anti-depressants) expected to have little effect. Increased levels of ethosuximide, lamotrigine, PB.	Decreased levels with enzyme inducers (rifampin). Increased levels with VPA. Increased seda-tion with other CNS depressants. Decreased effectiveness of warfarin, CBZ, metronidazole, oral contraceptives.

Questions

1. A 65-year-old 60-kg woman presents to the ambulatory care clinic 2 weeks after a frontotemporal craniotomy (for resection of a glioblastoma) for removal of her staples. She was started on phenytoin extended-release capsules 300 mg orally at bedtime, after receiving 1 g of phenytoin IV during her surgery. She has no history of seizures. Today, her LFTs were normal (AST 29 IU/L, ALT 30 IU/L, AlkPhos 40 IU/L, Tbili 1.0 mg/dL). Labs drawn yesterday afternoon: phenytoin = 5 µg/mL, albumin = 2.8 g/dL. She denies missing any doses of medication. A decision is made to increase her maintenance dosage of phenytoin. What most likely influenced this decision to change her phenytoin regimen?

   A. Her compliance
   B. Accounting for the albumin level when evaluating the phenytoin level
   C. Her phenytoin level was drawn at the wrong time
   D. Her LFTs
   E. Phenytoin levels in patients without a history of seizures have a lower targeted range (less than 10 µg/mL)

2. KM is a 20-year-old woman with a history of epilepsy and scoliosis. Her seizures have been controlled on a maintenance dosage of divalproex sodium. She is scheduled to undergo a spinal fusion, and will not be taking anything by mouth (NPO) for several days. Which factor should be taken into consideration for her postsurgical care?

   A. Avoid propoxyphene napsylate for pain relief as it can interact with her valproic acid therapy.
   B. Change her antiepileptic regimen to phenytoin immediately postoperatively, as phenytoin can be given IV.
   C. Convert her oral divalproex regimen to an equivalent IV regimen of valproic acid while she is NPO.
   D. Monitor peak levels of valproic acid postoperatively to evaluate whether additional doses are needed.
   E. Avoid doxycycline as it has decreased effectiveness when given with valproic acid.

HPI: BZ is a 24-year-old man s/p frontal craniotomy for resection of a meningioma. Prior to surgery, he was maintained on carbamazepine for his generalized seizures with good results. His carbamazepine level was 9 μg/mL (normal 4–12 μg/mL) prior to admission. Postoperatively, upon admission to the ICU, he had three generalized tonic-clonic seizures over 30 minutes. Though able to follow commands in the recovery room, he is now semiconscious.

PE: Vitals: BP 187/102 mm Hg, HR 118 beats/min, RR 24 breaths/min, T 38°C, Weight 74 kg. Allergy to sulfa = rash, shortness of breath (SOB).

Thought Questions

- What is the definition of status epilepticus (SE)?

- What are acute systemic concerns associated with status epilepticus?

- What are treatment options for BZ?

- What objective data should be monitored during status epilepticus?

Basic Science Review and Discussion

Status epilepticus occurs in approximately 50,000 patients per year in the United States, and 10% to 35% have no prior history of seizures. Risk factors include acute cerebral insult and drug overdose or withdrawal.

Status epilepticus is defined as "more than 30 minutes of either continuous seizure activity or two or more sequential seizures without full recovery of consciousness between seizures." SE is a medical emergency because it can lead to permanent brain damage. Mortality is as high as 10% in children and 25% in adults.

Early management should include evaluating airway patency and proper positioning of the patient to avoid aspiration. Vital signs and labs should be monitored and IV glucose given. If fever or meningeal signs are present, a lumbar puncture is mandatory to exclude bacterial meningitis. Severe hyperthermia (42° to 43°C) can increase the risk

for brain damage and should be managed with a cooling blanket. Fevers should resolve when seizures cease.

Drug therapy should be instituted immediately. IV **benzodiazepines** such as diazepam or lorazepam are effective and work rapidly for cessation of seizures. Diazepam has a higher level of **lipophilicity,** so although it works more quickly than lorazepam, it redistributes from the brain to other fatty tissues, causing both brain and serum levels to fall. Lorazepam is less lipid soluble and therefore has a longer duration of effect in the CNS, and is the preferred agent. Monitor for **respiratory depression** or hypotension. Seizure recurrence is as high as 50%, so a longer-acting antiepileptic must be added.

Either phenytoin or fosphenytoin is then administered. Fosphenytoin is a water-soluble prodrug of phenytoin and causes less hypotension and cardiac arrhythmias than phenytoin. **Cardiovascular status** should be carefully monitored, especially for hypotension and arrhythmias.

If SE continues, proceed to phenobarbital. Patients who receive phenobarbital after being treated with IV benzodiazepines should be carefully monitored for **respiratory depression** and hypotension as the effects are additive. Ventilatory support should be immediately available.

If SE has not resolved with the above algorithm, then proceed to general anesthesia, intubation, and respiratory support. Pentobarbital may then be administered with close supervision as moderate respiratory depression is expected. Vasopressors may also be necessary to maintain blood pressure. ECG monitoring is required.

Case Conclusion BZ is first given IV glucose and IV lorazepam. He continues to have generalized tonic-clonic seizures and his blood pressure decreases to 110/60 mm Hg as lorazepam is given. Per protocol, the medical team decides to continue with fosphenytoin, which is less frequently associated with hypotension than phenytoin. After the fosphenytoin is given, BZ ceases to seize and vital signs stabilize.

Thumbnail: Agents Used for Status Epilepticus

Drug class	Benzodiazepines	Phenytoin derivatives	Barbiturates
Prototypic agents	Diazepam (D), lorazepam (L)	Phenytoin, fosphenytoin	Phenobarbital (PB), pentobarbital (P)
Onset (min)	D: 1–3 L: 6–10	10–30	PB: 20–30 P: 1
Duration	D: 15–30 min L: 6–12 hr	24 hr	PB: > 48 hr P: 15 hr
MOA	Potentiates action of GABA	Blockade of neuronal sodium	Interferes with transmission of impulses
Adverse reactions	Hypotension, bradycardia, drowsiness, slurred speech, cardiac arrest	Drowsiness, dizziness, ataxia, diplopia, hypotension, rash, cardiac arrhythmias, nausea. Fosphenytoin has less incidence of hypotension and arrhythmias.	Hypotension, bradycardia, cardiac arrhythmias, dizziness, confusion, drowsiness, rash, nausea

Questions

1. A 22-year-old man is being treated for SE following a drug overdose. His current vital signs include an RR of 7 breaths/min. Respiratory depression is rarely seen in which of the following groups of agents used in the treatment of SE?

   A. Diazepam and lorazepam
   B. Diazepam and phenobarbital
   C. Phenobarbital and phenytoin
   D. Phenobarbital and pentobarbital
   E. Phenytoin and fosphenytoin

2. A 45-year-old woman is brought to the ED in SE following a head trauma. She began seizing in the ambulance 10 minutes ago and has been given lorazepam and phenytoin. In treating this patient, which of the following statements about management of SE is true?

   A. Diazepam has a higher level of lipophilicity, so onset time for the drug to act is slow.
   B. Fosphenytoin causes more hypotension and cardiac arrhythmias than phenytoin.
   C. If SE resolves after administering a benzodiazepine, then no further treatment is required.
   D. If repeated doses of either phenytoin or fosphenytoin do not cease seizures during SE, then the next agent used is pentobarbital.
   E. SE is defined as more than 60 minutes of continuous seizure activity or two or more sequential seizures without full recovery of consciousness between seizures.
   F. Lorazepam is less lipid soluble than diazepam and has a longer duration of effect in the CNS.
   G. A and E are both true.
   H. A, D, and E are all true.

HPI: CV is a 52-year-old woman brought into the ED by her husband complaining of chest pain, dizziness, SOB, and sweating. This is her third visit to the ED for chest pain in the past 2 years. On two previous visits it was concluded that she did not suffer an MI.

SH: Works full time as an office manager in the business district, but has been on medical leave for the past 4 weeks for "mental exhaustion" and is due to return to work in 2 days. Married for 25 years with two adult children living on the opposite side of the country. Drinks one to two cups of coffee daily and one large gin and tonic nightly; does not exercise.

PMH: Postmenopausal for 5 years. Migraine headaches (averages one per month; has had three in the past month); HTN.

General: Anxious-appearing female in obvious distress; sweating profusely; alert and coherent. Expresses fear of returning to work and shares that she has been reluctant to leave the house for the past year. Denies sadness or anhedonia. Admits to mid-nocturnal insomnia, increased weight (17 pounds in 2 months), low energy. Denies paranoia or hallucinations.

Medications: Hydrochlorothiazide/triamterene; diphenhydramine for sleep.

PE: Vitals: T 37.3°C, HR 108 beats/min, RR 22 breaths/min, BP 145/92 mm Hg. ECG: Sinus tachycardia; normal rhythm.

Labs: WNL.

Thought Questions

- What pharmacologic agents are used in maintenance treatment of anxiety disorders?

- What medications can be used for acute relief of anxiety or panic attacks?

- What pharmacologic options are available for patients with a history of substance abuse?

Basic Science Review and Discussion

The pharmacologic management of **generalized anxiety disorder (GAD)** and **panic disorder** often features the use of **benzodiazepines** and/or **selective serotonin reuptake inhibitor (SSRI)** antidepressants. While tricyclic antidepressants (TCAs) and monoamine oxidase (MAO) inhibitors were once popular for the long-term management of anxiety, their clinical utility has been overshadowed by the greater tolerability and acceptance of SSRIs. At the present time, SSRIs have received FDA approval for the treatment of GAD, panic disorder, obsessive-compulsive disorder (OCD), post-traumatic stress disorder (PTSD), and social phobia. Although not all agents are FDA approved for these disorders, all SSRIs are believed to be therapeutically effective for each of these indications. In general, clinicians have found that the SSRI should be started at relatively low doses to improve tolerability, but that the eventual effective dose may actually be slightly higher than average doses prescribed for major depression.

For the acute relief of anxiety or panic attacks, benzodiazepines are often useful, usually on an as-needed basis. Many clinicians are reluctant to prescribe these medications for an extended period of time (due to risks associated with **physiologic dependence,** withdrawal, or abuse), but for the relief of acute symptoms, benzodiazepines are a valuable therapeutic modality. Although a wide variety of benzodiazepines are currently available, they are all qualitatively similar in terms of their pharmacologic effects and side effect potential. Clonazepam and alprazolam are the two benzodiazepines used most commonly to treat anxiety disorders.

An additional psychotropic medication that may be worth considering specifically for GAD is buspirone. One major benefit of buspirone can be found in the virtual absence of dependence and abuse liability. Although it is not effective for the acute relief of anxiety or panic disorders (anxiolytic effects may take up to a week to be established), buspirone may be indicated for patients with a history of alcohol abuse or among those who fear physiologic and psychological dependence with benzodiazepines.

In summary, the pharmacologic management of GAD and panic disorder usually features maintenance with an SSRI and acute symptom relief with benzodiazepines (if necessary). The duration of maintenance treatment is highly variable with pharmacologic management, but it should be remembered that in most patients, GAD and panic disorders will be chronic and recurrent conditions.

Case Conclusion   After beginning another rule-out MI protocol, CV was given an IM injection of lorazepam to acutely control her anxiety and related somatic complaints. She was seen by her primary care provider the next day and ultimately diagnosed with panic disorder and agoraphobia. She was started on daily paroxetine therapy and instructed that she could use clonazepam as needed for extreme anxiety. In addition, she was counseled to diminish the use of alcohol to self-medicate. A referral for psychological counseling was given as well.

Thumbnail: Agents Used for Anxiety Disorders

	Benzodiazepines	SSRIs	Buspirone
Prototypic agent	Diazepam (D)	Fluoxetine (F)	Buspirone
Other agents	Clonazepam (C) Alprazolam (A) Lorazepam (L)	Paroxetine (P) Sertraline (S) Citalopram (C)	
MOA	Bind to components of GABA$_A$ receptors → facilitate inhibitory actions of GABA in CNS	Inhibit reuptake of serotonin	Partial agonist at 5HT$_{1A}$ brain receptors; anxiolytic action unknown
Indications	Anxiety disorders (especially A and C for panic and phobic disorders); sedation; seizure disorders; muscle relaxants (D); management of alcohol withdrawal	Depression, anxiety disorders (OCD, panic attacks, social phobias, etc.)	Generalized anxiety disorders (GAD)
Pharmacokinetics	Potency: C > A > L > D T½: L = A < C < D Hepatic metabolism	PO only; hepatic metabolism	PO only; hepatic metabolism
Adverse reactions	Cognitive impairment, sedation, amnesia, diminished motor skills	Sedation or insomnia; headache, nausea, appetite and weight changes, sexual dysfunction	Dizziness, headache, nausea
Warnings/precautions	Additive sedative effects with other CNS depressants (ethanol); tolerance and dependence may develop with prolonged use	**Serotonin syndrome** may occur with other serotonergic drugs (i.e. MAO inhibitors); SSRIs may inhibit CYP450 liver enzymes	

Questions

1. RM is a 25-year-old professional football player who was recently diagnosed with social phobic disorder. Although he has never missed a football game for this condition, he has experienced extreme anxiety in other public situations, failing to appear for numerous press conferences and community events. He is not interested in psychotherapy ("I don't have the time") and does not want to take any medication that may cause weight gain or addiction. What would be the best treatment option?

   A. Sertraline
   B. Paroxetine
   C. Buspirone
   D. Clonazepam
   E. Propranolol

2. JF is a 41-year-old man suffering from PTSD for the past 3 years, after his near death in an automobile accident. During this time, he has suffered from nightmares, jitteriness, irritability, and avoidance behavior, which has only been partially relieved for the last 3 months with a combination of trazodone and clonazepam. Tired of "feeling like a zombie" with the clonazepam, JF decides to abruptly discontinue this agent. What is the most likely consequence of this treatment action?

   A. Extreme sluggishness and ataxia within 24 hours
   B. Restlessness, blurred vision within 2 to 3 days
   C. Muscle tension and irritability within 5 to 6 days
   D. Grand mal seizures within 2 to 3 days
   E. Dizziness and paresthesias within 2 to 3 days

HPI: PM is a 39-year-old woman who arrives today at her gynecologist's office for her annual examination. When asked how she has been feeling, PM mentions that she has been "kind of down in the dumps" for the past month. She says that she feels very sad, particularly when she wakes up in the morning, and has missed 3 days of work during this time frame. ("I just don't have the energy to get up out of bed some days and I don't know why.") She also says that even when she does go to work, her concentration is poor and she has a hard time making decisions. PM also complains of occasional stress headaches and has noticed that she has returned to her old habit of binging on snack foods (she has gained approximately 7 pounds in the past month). She denies suicidality but does feel like giving up sometimes. Her PMH is significant for an acute episode of depression following the breakup of a long-term relationship 1 year ago. PM was previously successfully treated with sertraline but discontinued the medication 3 months ago because "it was interfering with my sex life."

Thought Questions

- What are the treatment options for depression?
- What are the main adverse effects of the various antidepressants?

Basic Science Review and Discussion

From a pathophysiologic perspective, a decrease in certain neurotransmitters (serotonin, norepinephrine and possibly dopamine) have been causally associated with depression through the indirect evidence that all approved antidepressants will increase the activity of one or more of these chemical messengers.

All of the current antidepressants agents are equally effective in the general depressed population, generating a therapeutic response in 60% to 70% of patients given a therapeutic trial. Generally, symptoms begin to improve within the first 2 weeks of treatment, and 4 weeks (or more) are required to observe optimal treatment outcomes.

Selective serotonin reuptake inhibitors (SSRIs) are the most popular treatment option due to safety in overdose situations, low side effect burden, and ease of administration (i.e., once-daily dosing with minimal titration required). SSRIs are also effective treatment for the management of anxiety disorders, a common psychiatric comorbidity among the depressed.

In general, SSRIs are regarded as "activating antidepressants" less likely to induce sedation or sluggishness than tricyclic antidepressants or trazodone. Many patients experience mild nausea or light sleep when they first start taking an SSRI, but these side effects usually abate after a few days of continued treatment. Sexual dysfunction, most commonly presenting as a difficulty achieving orgasm, is more problematic and frequently leads to discontinuation, particularly if the patient is uncomfortable discussing this condition with his or her physician. Sweating is another common and dose-dependent phenomenon, and bruxism may present on occasion as well.

The potential of SSRIs to inhibit liver enzymes and cause drug interactions is relatively well known, but there are important differences among the SSRIs in this regard. Paroxetine and fluoxetine have a particularly strong affinity for the CYP450 2D6 isoenzyme, elevating plasma concentrations of drugs such as narcotics and beta-blockers that are metabolized via this route. Fluvoxamine and norfluoxetine (the principal metabolite of fluoxetine) have a high affinity for the CYP450 3A4 isoenzyme, responsible for the metabolism of calcium channel blockers, antifungals, certain benzodiazepines (alprazolam and triazolam), and estrogen. Although it is true that sertraline and citalopram have a lower likelihood than other SSRIs of causing drug interactions, these reactions are somewhat unpredictable, and caution should be exercised whenever other medications are prescribed with an SSRI.

Because 25% of patients will stop SSRIs due to side effects and an additional 30% to 40% will fail to achieve a therapeutic response, other antidepressant alternatives are of great importance. Venlafaxine is a dual-action antidepressant that enhances serotonin activity at low doses and norepinephrine at higher doses. Preliminary evidence suggests that these multiple actions on neurotransmitters may confer therapeutic superiority over SSRIs for the management of severe or melancholic depression, but the risk of HTN with high-dose venlafaxine should not be overlooked.

Bupropion is another second-line agent, particularly for patients who are wary of the SSRIs' negative impact on sexual dysfunction. Because it appears to relieve depression through a completely different mechanism than SSRIs, enhancing norepinephrine or dopamine, it is often administered to patients who fail SSRIs or exhibit a partial response. The most common side effects encountered with bupropion are insomnia, jitteriness, and nausea. Bupropion is contraindicated in patients with a history of seizures or eating disorders.

Mirtazapine is another antidepressant with a unique mechanism of action, enhancing serotonin and norepinephrine in a manner quite complex and distinct from venlafaxine or tricyclics. Like venlafaxine, it may be effective for severe or treatment-resistant depression, though its widespread use has been hampered by a high incidence of sedation and weight gain. Similarly, the popularity of trazodone and nefazodone has been limited by the potent sedating properties of these agents. In addition, nefazodone has been implicated rarely with the development of liver failure and it is also a potent inhibitor of the CYP450 3A4 isoenzyme.

Case Conclusion   Given her favorable response to an SSRI in the past, sertraline would appear to be a logical choice for treatment of her latest episode, but her complaint of sexual dysfunction should be taken seriously, as this commonly leads to medication noncompliance. As all SSRI and venlafaxine are capable of inducing this side effect, bupropion is initiated and slowly titrated to effect. The activating properties of bupropion proved to be a notable benefit for this patient as her symptoms resolved within the first 3 weeks of receiving a therapeutic dose.

Thumbnail: Adverse Effects of Antidepressant Medications

Medication	Sedation	Agitation/ insomnia	Anticholinergic effects	Orthostasis	GI effects (nausea/diarrhea)	Sexual dysfunction	Weight gain
SSRIs							
Fluoxetine	+	++++	0/+	0/+	++++	++++	+
Sertraline	+	+++	0/+	0	+++	+++	+
Paroxetine	++	++	+	0	+++	++++	++
Citalopram	++	++	0/+	0	+++	++	+
Tricyclics							
Desipramine	++	+	++	+++	0/+	+	++
Nortriptyline	++	+	++	++	0/+	+	++
Amitriptyline	++++	0/+	++++	++++	0/+	++	+++
Imipramine	+++	0/+	+++	++++	0/+	++	++
Doxepin	++++	0/+	++++	++++	0/+	++	++
Others							
Bupropion	0	+++	+	0	+	0/+	0
Venlafaxine	++	++	+	0	+++	+++	+
Nefazodone	+++	+	+	++	++	0/+	0/+
Mirtazapine	++++	0	++	0/+	+	0/+	+++

0, negligible; +, very low; ++, low; +++, moderate; ++++, high.

Questions

1. RH is a 48-year-old man who had enjoyed an excellent response to paroxetine. Two months after starting the antidepressant, he mentions that he is no longer able to ejaculate and, though he has no interest in stopping the SSRI, wonders what can be done to preserve his marital relations. Which would be the best option at the present time?

   A. Change his paroxetine to sertraline.
   B. Reduce his paroxetine dose.
   C. Add bupropion.
   D. Add sildenafil.
   E. Encourage marital counseling.

2. EV is a 21-year-old college student suffering from an acute episode of major depressive disorder with severe symptomatology. Although her symptoms went into remission after 8 weeks of venlafaxine, she now complains of sudden dizziness, anxiety, and shooting pains in her legs. What is the most likely explanation for these complaints?

   A. Eosinophilia myalgia syndrome
   B. Serotonin syndrome
   C. SSRI withdrawal syndrome
   D. Stroke (cerebrovascular accident)
   E. Neuroleptic malignant syndrome

HPI: SH is a 32-year-old, moderately obese man brought into the ED by the police after attempting to cut himself with a piece of glass from his bathroom mirror. He said he had to cut himself in order to "let the evil out!" In the examination room, SH looked suspiciously at the interviewer and was muttering to himself. His PMH is significant for chronic schizophrenia, HTN, hyperlipidemia, and major depressive disorder. Medications include thioridazine, benztropine, paroxetine, atorvastatin, and metoprolol, although SH states he discontinued all his medications 3 weeks ago for fear he was being poisoned.

PE: On physical examination, he has noticeable cuts on his hands. During the interview, he demonstrated noticeable facial grimacing and lip smacking, a stooped posture, and sluggish gait.

Thought Questions

- What are the mechanisms of action of neuroleptics and atypical antipsychotics and how do they affect the positive and negative symptoms of schizophrenia?

- How are neuroleptics and atypical antipsychotics classified and how do they differ in potency, dosing range, and adverse effects?

- What are **extrapyramidal symptoms** (EPS) and what are the predisposing risk factors? What is the recommended treatment of choice?

- What is **neuroleptic malignancy syndrome** (NMS) and what are the predisposing risk factors? What is the recommended treatment of choice?

Basic Science Review and Discussion

Traditional **antipsychotics** or **neuroleptics** block the D_2 dopamine receptor and alleviate the positive symptoms of schizophrenia (e.g., hallucinations, delusions, thought dysfunction). These positive symptoms are due to excess dopamine in the mesolimbic pathway while the negative symptoms are due to deficiency of dopamine in the mesocortical pathway and frontal cortex (regulated by serotonin). Negative symptoms can include affective blunting, avolition, anhedonia, and memory impairment. Traditional neuroleptics have little effect on controlling negative symptoms or cognitive dysfunction associated with schizophrenia. Neuroleptics also block dopamine receptors in the nigrostriatal and tuberoinfundibular pathway in the brain and result in adverse effects such as movement disorders and hyperprolactinemia, respectively.

Atypical antipsychotic agents or "newer" agents alleviate both positive and negative symptoms. The atypical antipsychotics also improve cognitive deficits associated with schizophrenia. Although these agents are much safer, they have added cost and have been associated with their own class of adverse effects.

Traditional neuroleptics are classified in terms of potency or how strongly they bind to D_2 receptors. Low-potency agents have less affinity for D_2 receptors and therefore require high dosages to have equal effect as high-potency agents. They are, as a class, poorly tolerated due to unfavorable side effect profiles. They are associated with EPS, and **tardive dyskinesia** (TD) as well as muscarinic (M_1), histaminergic (H_1), and adrenergic (α_1 and α_2) side effects.

Extrapyramidal symptoms are common adverse effects of traditional neuroleptics, although they may still occur with atypical agents. Pseudoparkinsonism, akathisia, and acute dystonic reactions are the three early-onset types of EPS, whereas tardive dyskinesia, tardive dystonia, and tardive akathisia are late-onset EPS types that occur 6 months to 1 year after initiating treatment. High-potency antipsychotics at high doses have the greatest risk for inducing EPS. Atypical agents have a low risk for inducing EPS, and clozapine has been shown in limited cases to improve TD. The management of early-onset EPS symptoms includes drug discontinuation, dosage reduction of the antipsychotic agent, or switching to an agent with less risk for inducing EPS. Anticholinergic agents (diphenhydramine, benztropine) can be used to treat acute dystonic reactions, parkinsonism, and akathisia. Other agents such as amantadine, benzodiazepines, and propranolol also have been used.

Neuroleptic malignant syndrome is a rare but potentially fatal reaction associated with antipsychotic therapy. NMS can occur within hours or months after initiation of the drug and has a high mortality rate. The four cardinal features of NMS include (a) **hyperthermia**, (b) **muscular rigidity (lead-pipe rigidity)**, (c) **autonomic instability**, and (d) **altered consciousness**. Leukocytosis with or without a left shift, elevated creatinine phosphokinase, and metabolic acidosis may be present. Drug discontinuation, hydration, oxygenation, and fever reduction are key measures to reduce morbidity and mortality. Many pharmacologic agents (amantadine, bromocriptine, dantrolene) have been used for treatment of NMS with conflicting results.

Case Conclusion SH's symptoms are consistent with the diagnosis of uncontrolled chronic schizophrenia (paranoid type). Because SH is experiencing positive and negative symptoms and has evidence of EPS, he should be switched to an atypical antipsychotic agent. Clozapine is traditionally reserved for treatment-resistant patients and is not a first-line agent due to the risk of agranulocytosis. Olanzapine and quetiapine can be problematic due to weight gain and potential insulin resistance (if the patient has family history of diabetes mellitus type 2). Risperidone is also associated with a higher incidence of EPS symptoms compared with other atypical agents. In addition, SH is also taking paroxetine that can significantly elevate levels of risperidone. Therefore, ziprasidone would be the best choice for this patient.

Thumbnail: Agents for Schizophrenia

Available agents	Neuroleptics*		Atypical antipsychotics
	Phenothiazines	Nonphenothiazines	
	Chlorpromazine (L)	Loxapine (M)	Clozapine
	Thioridazine (L)	Molindone (M)	Risperidone
	Mesoridazine (L)	Haloperidol (H)	Quetiapine
	Perphenazine (M)	Thiothixene (H)	Olanzapine
	Trifluoperazine (M)		Ziprasidone
	Fluphenazine (H)		
MOA	General: Block primarily dopamine (D_2) receptors; have little affinity for serotonin 5-HT_{2A}. Also bind to α_1, M_1, H_1 receptors in varying degrees.		General: Binds with high affinity to serotonin 5-HT_2, dopamine (primarily D_2), histamine H_1, muscarinic M_1, α_1- and α_2-adrenergic receptors.
Pharmacokinetics			
Onset & duration	Oral: Peak levels approximately 1–4 hr for all agents; T½ 8–30 h.		Oral: Peak levels 1–8 hr (although therapeutic onset may take days); T½ 6–30 h
Elimination	Extensively metabolized by the liver with minimal amount of drug excreted in urine unchanged.		Metabolized by CYP450 via different isoenzymes. Use caution in hepatic impairment and elderly.
Adverse effects	Low potency agents: sedation, anticholinergic effects, orthostasis, ECG changes (QT_c prolongation, T-wave flattening, QRS widening). High potency: EPS, hyperprolactinemia. Overall, any of the side effects can occur in both low- and high-potency agents. Thioridazine: retinal pigmentation at high doses, sexual dysfunction.		EPS, TD, and NMS rare. All agents have potential to cause orthostasis, sedation, and weight gain. Clozapine: agranulocytosis, seizures, anticholinergic effects, constipation, sialorrhea. Risperidone: highest risk for inducing EPS among atypical agents; hyperprolactinemia. Olanzapine: glucose intolerance. Quetiapine: dizziness, cataracts, mild transient transaminase elevations. Ziprasidone: QT_c prolongation, nausea.
Drug interactions	Use caution when coadministered with drugs metabolized via the CYP450 system. Avoid concomitant use with drugs that have similar side effect profiles. Mesoridazine: contraindicated with drugs known to prolong QT_c interval.		Use caution when coadministered with drugs metabolized via the CYP450 system. Avoid concomitant use with drugs that have similar side effect profiles.

*H, high potency; M, medium potency; L, low potency.

Questions

1. A 20-year-old woman admitted to the inpatient psychiatric unit has been receiving an atypical antipsychotic for her chronic schizophrenia. She is unable to recollect the name of the medication but she does complain of galactorrhea. Which one of the following medications is most likely to cause galactorrhea?

   A. Olanzapine
   B. Quetiapine
   C. Risperidone
   D. Ziprasidone
   E. Clozapine

2. One of your patients comes to your clinic with complaints of insomnia. She has been stable on haloperidol for schizophrenia for the past 5 years and asks you to recommend something for sleep. Which one of the following hypnotic medications would interact with the efficacy of haloperidol in controlling her psychotic symptoms?

   A. Zaleplon
   B. Diphenhydramine
   C. Diazepam
   D. Zolpidem
   E. Trazodone

> **HPI:** DL is a 65-year-old widowed man who presents to the clinic complaining of difficulty sleeping for the past month. His mid-nocturnal awakening has dramatically improved since he started citalopram, but he still has much difficulty falling asleep. He reports getting only about 3 to 4 hours of sleep per night and feels fatigued during the day due to the lack of sleep. He reports that he has followed all of the sleep hygiene instructions you provided him at the last clinic visit but it has not helped. He has even tried over-the-counter medication for sleep without success. PMH: Major depressive disorder (6 months ago, currently in remission). Medications: Citalopram, famotidine, hydrocodone/acetaminophen as needed, diphenhydramine. SH: Denies using tobacco, alcohol, or illicit substances.

Thought Questions

- What pharmacologic agents are available to treat insomnia and what are their pharmacologic mechanisms of action to promote sleep?

- What characteristics should be evaluated in choosing a sedative-hypnotic agent for a patient?

Basic Science Review and Discussion

Several classes of pharmacologic agents are available for insomnia. **Barbiturates** are the oldest agents that have been used for insomnia and include pentobarbital, secobarbital, and amobarbital. Barbiturates are currently not recommended because of their high **abuse potential** (due to rapid development of tolerance) and lethal potential in overdose situations. Barbiturates potentiate the GABAergic-induced increase in chloride ion conductance at low doses, and at high doses they depress calcium-dependent action potentials. Caution should be exercised in patients with marked renal or liver dysfunction, severe respiratory disease, suicidal tendencies, or history of alcohol/drug abuse.

Nonbarbiturate sedative-hypnotics have a similar mechanism of action as barbiturates and have high potential for tolerance, abuse, dependence, overdose, and withdrawal reactions. Chloral hydrate is still commonly used today due to its efficacy as a short-term sedative hypnotic and low cost. Chloral hydrate should not be used in patients with severe renal, hepatic, or cardiac disease.

Benzodiazepines are widely used as sedative-hypnotics and have a safer overdose profile compared with barbiturate and nonbarbiturate agents. Depending on the patient's primary symptoms of insomnia, one benzodiazepine may be preferred over another. Agents with quick onset (triazolam, flurazepam, quazepam) may be used in patients with difficulty falling asleep, whereas patients who have frequent nocturnal awakenings may benefit from longer-acting agents (temazepam, flurazepam, quazepam, estazolam). **Tolerance** and dependence are also significant concerns with all benzodiazepines.

Over-the-counter agents are widely used among the general public. Essentially all of these nonprescription sleeping aids contain an ingredient with antihistaminic properties. Diphenhydramine is an antihistamine with high lipid solubility and central histaminic (H_1) blockade. This blockade results in a "hangover effect," and daytime residual drowsiness can be significant. It also has significant **anticholinergic** effects with accompanying side effects such as dry mouth, blurred vision, constipation, confusion, and memory problems. Cognitive effects may be greatly enhanced in the elderly and can result in anticholinergic delirium.

Antidepressant medications with sedating properties have been frequently used for insomnia. Although mirtazapine and nefazodone are still being used in patients with depression, trazodone is commonly used for the sole purpose of treating insomnia. Trazodone blocks serotonin 2A receptors and has significant sedating properties. The efficacy of trazodone as an antidepressant occurs at high doses but at lower doses it is safely used as a hypnotic. Mirtazapine and nefazodone also block serotonin 2A receptors and have occasionally been used as sedative-hypnotics.

The new sedative-hypnotics, zaleplon (a pyrazolopyridine) and zolpidem (an imidazopyridine), are rapidly becoming the drugs of choice in treating insomnia. These agents are structurally unrelated to the benzodiazepines but they act selectively at benzodiazepine omega-1 receptors involved in sedation. Conversely, they do not act at the benzodiazepine omega-2 receptors in the brain that regulate cognition, memory, and motor function. These agents also have rapid onset and short duration of action but bind to the benzodiazepine receptor differently than the benzodiazepines. Therefore, rebound insomnia, dependence, tolerance, and withdrawal symptoms are rare with these newer agents.

Zolpidem was the first omega-1 selective sedative-hypnotic to be marketed. Zaleplon is shorter acting and has faster onset of action compared with zolpidem. In patients with nocturnal awakenings, the drug has such a short duration of action that a dose can be repeated in the middle of the night. Although these newer selective agents have less potential for abuse, fatal overdose, and withdrawal reactions, caution should be exercised in high-risk patients.

In general, sedative-hypnotics should only be used for a short period of time (7 to 10 days) and patients should be reevaluated if they are to be taken for a longer period of time.

Case Conclusion Upon a thorough examination and interview, you have ruled out medical and pharmacologic agents as possible causes of DL's insomnia. His major depressive disorder may still be a contributing factor to his sleep problem, but at this time DL may benefit from a short-term use of a hypnotic. Upon further discussion, you decide to try one of the newer agents approved for insomnia. DL is prescribed zolpidem as needed for sleep.

Thumbnail: New Sedative-Hypnotics

Prototypic agent: Zolpidem.

Other agents: Zaleplon.

Clinical use: Short-term treatment for insomnia.

MOA: Nonbenzodiazepine hypnotic but binds to benzodiazepine omega-1 receptor in vitro. No muscle relaxant, anxiolytic, or anticonvulsant effects.

Pharmacokinetics

Absorption/distribution: Rapid oral absorption, peak serum levels in 1 to 2 hours.

Metabolism/elimination: Converted to inactive metabolites in liver; renal excretion.

Adverse effects: CNS depression, dizziness, headache, drowsiness, lethargy, nausea, dyspepsia, diarrhea.

Precautions: Tolerance and withdrawal reactions may still occur at high doses. Caution in patients with compromised respiratory function. Caution in elderly patients and in hepatic impairment.

Comments: Limit use to 7 to 10 days. Avoid alcohol.

Questions

1. A 40-year-old woman was recently prescribed a benzodiazepine for her short-term insomnia. After a few weeks of using the medication with success, she tried to discontinue the medication. Within a couple of days, she noticed worsening of her insomnia and significant jitteriness upon stopping her medication. Which one of the following medications would most likely cause her symptoms?

   A. Diazepam
   B. Triazolam
   C. Temazepam
   D. Estazolam
   E. Lorazepam

2. A 35-year-old man was recently started on an antidepressant medication to treat his acute major depressive episode. Which of the following medications is most likely the antidepressant medication that is contributing to his insomnia?

   A. Mirtazapine
   B. Nefazodone
   C. Trazodone
   D. Bupropion
   E. Paroxetine

> **HPI:** HP is a 32-year-old white woman who reports profuse sweating, irritability, and a rapid heart beat. HP has been unable to exercise over the past few weeks, complaining of tachycardia and decreased exercise tolerance. She also reports diaphoresis, which contributes to frequent nocturnal awakenings.
>
> **PE:** Vitals: BP 130/84 mm Hg, HR 120 beats/min, weight 125 pounds (143 pounds at last visit).

Thought Questions

■ What treatment options are available for Graves' hyperthyroidism?

■ What are the pharmacologic differences between each treatment approach?

■ What side effects are associated with the use of **thioamides**?

Basic Science Review and Discussion

Hyperthyroidism results in a **hypermetabolic state** due to an excess of thyroid hormones. Hyperthyroidism is more common in women (2%) than men (0.1%). Graves' disease is an autoimmune disorder that leads to hyperthyroidism, diffuse goiter, ophthalmopathy, dermopathy, and acropathy. Graves' disease is the most common cause of hyperthyroidism, more common than multi- or uninodular goiters.

Hyperthyroidism treatment involves partial or complete thyroidectomy, radioactive iodine (RAI) treatment, or thioamide therapy. There is no one best approach because treatment is often individualized.

The thioamides are often used as primary therapy for hyperthyroidism. They are also used as adjunctive therapy to achieve euthyroidism in patients prior to surgery or radioactive iodine therapy. The thioamides primarily inhibit thyroid hormone synthesis but do not affect existing thyroid hormone stores (which last approximately 30 days). Therefore, hyperthyroid symptoms may continue for 4 to 6 weeks after thioamide initiation. Other agents such as beta-blockers and iodides are used short term for symptomatic relief. Beta-blockers are used for 2 to 3 weeks or until cardiac symptoms have resolved. Thioamide treatment is typically continued for 12 months or longer to induce long-term spontaneous remission once the drug is discontinued. Because the thioamides do not alter the course of the disease process, spontaneous remission is often poor, and many patients require long-term thioamide therapy, often for many years.

During the hyperthyroid state, other drugs that are metabolized by the liver or eliminated renally may need to be adjusted because metabolism may be increased. Patients using drugs with a narrow therapeutic index such as digoxin, warfarin, and phenytoin should be monitored carefully because dosing adjustments will be necessary as the hyperthyroidism or hypermetabolic state resolves.

Other treatment options, besides thioamide therapy, involve RAI. The iodine 131 isotope is taken up by the thyroid gland and the radioactivity destroys the gland. RAI is safe, pain free, easy to administer, and very effective. RAI may result in euthyroidism but more frequently results in hypothyroidism requiring lifelong levothyroxine supplementation. RAI should never be given during pregnancy since it crosses the placenta.

Case Conclusion HP began methimazole therapy for her Graves' hyperthyroidism. She also began propranolol to help control her tachycardia and tremor. During this time HP should avoid excessive exercise or other sympathomimetic drugs until her symptoms of tachycardia have subsided. HP will return to the clinic for follow-up in 4 weeks. At that time, methimazole dose, tolerability, compliance, and thyroid function tests will be reassessed.

Thumbnail: Thioamides

Available agents: Prophylthiouracil (PTU) and methimazole.

MOA: Thioamides inhibit the synthesis of thyroid hormones by inhibiting thyroid peroxidase-catalyzed reactions to block iodine organification. Thioamides also block coupling of mono-iodothyronine and diiodothyronine. PTU also inhibits the peripheral conversion of T_4 to T_3.

Pharmacokinetics: PTU is rapidly absorbed. The oral bioavailability of 50% to 80% may be due to a large hepatic first-pass effect. Methimazole is completely absorbed. The duration of action for PTU is approximately 7 hours and therefore requires multiple daily doses (every 6 to 8 hours).

Adverse reactions: The most common adverse effect is maculopapular rash. Rarely, hepatitis, vasculitis, urticarial rash, and arthralgia have been observed. **Agranulocytosis** can occur in 0.3% to 0.6% of patients. Patients who develop agranulocytosis with one thioamide should not be switched to the alternate thioamide because there is a 50% cross-reactivity between the agents. Methimazole is contraindicated during pregnancy because scalp defects have been observed in infants born to mothers using methimazole.

Drug interactions: The thioamides do not directly interact with other drugs. Because the thioamides can affect thyroid hormone synthesis and therefore decrease clotting factor turnover, the thioamides may increase anticoagulant activity.

Questions

1. MJ is a 42-year-old woman who was recently diagnosed with Graves' disease and will be started on a thioamide and a beta-blocker. Which of the following characteristics regarding thioamides are true?

   A. Methimazole has a long T½ and may be dosed once daily.

   B. PTU can cause pretibial myxedema.

   C. Methimazole interacts with amiodarone therapy.

   D. PTU therapy typically induces spontaneous remission within 12 months.

2. JC is a 31-year-old woman with Graves' disease in her first trimester of pregnancy. Which of the following statements regarding PTU are true?

   A. PTU can increase the peripheral conversion of T_4 to T_3.

   B. PTU is safer to use in pregnancy since it is not teratogenic.

   C. PTU is used following surgery to prevent complications.

   D. PTU can be used during myxedema coma.

HPI: GM is a 68-year-old woman who presents to the general medicine clinic complaining of fatigue and weight gain. GM reports that she has felt sluggish and sleepy over the past 6 months. She also notes that she has gained weight despite no changes in her diet and has experienced some cold intolerance. GM's PMH is significant for AF s/p cardioversion 12 months ago, and RAI therapy for Graves' hyperthyroidism.

Labs: TSH 16.5 mIU/L, BP 110/76 mm Hg, HR 60 beats/min, weight 165 pounds (155 pounds at last visit), delayed deep tendon reflexes.

Thought Questions

- What are the signs and symptoms of hypothyroidism?

- What treatment options are available for hypothyroidism?

- What are the goals of drug therapy for hypothyroidism?

- What significant drug interactions are associated with the use of levothyroxine?

Basic Science Review and Discussion

Hypothyroidism is a relative deficiency in thyroid hormones. It manifests as a slowing down of all body functions or a decrease in metabolic rate. There are many causes for hypothyroidism, including Hashimoto's thyroiditis, drug-induced, radiation and radioactive iodine, dyshormonogenesis, congenital, and secondary causes (pituitary or hypothalamic disease). Hashimoto's thyroiditis is an immunologic disorder and is the most common cause for hypothyroidism in the United States.

The treatment of hypothyroidism involves replacing thyroid hormones. Levothyroxine (T_4) is the drug of choice. T_4 has a long half-life (7 days), which allows it to be dosed once daily. Older patients, patients with cardiac disease, or those with chronic hypothyroidism should be started at a lower dose. If cardiac symptoms develop, the dose should be reduced.

During pregnancy, thyroid requirements increase because of increased serum concentrations of **thyroxine-binding globulin** induced by estrogen. Typically, patients may require a 45% increase in dose. T_4 is safe to use during pregnancy because it does not cross the placenta. TSH levels should be checked every trimester and the dose should be changed back to prepregnancy dosing immediately following delivery.

Case Conclusion   GM began thyroid hormone therapy with T_4. Her dose was initiated at the lower-than-recommended dose because GM has a history of AF, which may increase her sensitivity to the cardiac effects of T_4. GM will return to the clinic in 4 to 6 weeks to assess her thyroid function and symptoms. Symptoms should begin to resolve in 2 to 3 weeks and should disappear by 6 weeks.

Thumbnail: Thyroid Hormone Preparations

Thyroid preparation	Content
Levothyroxine	T_4
Triiodothyronine or liothyronine	T_3
Liotrix	T_4 and T_3 (4:1 ratio)
Desiccated thyroid	Variable T_4 and T_3 content

Adverse Reactions Thyroxine toxicity may lead to restlessness, insomnia, nervousness, heat intolerance, palpitations, tachycardia, and weight loss. T_3 preparations are rapidly absorbed from the GI tract, leading to a high peak effect and resulting in **tachycardia and palpitations.** For this reason, T_3 preparations are not preferred and are used only in select patients. In addition, T_3 products often require multiple daily dosing, which can affect compliance. T_3 is sometimes used as a diagnostic agent in T_3 suppression tests. **Desic-cated thyroid** is a natural product derived from pork thyroid glands. Potency is based on iodine content without regard to con-sistency in the T_3 and T_4 content. Desiccated thyroid leads to unpredictable potency that can result in over- and understimula-tion. Today, desiccated thyroid products are obsolete and have no role in therapy.

Drug Interactions Various drugs can decrease T_4 absorption. Drugs such as aluminum hydroxide, ferrous sulfate, sucralfate, and calcium carbonate should be separated from T_4 administration by 1 to 2 hours. Bile acid sequestrants (cholestyramine and colestipol) must be separated from T_4 by at least 4 hours and preferably 6 hours. CYP450 enzyme inducing drugs such as phenytoin, carba-mazepine, rifampin, and phenobarbital can increase T_4 requirements.

Questions

1. CS is a 27-year-old woman who recently underwent a total thyroidectomy for papillary thyroid carcinoma and is now hypothyroid. Which of the following is the best therapy for hypothyroidism?

   A. Liothyronine
   B. Liotrix
   C. Desiccated thyroid
   D. T_4
   E. T_3

2. LM is a 65-year-old woman with AF, a seizure disorder, and latent tuberculosis infection. LM's medications include digoxin, rifampin, calcium carbonate, phenytoin, and warfarin. Which of the following drugs can interfere with the oral absorption of T_4?

   A. Digoxin
   B. Rifampin
   C. Calcium carbonate
   D. Phenytoin
   E. Warfarin

> HPI: AJ is a 27-year-old woman with type 1 diabetes diagnosed at age 11. She has not been seen by a health-care provider for 3 years. She is 5 feet 6 inches tall and weighs 60 kg. She takes 70/30 insulin twice daily, before breakfast and dinner. She self-monitors her blood glucose once a day; her FBG range is 200 to 250 mg/dL.
>
> Labs: Upon completing her laboratory work, you learn her HgbA1c is 9.5% (NI ≤ 6%).

Thought Questions

- What is your assessment of AJ's blood glucose control?

- What is the difference between the various insulin preparations?

- What insulin therapy would you consider for AJ to intensify her glucose control?

Basic Science Review and Discussion

Type 1 diabetes is characterized by a near-absolute insulin deficiency at diagnosis or soon thereafter. The beta cells of the pancreas are no longer able to secrete **insulin** due to autoimmune destruction. Therefore, people with type 1 diabetes require exogenous administration of insulin for survival. People with **type 2 diabetes** may require insulin therapy when diet, exercise, and the oral agents are no longer enough to provide adequate glucose control.

The insulin molecule consists of 51 amino acids arranged in two chains, an A chain (21 amino acids) and B chain (30 amino acids), that are linked by two disulfide bonds. **Proinsulin** is the insulin precursor that is first processed in the Golgi apparatus of the beta cell where it is processed and packaged into granules. Proinsulin, a single-chain 86-amino acid peptide, is cleaved into insulin and **C-peptide,** a connecting peptide. These are secreted in equimolar portions from the beta cell upon stimulation from glucose and other insulin secretagogues. C-peptide has no known physiologic function. Insulin exerts its effect on glucose metabolism by binding to insulin receptors throughout the body. Upon binding, insulin promotes the cellular uptake of glucose into fat and skeletal muscle and inhibits **hepatic glucose output,** thus lowering the blood glucose.

Normal, endogenous insulin secretion is characterized by a continuous basal insulin release and food-stimulated bursts of insulin. Exogenous insulin regimens should mimic physiologic insulin release as best as possible. Basal insulin secretion is about 50% of the body's total daily insulin requirement and prandial insulin approximately 40% to 60% (10% to 20% of daily insulin at each meal). This is referred to as the "basal/bolus" concept. The rapid and short-acting insulins serve as prandial insulin replacement, while the intermediate and long-acting insulins serve as basal insulin replacement. There are numerous types of insulin regimens, from one to two injections a day, to multiple daily injections or a continuous subcutaneous insulin infusion with an insulin pump. The sources of commercially available insulins are pork, human, and human analogues and are injected subcutaneously. The only exception is regular insulin, which can be used IV for hospitalized patients or patients on insulin infusions. Pork insulin is rarely used. The strength of commercially available insulins is 100 units per 1 mL (U-100).

Case Conclusion AJ is not in good glycemic control. Her HgbA1c and FBG are well above goal. For a patient with type 1 diabetes, generally it is not possible to achieve good glycemic control with a daily regimen of one to two injections. In order to achieve better glycemic control, a daily regimen of three to four injections should be initiated. This can be accomplished by using a short- or rapid-acting insulin before each meal (e.g., insulin lispro or aspart or regular insulin) and a longer-acting insulin (e.g., ultralente, insulin glargine) as basal insulin. AJ should also be instructed to self monitor her blood glucose more frequently, at least three to four times a day (e.g., premeal and bedtime with occasional 2-hour post-meal monitoring), in order to properly adjust her insulin regimen and detect any hypoglycemia. Because AJ has not been seen in the health-care system for 3 years, she also should be assessed for the standards of care set forth by the American Diabetes Association.

Thumbnail: Insulin Preparations

Insulin Preparation	Onset (hr)	Peak (hr)	Duration (hr)
Rapid-acting			
Insulin lispro	Within 15 min	½–1½	3–5
Insulin aspart	Within 10 min	1–3	3–5
Short-acting			
Regular	½–1	2–4	5–8
Intermediate-acting			
NPH	1–2	6–14	12+
Lente	1–3	6–14	12+
Long-acting			
Ultralente	6	18–24	24+
Insulin glargine	1½	Flat	24

Questions

1. RC is a 40-year-old woman with type 1 diabetes for 25 years. She takes four injections daily: insulin lispro before each meal and insulin glargine at bedtime. She states that she feels jittery, sweaty, and disoriented in the mid-afternoon two to three times a week; her blood glucose when she feels like this is 50 to 55 mg/dL. Her HgbA1c is 7.1%. Which of the following actions regarding her insulin regimen would be most appropriate?

   A. Do nothing. Her HgbA1c represents good glycemic control.
   B. Switch her to a twice-daily insulin regimen with 70/30 insulin.
   C. Increase her insulin glargine dose.
   D. Decrease her lunchtime insulin lispro dose.
   E. Increase her breakfast insulin lispro dose.

2. Which of the following are factors that can affect insulin absorption?

   A. Massage of injection site
   B. Exercise
   C. Heat
   D. Lipohypertrophy
   E. All of the above

HPI: DK is a 62-year-old woman with type 2 diabetes for 5 years. She has been treated with glyburide for 4 years. She follows dietary recommendations (low fat; distributes carbohydrates throughout her three meals a day) to the best of her ability and walks 30 minutes three times weekly. At a routine visit with her primary care provider, her FBG is 180 mg/dL. She does not monitor her blood glucose at home and does not have a glucose meter. She is a nonsmoker and her father has type 2 diabetes. Her only long-term diabetes complication is background diabetic retinopathy.

PE: Vitals: BP 138/84 mm Hg, 5 feet 4 inches tall, 157 pounds, body mass index (BMI) 27.

Labs: HgbA1c 9.0%; Cr 0.9 mg/dL; LFTs wnl.

Thought Questions

- What is your assessment of DK's blood glucose control?

- What are the pharmacologic options for her diabetes management?

- What are the contraindications to the various diabetes medications?

Basic Science Review and Discussion

Nearly 17 million Americans have diabetes, representing approximately 6% of the population. The majority of people with diabetes have type 2 diabetes, whereas approximately 1 million have type 1 diabetes. It is estimated that a third of people with type 2 diabetes are undiagnosed. Type 2 diabetes is a metabolic disorder involving a defect in insulin secretion and insulin action (i.e., insulin resistance), whereas type 1 diabetes is an autoimmune disorder associated with an absolute insulin deficiency.

The diagnostic criteria for diabetes are (a) symptoms of diabetes plus a casual plasma glucose concentration of ≥ 200 mg/dL (casual means any time of day without regard to meals); (b) FBG concentration of ≥ 126 mg/dL; or (c) 2-hour plasma glucose concentration of ≥ 200 mg/dL during an oral glucose tolerance test. All criteria must be confirmed on a subsequent day. The FBG is the most common criterion used due to its simplicity in measuring. Symptoms of hyperglycemia include polyuria, polydipsia, polyphagia, unexplained weight loss, blurred vision, and increased fatigue. A normal FBG concentration < 110 mg/dL and an FBG concentration > 110 mg/dL or < 126 mg/dL is defined as impaired fasting glucose (IFG).

The glycemic goals recommended by the American Diabetes Association (ADA) include the following: (a) premeal blood glucose of 80 to 120 mg/dL; (b) bedtime blood glucose of 100 to 140 mg/dL; and (c) HgbA1c of < 7% (the American Association of Clinical Endocrinologists recommends an HgbA1c of < 6.5%). The HgbA1c is the glycosylated hemoglobin, which represents the average blood glucose over

the past 2 to 3 months. The United Kingdom Prospective Diabetes Study (UKPDS) demonstrated that improved glycemic control lowers the risk for developing microvascular complications. In this landmark, multicenter trial of newly diagnosed type 2 diabetes patients, for every 1% decrease in the HgbA1c there was a 35% reduction in the risk of microvascular complications of diabetes (e.g., nephropathy, neuropathy, and retinopathy). The study demonstrated a trend in reducing cardiovascular events, but it was not statistically significant.

The current approach used by many clinicians for glycemic control in the management of diabetes is a stepped-care approach. The first step is lifestyle changes (e.g., diet and exercise). When diet and exercise are no longer enough to control the blood glucose, pharmacologic therapy is added. Monotherapy with oral antidiabetic agents is added to the diet and exercise plan as the second step. Six classes of oral agents for type 2 diabetes medications are available. In an overweight patient with type 2 diabetes, metformin is often considered the first-line agent because it does not cause hypoglycemia when used alone. Metformin decreases **hepatic glucose output** and does not cause weight gain, an advantage in an overweight patient with type 2 diabetes. However, sulfonylureas are still often used as oral monotherapy because they are still some of the most potent antidiabetics available. On the beta cell, insulin secretagogues (e.g., sulfonylureas) cause closure of the potassium channels, which results in a depolarization of the cell membrane and subsequent opening of the calcium channels. The increase in intracellular calcium leads to insulin secretion.

When a single oral agent is no longer enough to achieve the target glucose levels, combination oral therapy is used. The key to combination oral therapy is to add a second agent that has a different mechanism of action. Some patients may eventually require three oral agents and/or the initiation of insulin therapy to achieve glucose goals. The UKPDS demonstrated that 3 and 9 years after diagnosis of diabetes, 50% and 75% of patients will require combination therapy, respectively, which is consistent with the progressive decline in beta-cell function.

Case Conclusion   DK's HgbA1c of 9% and FBG of 180 mg/dL are both above the target glycemic goals set forth by the ADA. Because she has been on glyburide for 4 years and follows a diet/exercise plan, addition of a second oral agent would be indicated in this patient to lower her blood glucose. Metformin would be an appropriate choice in this overweight patient. Reinforcement of the diet and exercise plan is also important at this point. It is important to provide this patient with diabetes self-management education so that she can achieve her target metabolic goals. Self monitoring of blood glucose should be incorporated, especially since she is on a regimen that could cause hypoglycemia.

Thumbnail: Oral Agents for Diabetes

	Sulfonylureas	Meglitinides	Amino acid derivatives	Biguanides	Thiazolidinediones	Alpha-glucosidase inhibitors
Available agents	Acetohexamide Chlorpropamide Tolazamide Tolbutamide Glimepiride Glipizide Glyburide	Repalinide	Nateglinide	Metformin	Pioglitazone Rosiglitazone	Acarbose Miglitol
Primary MOA	Stimulate insulin secretion	Stimulate insulin secretion	Stimulate insulin secretion	Decrease hepatic glucose output	Decrease insulin resistance*	Delay carbohydrate absorption
Efficacy as monotherapy (HgbA1c ↓)	1.5%–2%	1.7%	0.5%	1.5%–2%	0.6%–1.5%	0.5%–1%
Pharmacokinetics						
Metabolism/ elimination	Acetohexamide, chlorpropamide, tolazamide, glyburide glimepiride: weakly active metabolites. Glipizide, tolbutamide: inactive metabolites.	Inactive metabolites	Predominantly inactive metabolites	Excreted unchanged in urine	Extensively metabolized in liver to metabolites	Acarbose: inactive metabolites. Miglitol: excreted unchanged in urine.
Adverse reactions	Hypoglycemia; weight gain	Hypoglycemia; weight gain	Hypoglycemia; weight gain	GI (nausea, cramping, diarrhea); lactic acidosis†	Fluid retention; anemia; weight gain	Abdominal pain; diarrhea; flatulence
Contraindications	Hepatic impairment; renal impairment (use caution; glipizide/tolbutamide preferred agents in renal impairment)	Hepatic impairment	Hepatic impairment	Renal impairment; CHF requiring drug therapy	Hepatic impairment (require bi-monthly LFT monitoring for first year; periodically thereafter)	Hepatic impairment; intestinal obstruction; other chronic intestinal diseases

*Due to delay in onset of effect, assessment of response should be at 3 months (using HgbA1c).

†Very rare side effect (~1 in 30,000 people); metformin should be temporarily withheld prior to any surgical procedure; it should be withheld at the time of (or prior to) a radiologic study involving the use of intravascular iodinated contrast dye and withheld 48 hours after the study and restarted after renal function has been found to be normal.

Questions

1. AK is a 55-year-old man diagnosed with diabetes 2 years ago. He has been following a diet and exercise program, but his HgbA1c is now 8.5%. BMI 20.2. Labs: Cr 1.6 mg/dL; LFTs wnl. Which of the following oral agents is most appropriate to initiate in this patient to obtain an HgbA1c of less than 7%?

   A. Metformin - biguanide
   B. Glipizide - sulfonylurea
   C. Nateglinide - amino acid derivative
   D. Chlorpropamide - sulfonylurea
   E. Acarbose - alpha glucosidase inhibitor

2. RJ has had type 2 diabetes for 10 years. His other medical problems include dyslipidemia, HTN, and retinopathy. He takes benazepril, simvastatin, and metformin. His BP is 120/70 mm Hg; LDL cholesterol 137 mg/dL; HgbA1c 7.8%. He had a dilated retinal eye examination 1.5 years ago. He has not had a pneumococcal vaccination and has never brought a urine sample into the lab. Which of the standards of care is in compliance according to the ADA guidelines?

   A. Blood pressure
   B. Eye exam visit
   C. LDL cholesterol
   D. HgbA1c
   E. Pneumococcal vaccination
   F. Microalbuminuria test

HPI: JL is a 55-year-old man s/p MI 3 years ago. He was placed on cholesterol-lowering therapy following his MI. He currently takes simvastatin to control his cholesterol. He finds it difficult to incorporate any physical activity in his daily routine and does not attempt to reduce his cholesterol/fat intake. His most recent lipid panel is total cholesterol 206 mg/dL; triglyericides 180 mg/dL; high density lipoprotein 35 mg/dL; low density lipoprotein 135 mg/dL.

Thought Questions

- What is your assessment of JL's lipid profile?

- Would you modify his current lipid-lowering therapy? If so, how?

- What are the common side effects associated with lipid-lowering medications?

- What are the common drug interactions with lipid-lowering medications?

Basic Science Review and Discussion

Coronary heart disease (CHD) is one of the leading causes of morbidity and mortality in the United States. Hyperlipidemia is a major risk factor for atherosclerosis and CHD. Hyperlipidemia is defined as an elevation in blood cholesterol or triglycerides (TG). Lipids are primarily transported in the body by three major lipoproteins: **low-density (LDL), very-low-density (VLDL),** and **high-density lipoproteins (HDL).** Cholesteryl esters and TG are carried by the lipoproteins, which vary in size and composition of cholesterol and TG. Cholesterol is used to form cell membranes and is the precursor to bile acids and steroid hormones.

Although several lipoproteins are considered to play a role in atherogenesis [VLDL, LDL and Lp(a)], LDL cholesterol (LDL-C) is the primary target of therapy. The risk of CHD is inversely related to levels of HDL, because HDL is responsible for reverse cholesterol transport. Lipoprotein disorders can involve abnormalities in lipid metabolism (e.g., synthesis, transport, and catabolism). Attainment of a lipid profile must be made after a 9- to 12-hour fast.

In addition to the level of LDL-C, the following are major risk factors for CHD: (a) cigarette smoking; (b) HTN (blood pressure $\geq$ 140/90 mm Hg or on antihypertensive medication); (c) low HDL cholesterol ($<$ 40 mg/dL); (d) family history of premature CHD (CHD in male first-degree relative $<$ 55 years of age or CHD in female first-degree relative $<$ 65 years of age); and (e) age (men $\geq$ 45 years; women $\geq$ 55 years).

Four main classes of lipid-lowering medications are available: HMG CoA reductase inhibitors (otherwise known as statins), bile acid sequestrants, nicotinic acid, and fibric acids.

Case Conclusion   Because JL already has CHD (s/p MI) and his LDL-C goal is more than 100 mg/dL, his current therapy is inadequate. Lifestyles changes should be emphasized to him, including reduction of saturated fat and cholesterol and physical activity as tolerated. Physical activity will be beneficial in raising the HDL-C in this patient. In addition, his simvastatin dose should be increased. LDL-C reduction with statins is dose-dependent. In general, a doubling of the dose will result in an additional 6% lowering of the LDL-C. If he is already taking the maximum dose, combination drug therapy should be instituted.

Thumbnail: Agents for Hyperlipidemia

Drug class	MOA	Lipid effects	Adverse reactions	Metabolism	Drug interactions	Contraindications/ precautions
HMG CoA reductase inhibitors (statins) Atorvastatin Fluvastatin Lovastatin Pravastatin Simvastatin	Inhibit rate-limiting step in cholesterol synthesis	LDL ↓ 18%-55% HDL ↑ 5%-15% TG ↓ 7%-30%	Myopathy (rare) ↑ LFTs (rare)	All via CYP450, although the specific isoenzyme is drug specific.	Macrolide antibiotics Cyclosporine Digoxin Nefazodone Azole antifungals HIV protease inhibitors Amiodarone Warfarin Fibric acids Niacin	Liver disease; pregnancy and lactation
Bile acid sequestrants Cholestyramine Colestipol Colesevalam	Bind to bile acids in gut	LDL ↓ 15%-30% HDL ↑ 30% TG no change or ↑	GI: constipation, bloating, abdominal pain	None (not systemically absorbed)	↓ bioavailability of coadministered drugs; separate other drugs at least 1 hr before or 4–6 hr after	Complete biliary obstruction; severely elevated TG
Nicotinic acid	Inhibit VLDL secretion	LDL ↓ 5%–25% HDL ↑ 15%–35% TG ↓ 20%–50%	Flushing; ↑ blood sugar and uric acid; GI upset; liver toxicity	88% excreted as unchanged drug and nicotinuric acid	Statins	Liver disease; active peptic ulcer disease (PUD); arterial bleeding; caution use in diabetes; and gout
Fibric acids Clofibrate Gemfibrozil Fenofibrate	Increase VLDL catabolism; PPAR$_\alpha$ agonist	LDL ↓ 5–20% HDL ↑ 10%–20% TG ↓ 20%-50%	GI upset, dyspepsia, gallstones, ↑ LFTs, myopathy	Non-CYP450 metabolism	Warfarin Cyclosporine Statins	Liver or severe renal disease; primary biliary cirrhosis; preexisting gallbladder disease

PPAR$_\alpha$: peroxisome proliferator activated receptor.

Questions

1. RM had his dose of lovastatin increased since his LDL-C was above his goal. How soon should his response to the higher dose be assessed?

   A. 1 week
   B. 2 weeks
   C. 3 weeks
   D. 4 weeks
   E. 6 weeks

2. PJ is a 60-year-old woman with a history of an abdominal aortic aneurysm who is taking niacin for her dyslipidemia. Her LDL-C is 120 mg/dL, so a statin is added to her therapy. Which of the following are true for statins?

   A. Baseline LFTs should be checked prior to initiation.
   B. Generally taken at dinner or bedtime.
   C. Statins interact with cyclosporine.
   D. Statins interact with azole antifungals.
   E. Statins interact with niacin and fibrates.
   F. All of the above.

> **HPI:**   KG is a 39-year-old woman with asthma on fluticasone and albuterol complaining of SOB associated with exercise. Three months ago she started an aerobic exercise program that has been hampered by chest tightness and SOB shortly after she begins running. She admits to poor compliance with her corticosteroid inhaler and requests an oral medication to control her asthma symptoms. Her PMH is significant for mild, persistent asthma for 35 years and allergic rhinitis. Her medications include fluticasone and albuterol inhalers and fexofenadine. Pulmonary function tests (PFTs) reveal her forced expiratory volume in the first second (FEV_1) = 89% of predicted.

Thought Questions

- What general classes of medications are appropriate for the treatment of mild persistent asthma?

- Which medications are effective for exercise-induced bronchospasm (EIB)?

- What adverse effects are associated with inhaled corticosteroid therapy?

Basic Science Review and Discussion

Asthma is a chronic inflammatory disease of the airways afflicting an estimated 15 million people in the United States (approximately 6% of the population), nearly 5 million of whom are under the age of 18. Symptoms of asthma include recurrent wheezing, difficulty breathing, chest tightness, and cough (particularly at night). Pharmacotherapy for asthma consists of quick-relief (rescue) and long-term control (maintenance) medications. Quick-relief medications are used to provide rapid relief of asthma symptoms (wheezing, cough, and SOB) and include short-acting inhaled β_2-agonists and systemic corticosteroids. Long-term control medications are taken on a daily basis to achieve and maintain control of persistent asthma and include anti-inflammatory agents (inhaled corticosteroids, mast cell stabilizers), long-acting β_2-agonists, methylxanthines, and leukotriene modifiers.

The goal of EIB treatment is to allow patients to exercise (including vigorous activities) without experiencing symptoms of bronchospasm. Recommended treatments consist of medications taken as needed just prior to exercise to prevent symptoms or those taken long term on a daily basis to decrease inflammation and airway hyperresponsiveness. Medications taken immediately before exercise include β_2-agonists and mast cell stabilizing agents. Inhaled β_2-agonists are the mainstay of treatment and are more than 80% effective in preventing EIB if administered prophylactically. Short-acting inhaled β_2-agonists (albuterol, bitolterol, pirbuterol) administered 5–15 minutes before exercise are generally effective for 2 to 3 hours. Long-acting agents (salmeterol, formoterol) offer protection for up to 12 hours. The mast cell stabilizing agents (cromolyn, nedocromil) when taken 10 to 15 minutes before exercise are also effective alternatives.

Patients who experience symptoms more than twice weekly have persistent asthma, and should be managed with a long-term control medication with anti-inflammatory activity. In general, inhaled corticosteroids are well tolerated. Local reactions including cough, dysphonia (hoarseness), and oral candidiasis (thrush) are the most commonly observed adverse effects. These can be minimized by administering the drug with a spacer device and by rinsing the oral cavity with water after inhalation. Systemic adverse effects associated with corticosteroids (adrenal suppression, osteoporosis, growth suppression, ocular toxicity, dermal thinning, easy bruising) are significantly less likely to occur with the inhaled route of administration. Although higher doses of inhaled corticosteroids increase the risk for systemic adverse effects, these risks are far less than would be seen with oral administration of corticosteroids. When prescribed at the recommended doses, the superior effectiveness of inhaled corticosteroids outweighs the minimal risks for serious adverse effects.

> **Case Conclusion**   Because KG is poorly compliant with her inhaled corticosteroid therapy, she is started on daily montelukast to control her mild persistent asthma and EIB. She is also instructed to use her albuterol inhaler 15 minutes before exercise to provide additional protection against EIB.

Thumbnail: Agents for Asthma

Class/specific agent	MOA	Adverse reactions	Comments
β_2-agonists (inhaled)			
Short-acting • Albuterol • Bitolterol • Pirbuterol	β_2-selective adrenergic agonists that induce bronchodilation through activation of adenylate cyclase, causing an increase in cyclic AMP levels and resulting in smooth muscle relaxation in the airways.	Tachycardia, skeletal muscle tremor, hypokalemia, prolonged QT_c interval (in overdose).	**Onset of action:** 5–15 min **Duration of action:** 2–3 hr Nonselective agents (epinephrine, isoproterenol, metaproterenol) are not recommended due to their potential for excessive cardiac stimulation. Oral agents are less preferred due to the slower onset of action (30–60 min) and higher incidence of systemic side effects.
Long-acting • Formoterol • Salmeterol			**Onset of action:** 15 min (formoterol); 15–30 min (salmeterol) **Duration of action:** 12 hr
Mast cell stabilizers (inhaled)			
• Cromolyn • Nedocromil	Work topically on lung mucosa. Block early and late reaction to allergen. Stabilize mast cell membranes and inhibit activation and release of inflammatory mediators from eosinophils and epithelial cells, inhibiting bronchoconstriction caused by exercise and cold dry air.	Poorly absorbed so adverse effects usually localized: cough, mouth dryness, throat irritation, metallic taste (15%–20%) with nedocromil.	**Onset of action:** 10–15 min **Duration of action:** 1–2 hr
Corticosteroids (inhaled)			
• Beclomethasone • Budesonide • Flunisolide • Fluticasone • Triamcinolone	Block late reaction to allergen and reduce airway hyper-responsiveness. Inhibit production of cytokines responsible for initiation of inflammatory cascade.	Cough, dysphonia, oral candidiasis (thrush). High doses may cause systemic effects (e.g., adrenal and growth suppression, osteoporosis, skin thinning, and cataracts).	**Onset of action:** 7–14 days; full effect may not be realized for 6–8 wk. Adverse effects minimized by administering with a spacer and by rinsing the oral cavity with water after inhalation.
Leukotriene modifiers			
Leukotriene receptor antagonists • Montelukast • Zafirlukast	Selective, competitive inhibitor of the leukotriene D_4 (LTD_4) receptor. Inhibition of LTD_4 reduces bronchoconstriction, airway hyperresponsiveness, mucosal edema, and mucus production.	Headache, abdominal pain, hepatotoxicity (~2%), Churg-Strauss syndrome (rare).	Oral medications administered once (montelukast) or twice (zafirlukast) daily.
5-lipoxygenase inhibitor • Zileuton	Inhibitor of the 5-lipoxygenase enzyme necessary for the biosynthesis of leukotrienes including LTD_4.	Headache, hepatotoxicity (12%) Abdominal pain, nausea, Churg-Strauss syndrome (rare).	Oral medication administered four times daily. Regular monitoring for hepatotoxicity is necessary.

Questions

1. JC is a 14-year-old boy with a 7-year history of mild-intermittent asthma who complains of SOB, cough, and poor endurance during football practice. Other than this EIB, his asthma has been well controlled for the past several years with only "as needed" β_2-agonist therapy for asthma symptoms. He has not needed to use his rescue inhaler (albuterol) for nearly a year. PFTs reveal his $FEV_1 = 95\%$ of predicted. Which of the following is the best treatment for JC?

   A. Administer albuterol aerosol 5 to 15 minutes before exercise.
   B. Administer oral albuterol 5 to 15 minutes before exercise.
   C. Administer albuterol aerosol every 6 hours during football season.
   D. Administer epinephrine aerosol 5 to 15 minutes before exercise.
   E. Initiate high-dose inhaled corticosteroid therapy.

2. A 32-year-old woman receiving beclomethasone eight puffs twice daily for moderate persistent asthma complains of white spots on her tongue and hard palate and pain on swallowing. Her asthma control has been excellent and she has no other medical problems. The most appropriate change in her asthma therapy would be to:

   A. Discontinue beclomethasone.
   B. Change the beclomethasone inhaler to two puffs four times daily.
   C. Change the beclomethasone inhaler to a flunisolide inhaler.
   D. Instruct the patient to use the beclomethasone inhaler with a spacer.
   E. Change the beclomethasone inhaler to oral prednisone.

HPI: LR is a 62-year-old woman who presents to the emergency room today with complaints of increasing SOB, fever, and increasing production of purulent sputum over the past 2 days. Her PMH includes chronic bronchitis and hypothyroidism. She has been smoking one pack of cigarettes per day for the past 45 years.

PE: Her chest examination is notable for decreased breath sounds throughout, bilateral crackles at the bases, and diffuse expiratory wheezing.

The patient is diagnosed with an acute exacerbation of COPD and started on oxygen via face mask with a target oxygen saturation (SaO_2) of > 90%.

Thought Questions

- Which bronchodilators are indicated in the management of acute exacerbations of COPD?

- Are systemic corticosteroids and antibiotics warranted for the treatment of COPD?

Basic Science Review and Discussion

Chronic obstructive pulmonary disease is a respiratory condition characterized by irreversible airway obstruction caused by chronic bronchitis or emphysema. The major symptoms of COPD include chronic cough, increased sputum production, and dyspnea. The vast majority of patients with COPD are those who are current or former heavy smokers. Other risk factors for the development of COPD include occupational exposure (dusts, chemicals) and rare genetic disorders (α_1-antitrypsin deficiency). The medical management of COPD includes pharmacotherapy (bronchodilators, corticosteroids, and antibiotics) in combination with interventions to reduce risk factors for disease progression (e.g., smoking cessation). Some patients require long-term administration of supplemental oxygen.

LR has symptoms consistent with an acute exacerbation of COPD, including worsening dyspnea, increased production of purulent sputum, and acute respiratory acidosis. The use of supplemental oxygen with careful monitoring of arterial blood gases is recommended in patients presenting with hypoxemia. Bronchodilator therapy should be initiated to alleviate airflow obstruction and improve oxygenation. Both short-acting inhaled β_2-agonists (e.g., albuterol) and anticholinergic agents (e.g., ipratropium) are effective in patients with acute exacerbations of COPD. Combination therapy with inhaled short-acting β_2-agonists and anticholinergic agents is recommended in patients who fail to respond to maximal doses of either agent alone. Other bronchodilators, including methylxanthines (aminophylline, theophylline) and systemic β_2-agonists, are not generally recommended due to an increased risk for adverse effects. Patients should be continually assessed to determine the need for additional medication or more aggressive respiratory support (e.g., mechanical ventilation). Because bacterial respiratory infections also may precipitate acute exacerbations of COPD, antibiotics may be warranted.

In addition to the above measures, systemic corticosteroids are used to improve pulmonary function and provide symptomatic relief. Treatment durations in excess of 2 weeks are associated with increased corticosteroid-related adverse effects. The use of topical, inhaled corticosteroids in the acute management of COPD exacerbation is not appropriate.

Case Conclusion Because LR is in severe respiratory distress, she is started on albuterol and ipratropium. She is also given oral prednisone to hasten improvement of her pulmonary function and doxycycline for treatment of a suspected respiratory bacterial infection. She also will be strongly advised to quit smoking.

Thumbnail: Short-Acting Inhaled Bronchodilators

Prototypical agents: Albuterol (short-acting β_2-agonist); ipratropium (anticholinergic)

Clinical usage: Short-acting inhaled bronchodilators are indicated for the treatment of bronchospasm associated with obstructive pulmonary disorders.

	Albuterol	Ipratropium
MOA	Selective β_2-adrenergic agonist that induces bronchodilation through activation of adenylate cyclase causing an increase in cyclic AMP levels, resulting in smooth muscle relaxation in the airways.	A synthetic quaternary ammonium analogue of atropine that antagonizes smooth muscle contraction in the airways mediated by the release of acetylcholine from the vagus nerve.
Onset of action	2–15 min	< 15 min
Duration of action	2–6 hr	3–6 hr
Absorption	Slowly absorbed across the respiratory tract but < 20% of an inhaled dose reaches the airways. The fraction of the dose that is swallowed is rapidly and completely absorbed from the GI tract.	Poor systemic absorption from the pulmonary and GI tract.
Distribution	Appears to cross the blood–brain barrier and placenta	Poorly crosses the blood–brain barrier
Elimination	Undergoes extensive hepatic metabolism to inactive compounds that are eliminated primarily in urine (90%) and to a lesser extent in feces (10%). $T^{1/2} = 2.7$–6 hr	Metabolized via ester hydrolysis to inactive compounds. Approximately 50% of the administered dose is excreted unchanged in urine. $T^{1/2} = 2$ hr

Questions

1. PJ is 68-year-old man with mild COPD and HTN seen in the clinic today for increasing dyspnea (associated with exertion), cough, and clear sputum production over the past 3 months. His current medications include hydro-chlorothiazide and albuterol inhaler. The patient reports using his albuterol inhaler several times daily with only minimal symptomatic improvement. The most appropriate change in COPD therapy would be to:

   A. Add a corticosteroid inhaler.
   B. Start low-dose prednisone.
   C. Add an ipratropium inhaler.
   D. Start prophylactic antibiotic therapy.
   E. Start antitussive therapy (codeine or dextromethorphan).

2. DD is a 70-year-old woman admitted to the hospital for exacerbation of her COPD. She is currently intubated and receiving high-dose albuterol therapy by continuous nebulization. Which of the following adverse effects may be associated with this treatment?

   A. HTN
   B. Bradycardia
   C. Somnolence
   D. Hypoglycemia
   E. Hypokalemia

> **HPI:** AL is a 23-year-old woman with no medical conditions, who comes into the clinic requesting medication for hay fever. She has been experiencing frequent sneezing, watery itchy eyes, and congestion. She works at a law firm during the day and would prefer a quick-acting agent that does not cause sedation.

Thought Questions

- What is the pharmacology of antihistamines?

- What are the differences between first- and second-generation antihistamines?

- Other than allergies and allergic reactions, what other conditions are antihistamines used for?

- What side effects are associated with antihistaminic treatments?

Basic Science Review and Discussion

Histamine is an endogenous substance that activates histamine H_1, H_2, and H_3 receptors, and its principal pharmacologic effects involve exocrine glands, extravascular smooth muscles, and the cardiovascular system. H_1 receptor stimulation increases inositol-1,4,5-triphosphate, which increases intracellular calcium, resulting in vasoconstriction. Activation of H_2 receptors increases intracellular cAMP, which mediates gastric acid secretions and cardiovascular effects. H_3 receptor stimulation may be involved in feedback inhibition of histamine synthesis and release.

In allergic conditions, histamine released from mast cells, basophils, and other cells bind to and activate specific H_1 receptors in the nose, eyes, respiratory tract, and skin, causing characteristic symptoms of edema, **wheal and flare** reactions, itching, rhinorrhea, and lacrimation. Histamine also stimulates nerve endings, causing pruritus. The action of histamine on H_1 receptors in the microcirculation

increases intracellular calcium. This results in endothelial cellular constriction and increased permeability between cells, permitting the transudation of fluids and small proteins into the extravascular space.

Antihistamines are primarily H_1-receptor competitive antagonists with negligible effects on H_2 and H_3 receptors. They do not directly alter the effects of histamine or prevent histamine release, but suppress histamine-induced effects by preventing access of histamine to H_1 receptor sites. Aside from antihistaminic effects, however, first-generation antihistamines also possess **anticholinergic** properties that account for their utility in conditions such as emesis and parkinsonian symptoms. Antiemetic actions of antihistamines result from central anticholinergic and CNS depressant properties. Scopolamine, an anticholinergic agent, is often used for motion sickness and nausea. The antimuscarinic actions of antihistamines reduce antipsychotic **drug-induced parkinsonism** by inhibiting acetylcholine.

Muscarinic effects, mediated by acetylcholine, the primary transmitter of the autonomic nervous system ganglia, are inhibited by the anticholinergic effects exerted by antihistamines. Anticholinergic side effects include dry mouth, urinary retention, blurred vision, and constipation. Because first-generation antihistamines also distribute into the CNS, sedation is a prominent side effect. The development of second-generation antihistamines, such as loratadine and fexofenadine, lack anticholinergic activity and do not distribute into the CNS (Table 31-1). Hence, they are not typically associated with sedation and do not possess antiemetic properties.

> **Case Conclusion** AL is prescribed loratadine, a nonsedating antihistamine, to be taken once daily. She is advised not to use it on an as-needed basis but to take it daily to effectively prevent symptoms.

Table 31-1 Characteristics of H$_1$ antihistaminic agents

	Antihistaminic activity	Anticholinergic activity	Sedative effects	Antiemetic activity
First-generation antihistamines				
Diphenhydramine	Low to moderate	High	High	Moderate to high
Tripelennamine	Low to moderate	Low to none	Moderate	
Brompheniramine	High	Moderate	Low	
Chlorpheniramine	Moderate	Moderate	Low	
Promethazine	High	High	High	Very high
Hydroxyzine	Moderate to high	Moderate	High	High
Cyproheptadine	Moderate	Moderate	Low	
Second-generation antihistamines				
Cetirizine	Moderate to high	Low to none	Low to none	Low
Fexofenadine	Moderate to high	Low to none	Low to none	Low
Loratadine	Moderate to high	Low to none	Low to none	Low

Thumbnail: Antihistamines

Prototypical agent: Diphenhydramine. Other first-generation antihistamines include chlorpheniramine, clemastine, promethazine, and cyproheptadine. Second-generation antihistamines—loratadine, cetirizine, and fexofenadine—were developed to circumvent anticholinergic and sedative side effects.

Clinical uses: Symptomatic relief of seasonal allergies, nausea and vomiting, motion sickness, transfusion reactions, pruritis, edema, and urticaria associated with allergic reactions.

MOA: Competitive antagonism of the smooth muscle stimulating actions of histamine on H$_1$ receptors. The central anticholinergic activity of antihistamines reduces symptoms of emesis and counteracts EPS associated with antipsychotic treatment.

Pharmacokinetics

Absorption: Antihistamines are well absorbed. Approximately 40% to 60% reaches systemic circulation with oral dosing. Onset of action is rapid, 15 to 30 minutes. Onset of action for transdermal scopalamine discs is 4 hours.

Distribution: Widely distributed.

Elimination: Primarily hepatic metabolism.

Adverse reactions: CNS depression and anticholinergic side effects are most prevalent. They include sedation, dry mouth, blurred vision, constipation, dizziness, and fatigue. Caution should be used in patients with closed-angle glaucoma, prostatic hyperplasia, and asthma or COPD. Geriatric patients may be more sensitive to the adverse effects of antihistamines and may experience a greater degree of dizziness and sedation. Additionally, both geriatric and pediatric patients may experience paradoxic hyperexcitability.

Drug interactions: Additive CNS depressant effects may occur when antihistamines are administered concomitantly with other CNS depressants, including barbiturates, benzodiazepines, alcohol, and other sedatives. Additive anticholinergic effect also may occur when used in combination with other anticholinergic agents.

Questions

1. GG is a 42-year-old man who has been on perphenazine as maintenance therapy for schizophrenia diagnosed at age 25. His mother is concerned because she has noticed abnormal posturing and stiffness in the movements of the body and face over the past few months. Which agent would be most appropriate to reverse and prevent further dystonic symptoms due to GG's antipsychotic therapy?

   A. Tripelennamine
   B. Diphenhydramine
   C. Brompheniramine
   D. Cetirizine
   E. Cyproheptadine

2. DL is an 82-year-old woman who is planning on celebrating her wedding anniversary aboard a cruise ship to Alaska. She wants to know what to take for prevention of seasickness. The cruise departs in 1 week. Which agent should she take to prevent nausea?

   A. Meclizine 1 hour prior to boarding and on an as-needed basis thereafter
   B. Chlorpheniramine 1 hour prior to boarding and every 6 hours thereafter
   C. Loratadine to avoid sedative side effects
   D. Scopalamine disc 30 to 60 minutes prior to boarding
   E. Scopalamine disc 4 hours prior to boarding

HPI: KD is a 74-year-old African-American man with diabetes mellitus and HTN who presents to the clinic for a routine eye examination. **Intraocular pressure** (IOP) = 39 mm Hg (normal 10–20 mm Hg) in the right eye (OD) and 25 mm Hg in the left eye (OS).

PE: Ophthalmoscopy reveals slight cupping of the optic disc OD. Visual field examination appears normal. The patient denies any decrease in visual acuity or pain. Current medications include metformin, fosinopril, and glyburide.

Thought Questions

- How do patients with **primary open-angle glaucoma** (POAG) usually present?

- What are the risk factors for POAG?

- What are the main factors to consider in determining the drug of choice for patients diagnosed with POAG?

Basic Science Review and Discussion

Primary open-angle glaucoma is usually asymptomatic upon initial presentation. Elevated IOP is frequently unaccompanied by pain or loss of vision. As the disease progresses, gradual nerve damage leads to cupping of the optic disc (an increase in cup-disc ratio) and subsequent visual field defects. This eventually results in loss of peripheral vision and even blindness. An IOP of greater than 21 mm Hg without changes in visual fields and optic discs is defined as ocular hypertension. Medical therapy for patients with ocular hypertension is debatable. However, treatment should be considered for patients over 50 years of age with an IOP greater than 30 mm Hg because older people are at higher risk for optic nerve damage with decreased vascular perfusion. Conversely, in rare cases some patients with normal IOP may have glaucomatous damage, and also should be treated.

Risk factors associated with POAG include advanced age, family history, race (Caucasian and African American), myopia, HTN, diabetes mellitus, and vascular diseases. Drugs associated with increasing IOP include topical and systemic corticosteroids, anticholinergic agents, amphetamines, and tricyclic antidepressants.

Although an increase in IOP alone does not lead to a definitive diagnosis of glaucoma, elevated IOP is associated with an elevated risk of disease progression. Hence, medications currently used to treat glaucoma target the reduction of IOP by either decreasing inflow (formation of aqueous humor) or increasing outflow (elimination of aqueous humor). Determination of the drug of choice for each patient is based on the concomitant disease states and the side effect profile of each medication class. Because glaucoma is a silent disease throughout its early stages, noncompliance to therapy is prevalent. This is especially notable in medications with bothersome side effects. Topical **beta-blockers** have been favored as a class due to their minimal local adverse effects. However, they should be used with caution in patients with a history of reactive airway disease or cardiovascular diseases. **Prostaglandin analogues** have gained popularity in recent years because of their convenient dosing frequency and minimal local and systemic side effects. Brimonidine, an α_2-receptor agonist, also lacks significant local irritation, although its predecessor, apraclonidine, is no longer used due to problems with tachyphylaxis. Topical **carbonic anhydrase inhibitors** are very effective IOP-reducing agents; however, they should be used with caution in patients with sulfa allergy. Topical miotic and mydriatic agents have fallen out of favor due to their bothersome local and systemic adverse effects. Secondary to their serious side effect profiles, oral carbonic anhydrase inhibitors and oral **cholinergic agents** are currently reserved as last-line therapies. Upon the failure of medical therapy, surgical options may be considered.

Case Conclusion   Because KM is newly diagnosed with open-angle glaucoma, first-line therapy can include a beta-blocker or a prostaglandin analogue. Although KM has diabetes, beta-blockers would not be an absolute contraindication. However, for ease of administration, KM is started on a trial of latanoprost in the right eye. If the IOP improves by the next follow-up visit, treatment will also start on the left eye.

Thumbnail: Agents for Primary Open-Angle Glaucoma

Drugs	MOA	Common side effects
Beta-adrenergic blockers Betaxolol Carteolol Levobunolol Metipranolol Timolol	Decrease aqueous inflow	Stinging, dry eyes, blurred vision, blepharitis
Sympathomimetics **Alpha/beta agonist** Epinephrine Dipivefrin	Increase aqueous outflow	Tearing, burning, conjunctival hyperemia, mydriasis, blurred vision, pigment deposition in conjunctiva and cornea, precipitation of narrow-angle glaucoma
α_2-agonists Apraclonidine Brimonidine	Decrease aqueous inflow	Allergic reactions (edema, foreign object sensation, hyperemia, itching, eyelid discomfort)
Parasympathomimetics **(direct acting)** Pilocarpine Carbachol	Increase aqueous outflow	Miosis, accommodative spasm, constriction of visual field, retinal tears, cataracts, periorbital pain, precipitation of angle-closure glaucoma (at high doses)
Carbonic anhydrase inhibitors Dorzolamide Brinzolamide	Decrease aqueous inflow	Ocular burning and stinging, transient blurry vision, itching, conjunctivitis, superficial punctate keratitis, tearing, photophobia
Prostaglandin analogues Latanoprost Bimatoprost Unoprostone Travoprost	Increase aqueous outflow	Blurry vision, conjunctival hyperemia, iris pigmentation, increase in eyelash length and coarseness

Questions

1. AK is a 65-year-old white woman with asthma, HTN, arrhythmias, and a history of sulfa allergy who presents to the eye clinic for a routine eye examination. IOP = 29 mm Hg OD and 31 mm Hg OS at 8:30 A.M. Ophthalmoscopy reveals cupping of optic disc OS > OD. A diagnosis of POAG is made. Which of the following is the best initial therapy for AK?

    A. Timolol
    B. Epinephrine
    C. Pilocarpine
    D. Dorzolamide
    E. Latanoprost

2. JC is a 56-year-old African-American man who presents to the eye clinic for a glaucoma follow-up visit. IOP = 28 mm Hg OD and 31 mm Hg OS. JC is currently on latanoprost and brimonidine. JC admits to poor compliance with his eyedrops, stating that they "burn my eyes and make them very red and itchy all day." Which of the following is the best management for JC?

    A. Discontinue glaucoma therapy to give the patient a drug holiday.
    B. Add tetrahydrozoline (Visine®) to current regimen.
    C. Replace latanoprost with bimatoprost.
    D. Replace brimonidine with brinzolamide.
    E. Replace brimonidine with dipivefrin.

HPI: AC is a 45-year-old woman who presents to the ED with nausea, vomiting, diaphoresis, and a severely red and painful right eye with "steamy"-appearing cornea.

PE: Upon examination, AC has poor pupil response to light. IOP is 50 mm Hg OD and 22 mm Hg OS.

Thought Questions

- How do patients with angle-closure glaucoma usually present?

- Which medications may precipitate an acute attack of angle-closure glaucoma?

- What are the treatment options for angle-closure glaucoma?

Basic Science Review and Discussion

Dilation of the pupil in the preexisting narrow anterior chamber may cause the iris to block aqueous humor outflow via the anterior chamber. This leads to an abrupt increase in IOP, resulting in an acute attack of angle-closure glaucoma. Signs and symptoms include blurred vision (often with colored halos around the light), severe ocular pain, red conjunctiva, diaphoresis, and nausea/vomiting. The cornea may appear cloudy due to edema. Upon presentation, the IOP is frequently above 50 mm Hg.

Any agents with **anticholinergic** effects, which may dilate the pupil, should be used with caution in patients predis-posed to angle-closure glaucoma. Strong **miotic agents** also should be avoided because they may lead to pupillary block. Other agents associated with inducing angle-closure glaucoma in rare cases include adrenergics, tricyclic antidepressants, MOA inhibitors, acetazolamide, and amphetamines.

Angle-closure glaucoma is a medical emergency that can lead to permanent damage to vision and blindness if not treated promptly. Medical management is used initially to rapidly reduce the IOP, although surgical intervention is necessary for a permanent cure. Management includes combination therapy with PO/IV acetazolamide, topical beta-blockers, PO/IV hyperosmotic agents, and pilocarpine. **Hyperosmotic agents** lower the IOP by creating an osmotic gradient between the plasma and aqueous humor from the anterior chamber of the eye. Available agents include glycerin, urea, mannitol, isosorbide, and ethyl alcohol. Common side effects of hyperosmotic agents are headache, nausea, vomiting, diuresis, and dehydration. However, patients should not be given fluids, which antagonize the effect of the hyperosmotic agent. When the IOP has been reduced to levels at which surgery can be performed, laser peripheral iridotomy is used to create a hole in the peripheral iris to relieve pupillary block.

Case Conclusion AC is started on combination therapy with glycerin, pilocarpine 2%, timolol, and acetazolamide to rapidly reduce the IOP. After the IOP has stabilized, AC is taken to surgery for laser peripheral iridotomy.

Thumbnail: Agents for Angle-Closure Glaucoma

Hyperosmotic agent	Route	Comments
Glycerin 50%	PO	Drug of choice among oral agents; use with caution in diabetic patients
Mannitol 20%	IV	Drug of choice among intravascular agents; more effective for glaucoma with inflammation than urea or glycerol
Urea 30%	IV	Contraindicated in patients with renal disease; caution in hepatic impairment
Isosorbide 45%	PO	Safe to use in diabetic patients (not metabolized to provide calories)
Ethyl alcohol 50%	PO	Effective in emergency situations when other agents are unavailable

Questions

1. KW is a 79-year-old woman who presents to the ED complaining of severe ocular pain, redness, blurred vision, headache, nausea, and vomiting. The cornea appears cloudy. IOP = 55 mm Hg OD and 19 mm Hg OS. Slit-lamp examination reveals inflammatory cells floating in the aqueous humor. A diagnosis of acute angle-closure glaucoma accompanied by uveitis is made. Which hyperosmotic agent would be the best choice for KW?

   A. Glycerin
   B. Mannitol
   C. Urea
   D. Isosorbide
   E. Ethyl alcohol

2. TK is a 67-year-old diabetic man who presents to the ED with a severe headache, a very red right eye, ocular pain, blurry vision, and a "steamy" cornea. IOP = 88 mm Hg OD and 25 mm Hg OS. Labs indicate glucose 250 mg/dL, Cr 1.9 mg/dL. A diagnosis of acute angle-closure glaucoma is made. How should TK be managed?

   A. TK should be given pilocarpine 10% every 5 minutes and mannitol 20% IV to reduce the IOP immediately.
   B. TK should be given pilocarpine 4% and timolol 0.5% to reduce the IOP.
   C. TK should be given 45% isosorbide orally and acetazolamide 500 mg IV to reduce the IOP.
   D. TK should be transferred directly to the operating room for emergency laser peripheral iridotomy due to the extremely elevated IOP.
   E. Both B and C.

> **HPI:** JL is a 23-year-old woman who complains of severe abdominal cramping, heavy menstrual flow, headache, and irritability during the first few days of her menstrual cycle. Last month her doctor started her on a 21-day monophasic combined oral contraceptive (COC) containing ethinyl estradiol (EE), and levonorgestrel (LNG). After completing two cycles, she states that her cramping and flow have improved, but she is experiencing break-through bleeding (BTB) around day 17 of her cycle, her acne has worsened, and she is considering stopping her pills. Her PMH is significant for a seizure disorder.

Thought Questions

- How do mono- and triphasic COCs differ?

- Aside from COC pills, what other formulations are available?

- What drugs and disease states would preclude the use of a particular contraceptive?

- What are some possible reasons that JL is having BTB?

Basic Science Review and Discussion

Monophasic formulations contain a constant dose of estrogen and progestin. **Triphasic** formulations contain varying doses of progestin (generally increasing) every 7 days, and either a stable or a variable amount of estrogen every 7 days. Typically the total progestin amount per cycle in monophasics is greater than that of triphasics. Estrogen content per cycle is similar between the two.

Patients who have contraindications to estrogen or who experience intolerable side effects are good candidates for progestin-only contraceptives. Progestin-only pills are less effective than COC pills, and are associated with a greater incidence of dysmenorrhea, amenorrhea, irregular menses, and BTB. Use of non-oral formulations may be desirable in individuals who forget to take their pills on a daily basis or who are noncompliant. Options include an intramuscular injectable (depo-medroxyprogesterone acetate [DMPA], Depo-Provera®), a surgically placed subdermal implant (LNG, Norplant®), and a surgically placed intrauterine system (LNG, Mirena®). DMPA has been linked to reversible bone loss. Estrogen is also available as a transdermal patch, a vaginal ring, and a monthly IM injectable. These nonoral routes allow for lower doses of hormones to be used and bypass first-pass metabolism, thereby limiting the production of factors produced by the liver (e.g., fibrinogen, C-reactive protein).

Contraceptive efficacy can be decreased when taken concurrently with drugs that increase the metabolism of hormones (e.g., CYP450 inducers). Similarly, drugs that reduce enterohepatic recycling of COCs (e.g., tetracycline, penicillins) can also reduce efficacy.

There are a variety of contraindications to contraceptive use. A family history of breast cancer does not preclude the use of COCs. In general, COC use does not increase the risk for breast cancer and may diminish the risk for endometrial, colorectal, and ovarian cancer. COC use is not recommended, however, in patients who have a current or past history of breast, hepatic, or cervical cancer. COC use may increase the risk for cervical dysplasia and cancer with more than 1 year of use. It also may increase the risk for hepatic cancer and gallbladder disease. Benefits of short-term COC use may include improved cycle regularity, less dysmenorrhea, fewer premenstrual symptoms, less irregular bleeding and blood loss, reduced risk for ectopic pregnancy and functional ovarian cysts, and possible reduction in acne. Long-term benefits of COC use may include a reduced risk for pelvic inflammatory disease (PID), benign breast disease, and improved bone mineral density and lipid profile ($\uparrow$ HDL).

Once initiated, patients should be monitored for side effects of COCs. BTB is a common reason for drug discontinuation. Generally, spotting and BTB diminish after the third cycle of use. BTB that extends beyond the third cycle may be due to patient noncompliance, insufficient estrogen dose (if occurring between days 1 and 9), insufficient progestin dose (if occurring between days 10 and 21), or a drug interaction that is reducing the amount of circulating estrogen/progestin. Newer COCs that employ very low doses of hormones are associated with fewer side effects overall, but may increase the risk for BTB due to endometrial instability.

> **Case Conclusion** JL is experiencing BTB during days 10 to 21 of her cycle, which may be due to progestin deficiency. Her acne also has worsened, which is most likely due to the high androgenicity of LNG. Although she has only completed two cycles of pills, and BTB tends to diminish after three cycles, she can be switched to another pill with more progestational/less androgenic activity.

Thumbnail: Oral Contraception

MOA

COCs decrease ovulation and sperm and egg transport and implantation. The estrogen component alters FSH (follicle stimulating hormone) and LH (leutinizing hormone) release, accelerates egg transport, and alters the endometrium so that it is unsuitable for implantation. Progestins alter FSH and LH release, thicken cervical mucous to reduce sperm and egg transport, inhibit enzymes necessary for fertilization, and also alter the endometrium so that it is unsuitable for implantation.

Common estrogenic side effects

Estrogen excess:

Nausea, vomiting

Fluid retention, weight gain, edema

↑ breast size or tenderness

Skin discoloration (cholasma)

White or yellowish vaginal discharge

Hypertension

Cyclic headache

Heavy flow, hypermenorrhea

Increased risk thrombus, blood clot

Estrogen deficiency:

BTB days 1–9

Vasomotor symptoms

Nervousness, irritability

Decreased libido

Atrophic vaginitis

Common progestational side effects

Progestin excess (also see androgenic effects):

Dysmenorrhea, amenorrhea

Hypertension

Candida vaginitis

Breast tenderness

Androgenic side effects (excess):

↑ LDL, ↓ HDL cholesterol

↑ appetite, weight gain

↑ acne, oily skin, hirsutism, hair loss

↑ tenderness

↑ depression, fatigue

↓ libido

Progestin deficiency:

BTB days 10–21

Amenorrhea

Heavy flow/clots

Questions

1. RM is a 35-year-old woman who severely tore her anterior cruciate ligament (ACL) in a skiing accident and is having major surgery in 2 months, followed by an additional 2 months of bed rest and reduced mobility. She has been taking COC pills for the past 4 years. Which of the following would be good advice for RM?

   A. Initiate aspririn 1 month prior to surgery.
   B. Initiate warfarin 1 month prior to surgery.
   C. Maintain COC use before and after the surgery.
   D. Discontinue COC use 1 month prior to surgery and reinitiate immediately after.
   E. Discontinue COC use 1 month prior to surgery and reinitiate after the patient is able to ambulate.

2. LN would like to initiate a contraceptive for the next 2 years. Her only specification is that she would like to use a contraceptive method that does not delay her fertility once she discontinues its use. A prolonged delay in fertility postdiscontinuation has been observed with which of the following?

   A. COC pills
   B. Depo-Provera® (progestin injectable every 3 months)
   C. Norplant® (progestin subdermal implant)
   D. Minera® (progestin IUD)
   E. Vaginal ring

HPI: ED is a 50-year-old woman who complains of intolerable hot flashes, irritability, and insomnia over the past few months. She also states that sexual intercourse has become less desirable due to vaginal irritation and dryness. She began having irregular menses over a year ago and her last menstrual period was 4 months ago. Her follicle stimulating hormone (FSH) level is 35 pg/mL and her bone mineral density (BMD) T score is −1.8. Her PMH is significant for AF and systemic lupus erythematosus (last flare 13 years ago). Her current medications are warfarin and digoxin. She used chronic low doses of corticosteroids between the ages of 25 to 37.

Thought Questions

- What types of hormone replacement products are available, how are they taken, and what symptoms are they likely to improve?

- What are some of the risks and benefits of short-term (1 to 4 years) versus long-term (5 or more years) hormone replacement therapy (HRT)?

- What factors have likely contributed to ED's low BMD T score?

- What other pharmacotherapeutic options should be considered for ED's osteopenia?

Basic Science Review and Discussion

Hormone replacement therapy restores premenopausal levels of circulating estrogen to reduce symptoms of hot flashes, insomnia, fatigue, irritability, nervousness, depression, vaginal atrophy, vaginal dryness, and poor concentration. In women with an intact uterus, a combination of estrogen and progesterone is necessary to reduce the risk for **endometrial hyperplasia** and endometrial cancer. Estrogen alone can be used in women who have had a hysterectomy. Progesterone alone is generally not used to relieve menopausal symptoms, unless there is an absolute contraindication to estrogen. Similar to oral contraceptives, pill formulations may contain estrogen, progesterone, or a fixed combination of both. Pills taken in a continuous fashion (i.e., every day) minimize the side effect of BTB. Cyclic treatment, daily estrogen with progesterone added during the last 12 to 14 days of the cycle, or continuous use of both for 3 weeks with 1 week off leads to regular withdrawal bleeding. Estrogen/progestin combination pills are only given in a continuous fashion. Both oral and transdermal formulations achieve systemic distribution and are useful in reducing hot flashes, vaginal dryness/atrophy, and osteoporosis. Oral estrogens are likely to improve the lipid profile, while transdermal formulations that bypass first-pass metabolism are less likely to increase HDL and TG and lower LDL. With both oral and transdermal formulations, concomitant use with a progestin is required in women with an intact uterus. Vaginal estrogen rings, creams, and tablets are generally used for vaginal atrophy and dryness only. However, vaginal estrogen is unlikely to improve hot flashes, osteoporosis, or cholesterol profile and does not require the concurrent use of a progestin in women with an intact uterus.

The combination of conjugated equine estrogen (CEE) and medroxyprogesterone acetate (MPA) for short-term administration is generally effective for relieving hot flashes. Because most hot flashes resolve in 1 to 3 years, short-term use may be all that is needed, and can significantly improve quality of life. Short-term use, however, may increase the risk for cardiovascular events due to thrombogenesis and coronary heart disease, and should generally be avoided in women with preexisting cardiovascular disease, prior history of blood clots, or any condition that increases the risk for thrombotic events. With each year of use the risk for breast cancer and gallbladder disease increases. Long-term use decreases the risk for colon cancer and hip fracture. The side effects, contraindications, and drug interactions with HRT are similar to those for oral contraception (see Case 34).

Peak BMD is generally achieved in a woman's mid-thirties and then gradually declines, with 30% of bone loss occurring after menopause in the absence of HRT. A BMD T score of −1 or higher is considered normal. A score of −1 to −2.5 indicates osteopenia, and a score of −2.5 or lower indicates osteoporosis. Therefore, ED has osteopenia. ED's previous chronic use of steroids is likely to have contributed to her reduced BMD. Steroids increase renal calcium excretion and bone resorption by parathyroid hormone. They also decrease bone collagen synthesis.

Reduction of the risk for vertebral and nonvertebral (e.g., hip) fractures may include the use of daily vitamin D and elemental calcium, **selective estrogen receptor modulators** (SERMs), **bisphosphonates,** calcitonin, and parathyroid hormone. Among the SERMs, raloxifene is preferred over tamoxifen for osteoporosis treatment. Raloxifene acts as an estrogen agonist on bone and lipid metabolism and an antagonist on the breast and endometrium. Tamoxifen acts as an agonist on bone, a partial agonist on the endometrium, and an antagonist on the breast. Raloxifene increases the risk for hot flashes and thromboembolic disease. Bisphosphonates (alendronate, risidronate) inhibit bone resorption by inhibiting osteoclast activity. Esophageal irritation and ulceration have been observed more commonly following the use of alendronate, necessitating that patients remain in an upright position for 30 minutes after taking the drug. Nondrug treatments for osteoporosis should include exercise, smoking cessation, and a balanced diet.

Case Conclusion Because ED has a history of AF, and is at increased risk for blood clots, she should avoid oral hormonal formulations. Pill formulations are metabolized by the liver and may increase the production of fibrinogen, C-reactive protein, TG, renin substrate, sex-hormone binding globulin (SHBG), thyroid binding globulin (TBG), cortisol binding globulin (CBG), and biliary cholesterol saturation. ED is a candidate for a transdermal estrogen/progestin or a transdermal estrogen with oral progesterone. Vaginal products could be used to relieve symptoms of vaginal atrophy, but are unlikely to significantly alleviate her hot flashes. She should also be started on a bisphosphonate, which will reduce her future risk for fractures and not increase her risk for thrombosis or worsen her hot flashes.

Thumbnail: Hormone Replacement Therapy

MOA: HRT restores premenopausal levels of circulating estrogen to reduce symptoms of hot flashes, insomnia, fatigue, irritability, nervousness, depression, vaginal atrophy, vaginal dryness, and poor concentration.

See Thumbnail: Oral Contraception (Case 34) for additional information regarding side effects.

Questions

1. MJ is experiencing multiple menopausal symptoms (insomnia, hot flashes, vaginal atrophy). She would like to initiate a hormone replacement product. She has not had a hysterectomy, but does have a history of HTN and hypertriglyceridemia. Which of the following combinations would be a good choice for MJ?

   A. Oral estrogen
   B. Oral estrogen/oral progesterone
   C. Transdermal estrogen/oral progesterone
   D. Transdermal estrogen/vaginal progesterone
   E. Vaginal estrogen/vaginal progesterone

2. The addition of testosterone to an HRT regimen is likely to have which effects?

   A. Reduce BMD
   B. Worsen hot flashes
   C. Worsen psychological symptoms
   D. Worsen sex drive and libido
   E. Worsen lipid profile

HPI: PH, a 28-year-old G1P0 woman presents to labor and delivery at 36 weeks' gestation with elevated blood pressures and proteinuria, and receives a diagnosis of preeclampsia. She has a mild headache, but no right upper quadrant (RUQ) pain or visual symptoms.

PE: On physical examination she has 2+ pitting edema in her lower extremities and her hands are swollen. Lung and abdominal examination yields benign results, and she has brisk 3+ deep tendon reflexes (DTRs), but no clonus. Her fetus has a reassuring fetal heart tracing, and examination shows that her cervix is closed and noneffaced.

Labs: Laboratory tests include a CBC, type and screen, AST, ALT, and Cr. As part of her treatment, the plan is made to induce her labor.

Thought Questions

- What agents are available for labor induction?
- What are the nonpharmacologic ways to induce labor?

Basic Science Review and Discussion

The actual initiation of labor in humans has not been well elucidated. It seemingly involves key input from both the mother and the fetus. Because not all of the aspects of labor are well understood, it is not always successful when induced. Patients undergoing induction can be thought of in two groups: those with a favorable cervix, and those without. The latter group should often undergo cervical ripening. This can be accomplished with prostaglandin agents, most commonly PGE_2 (dinoprostone) in gel or suppository form or PGE_{1M} (misoprostol) in tablet form used orally or vaginally. These prostaglandins can initiate uterine contractions throughout pregnancy, and can be used for pregnancy termination as well. They are also used, in addition to $PGF_{2\alpha}$ and methylergonovine, to treat postpartum hemorrhage. In the setting of an unfavorable cervix, the prostaglandins also affect collagenases in the cervix and enhance breakdown of the collagen matrix of the cervix, leading to softening or ripening of the cervix.

Cervical ripening is also accomplished in nonpharmacologic ways such as slow dilation of the cervix with an intracervical Foley catheter balloon or with laminaria tents. The laminaria are composed of seaweed and, as they absorb the fluid from the vagina and surrounding tissues, slowly expand over time. They are used more commonly in preparing the cervix for abortion than induction of labor. Acupuncture also has been cited in both cervical ripening and labor induction.

Once the cervix has been ripened, or in patients who present with a favorable, soft cervix, labor induction can proceed with IV oxytocin (Pitocin®). This is a synthesized form of the same peptide composed of nine amino acids that is synthesized by the hypothalamus and secreted by the posterior pituitary. Although it will cause contractions beyond the late second trimester of pregnancy, these contractions do not always lead to labor. Labor also can be initiated or augmented by rupture of the amniotic and chorionic membranes, which is thought to up-regulate oxytocin receptors on the uterus and release prostaglandins. Nipple stimulation causes the increased release of oxytocin from the posterior pituitary and can be used to initiate contractions as well.

Case Conclusion PH is begun on magnesium sulfate for seizure prophylaxis in the setting of preeclampsia and given two doses of vaginal misoprostol. After the second dose, she begins to have mild contractions, and upon reexamination her cervix is now 1 cm dilated and 75% effaced. IV oxytocin is begun and 4 hours later she is in active labor. Over the ensuing 6 hours she progresses to fully dilated and delivers a 6-pound boy with the assistance of forceps.

Thumbnail: Uterotonic Agents Used for Induction of Labor

Prototypical agent: Oxytocin, PGE_2

Clinical use: Induction of labor, to curtail bleeding postpartum, primarily responsible for dramatic decrease in maternal death secondary to postpartum hemorrhage.

MOA: Synthetic oxytocin is identical to natural oxytocin and binds to the oxytocin receptor on the uterine myometrium, causing contractions. Prostaglandins are also naturally synthesized by the body and cause uterine contractions.

Pharmacokinetics

Absorption: Oxytocin can be given IV or IM. Prostaglandins are well absorbed orally or transmucosally, so are commonly given per rectum or per vagina.

Adverse reactions: In induction of labor, both of these uterotonic agents can cause too frequent contractions, leading to uterine hypertonus, tetanic contractions, fetal distress, and uterine rupture.

Drug interactions: The only drug interaction is additive uterotonic effects.

Questions

1. PH, the patient in the case above, has a postpartum hemorrhage after her delivery. Which of the following regimens can be used to stop the excessive bleeding?

   A. PGE_{1M}, $PGF_{2\alpha}$, oxytocin, methergine
   B. PGE_2, PGE_{1M}, $PGF_{2\alpha}$, oxytocin, heparin
   C. Heparin, IV estrogen, PGE_{1M}, $PGF_{2\alpha}$, oxytocin
   D. IV estrogen, $PGF_{2\alpha}$, oxytocin, methergine
   E. PGE_2, PGE_{1M}, $PGF_{2\alpha}$, IV estrogen

2. A 34-year-old woman presents for labor induction. Her history is of two prior vaginal deliveries, and examination shows that her cervix is dilated 3 cm and 75% effaced. Which of the following would be the best agent for labor induction?

   A. $PGF_{2\alpha}$
   B. PGE_{1M}
   C. PGE_2
   D. Laminaria tents
   E. Oxytocin

HPI: PC is a 28-year-old G2P1 woman who presents at 29 3/7 weeks' gestation with recurrent contractions every 3 to 4 minutes. She notes no bleeding or leakage of fluid, and her fetus is active. On examination, her cervix is dilated 1 cm and 50% effaced and the fetal heart tracing is reassuring. She is given a dose of SC terbutaline, which initially stops her contractions, but they return 20 minutes later. She is admitted to labor and delivery for further tocolysis. However, the terbutaline made her heart race and gave her nausea and vomiting, and she asks if there is another medication that can be used to stop the contractions.

Thought Questions

- What is terbutaline's MOA?

- What other agents can be used as tocolytics (to stop contractions)?

- What are the indications and contraindications for the different tocolytics?

Basic Science Review and Discussion

The physiology and pharmacology of labor can be confusing. This is a result of both its intricacy as well as the fact that it is difficult to study in humans. Uterine myometrial (smooth muscle cells) contractions can result from stimulation via oxytocin or prostaglandins and is mediated by calcium ion flux and concentrations similar to other smooth muscle. In the setting of preterm labor, the goal is to stop these contractions in order to halt the progress of labor for the sake of the fetus. If one considers the simple approach to labor above, we see how the agents to stop uterine contractions (tocolytics) were derived. These include agents that interfere with the action of oxytocin, prostaglandins, and calcium.

Beta-Agonists The only FDA-approved tocolytic class is the beta-agonists, including IV ritodrine and SC or PO terbutaline. The beta-agonists work by binding to the β_2-receptor whose action is mediated by a G protein and leads both to decreased intracellular calcium concentrations and inhibition of the phosphorylation of myosin light-chain kinase. These two events both lead to muscle fiber relaxation. The first drug studied was IV ritodrine, but the more commonly used medication now is terbutaline. SC terbutaline is commonly used on labor and delivery in the short-term setting to see if contractions can be stopped. It has been used long term given by a pump, but has not been shown to be effective. Similarly, oral forms of terbutaline have been used to diminish contractions, but other than for patient reassurance, these long-term therapies have not been shown to change outcomes or decrease the rate of preterm labor and delivery. Beta-agonists cause tachycardia and flushing, and when used over the long term can cause pulmonary edema.

Calcium Antagonists Two commonly used tocolytics are IV magnesium sulfate and PO calcium channel blockers, classically, nifedipine. As shown in Figure 37-1, calcium is the key ion both in terms of its gradient and intracellular concentration that drives smooth muscle contraction. Thus, by interfering with calcium via calcium channel blockers, smooth muscle relaxation is promoted. Nifedipine, first used as an antihypertensive because it profoundly reduces systemic vascular resistance by relaxing the smooth muscle lining arteriole walls, can be used both in the immediate setting of labor and delivery and long term for patients who continue to contract. Because it can cause sudden drops in blood pressure, headaches are one of the most severe side effects, and patients also experience tachycardia and flushing. Magnesium sulfate ($MgSO_4$), a divalent cation similar to calcium, interferes with calcium's activity both at the membrane receptor level as well as intracellularly. Because magnesium levels need to be kept continuously high and it is excreted so rapidly by the kidneys, it is generally used IV or given via frequent IM injections. Side effects from $MgSO_4$ include flushing, fatigue, nausea, and diplopia. At toxic levels, $MgSO_4$ can cause, with increasing levels, absent reflexes, respiratory depression and failure, and cardiac arrest. One advantage of the worsening symptoms with increasing levels is that toxicity can be screened for by checking DTRs; if they are present, cardiopulmonary arrest should not be seen.

Prostaglandin Inhibitors One of the most important inhibitors of prostaglandins are the NSAIDs. Among these, indomethacin has been used for preterm labor and has been found to be at least as good as the other agents. However, because of studies exhibiting several fetal effects, including intraventricular hemorrhage (IVH), decreased renal function, and early closure of the ductus arteriosus, many practitioners are loathe to use it. Most commonly, indomethacin is used for uterine contraction prophylaxis in the setting of surgery involving the uterus in the second trimester, such as cerclage placement or for fetal surgery.

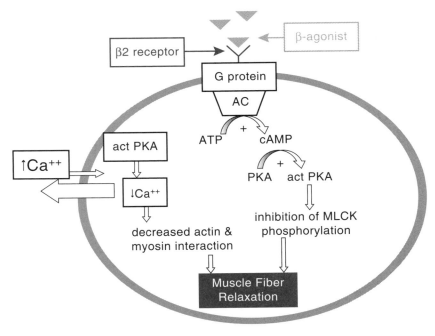

AC   Adenylyl Cyclase   **PKA**   Protein Kinase A
ATP   Adenosine Triphosphate   **act PKA**   activated PKA
cAMP   cyclic adenosine monophosphate   **MLCK**   myosin light chain kinase

CA⁺⁺   Calcium ions

Figure 37-1 Pathways of β-agonist stimulation of $β_2$-receptor leading to muscle fiber relaxation.

Oxytocin Receptor Antagonists   Because labor is mediated by increasing release of oxytocin from the posterior pituitary, it was thought that the oxytocin receptor antagonists (Antociban®) would become the leading tocolytic drugs. This has not been borne out by clinical trials. They seem to work as well as some of the other agents, but certainly not better. This may be a result of the multifactorial etiology of labor, so while oxytocin's activity is being inhibited, labor is being precipitated by other means.

Case Conclusion   Because of her reaction to the terbutaline, PC is placed on IV $MgSO_4$. Her contractions abate and she continues on the medication for the next 48 hours. At that time, the medication is discontinued and she remains acontractile. She is discharged to home, but presents 2 weeks later with stronger contractions. On her second admission, the $MgSO_4$ is unable to stop her labor and she delivers a 32-week infant weighing 1400 g. She is quite concerned about her infant, but he does well in the neonatal intensive care unit and is discharged home on day of life 23.

Thumbnail: Tocolytic Agents

	Agent				
	Beta-agonists: ritodrine (IV, SQ, PO), terbutaline (SQ, PO)	Magnesium sulfate (IV)	Calcium channel blockers (PO)	NSAIDs: indomethacin [PO, per vagina (PV), per rectum (PR)]	Oxytocin receptor antagonists
Clinical indications	Preterm labor, uterine hyperstimulation, prevent contractions from uterine manipulation and surgery in pregnancy	Preterm labor, seizure prophylaxis in pre-eclampsia	Preterm labor, HTN	Preterm labor, prevent contractions from uterine manipulation and surgery in pregnancy	Preterm labor
MOA	β_2-receptor stimulation, decreasing Ca^{2+}, decreasing phosphorylation of myosin light-chain kinase	A divalent cation, it interferes with calcium receptors and channels both on the membrane and intracellular	Block Ca^{2+} transport across the cell membrane	Block the synthesis of prostaglandins	Block the action of oxytocin at the receptor level
Absorption/ distribution	Well absorbed PO, faster when given SC	Well absorbed PO, but usually given IV	Well absorbed PO or sublingually	Well absorbed PO, PV, PR	IV
Adverse reactions	Tachycardia, palpitations, flushing, anxiety, pulmonary edema	Diplopia, fatigue, flushing, pulmonary edema. Toxic levels: absent DTRs, respiratory depression and failure, cardiac arrest	Headaches, tachycardia, flushing	Bleeding Fetal effects: premature closure of ductus arteriosus, decreased renal function; in preterm infants, increased IVH	Minimal
Contraindications	Cardiac disease, any clinical situation where you do not want tachycardia to mask bleeding/hypotension	Myasthenia gravis	Cardiac disease, hypotension	Renal disease, PUD/ gastritis, bleeding diatheses	None known

Questions

1. A 42-year-old G3P2 woman with a history of a three-vessel coronary artery bypass graft (CABG) now presents to labor and delivery at 27 weeks of gestation with frequent contractions in preterm labor. Which of the following lists the medications in likely order of safety, from safest to most dangerous, for her?

   A. Oxytocin antagonist, indomethacin, $MgSO_4$, terbutaline, nifedipine

   B. $MgSO_4$, oxytocin antagonist, indomethacin, terbutaline, nifedipine

   C. $MgSO_4$, oxytocin antagonist, terbutaline, nifedipine, indomethacin

   D. Nifedipine, indomethacin, $MgSO_4$, oxytocin antagonist, terbutaline

   E. Indomethacin, $MgSO_4$, terbutaline, nifedipine, oxytocin antagonist

2. A patient presents for her second admission with preterm contractions and possible preterm labor. She is at 32 weeks of gestation and claims to have been contracting pretty regularly since her last admission. Examination shows that her cervix is dilated 1 cm and 25% effaced. Which of the following preparations is best used long term for this patient?

   A. SQ terbutaline

   B. $MgSO_4$

   C. PO nifedipine

   D. IV ritodrine

   E. PO oxytocin receptor antagonist

HPI: MP is a 28-year-old female graduate student who was admitted to the hospital for extreme abdominal pain accompanied by a temperature of 38.8°C. She reports 5 months of episodic diarrhea with abdominal pain that is relieved upon defecation. Three weeks prior to admission, MP notes that the diarrhea frequency has increased to 10 to 15 episodes per day. She also says that bright red blood appears in her stools.

PE: Sigmoidoscopy revealed edematous, granular, friable mucosa with symmetrical continuous ulceration occurring in the colon. Stool cultures are negative.

Thought Questions

- What distinguishes the two major types of inflammatory bowel disease (IBD)?

- What therapeutic options are available for mild to moderate ulcerative colitis? For severe ulcerative colitis?

- When would you consider different routes of administration of corticosteroids?

- What are some important adverse reactions to corticosteroids?

Basic Science Review and Discussion

Inflammatory bowel disease is divided into two major gastrointestinal disorders: **ulcerative colitis (UC)** and **Crohn's disease.** Both diseases are chronic and tend to be characterized by periods of exacerbations and remissions. Major differences between UC and Crohn's disease are differentiated by anatomic location and distribution. UC occurs in the colon and rectum, whereas Crohn's disease can occur throughout the gastrointestinal tract. UC tends to be continuous, diffuse, and mucosal; Crohn's appears segmental, focal, and transmural. Fissures, strictures, abdominal masses, and pain are commonly associated with Crohn's. Classical symptoms of UC include chronic diarrhea with tenesmus, rectal bleeding, and abdominal pain.

The goals of therapy for ulcerative colitis are to induce remission of the gastrointestinal inflammatory process, to relieve symptoms, and to maintain remission. The two most frequent anti-inflammatory medications used for achieving remission are **corticosteroids** and **sulfasalazine** (an aminosalicylate). Choice of therapy is determined based on severity of disease as well as the anatomic location of inflammation (Table 38-1).

Corticosteroids should only be used during acute exacerbations of ulcerative colitis. The total duration of therapy should not exceed 4 to 8 weeks. Many different corticosteroids are available and differ in anti-inflammatory potency and mineralocorticoid activity (Table 38-2). Choosing a corticosteroid and route of administration depends on the clinical presentation.

Although steroids are effective in achieving remission of ulcerative colitis through their anti-inflammatory properties, they do not change the underlying disease process. In comparison with sulfasalazine or other aminosalicylates, corticosteroids seem to have a faster onset of action and induce remission in 2 to 4 weeks. Parenteral corticosteroids are indicated for severe ulcerative colitis. Once a response is achieved, IV corticosteroids should be converted to oral therapy. However, if there is no response from IV corticosteroids within 72 hours, surgery may be indicated.

Topical corticosteroid use is limited to disease located in the distal colon or rectum. Topical steroids are available for use as suppositories, enemas, or foams. The advantage of using topical steroids in acute mild to moderate disease is that it provides higher doses localized to the affected area. Although it was thought that topical therapy would decrease systemic effects of steroids, extensive anastomoses in the rectal area may lead to significant systemic absorption.

Table 38-1 Treatment based on severity of disease

	Mild to moderate	Severe
Characteristics	< 4 stools/day ± blood in stools No systemic symptoms Normal ESR	> 6 stools/day with blood in stools Toxicity present (fever, tachycardia, anemia) Elevated ESR
Distal colitis therapy	Aminosalicylate (PO/PR) Corticosteroid (PR)	Corticosteroid (PO/PR)
Extensive colitis therapy	Aminosalicylate (PO)	Corticosteroid (PO/IV)

Table 38-2 Corticosteroids

Drug	Route	Equivalent anti-inflammatory dose (mg)	Anti-inflammatory potency	Mineralocorticoid activity
Hydrocortisone	IV, PR	20	1	1
Prednisolone	PO, IV	5	4	0.8
Prednisone	PO	5	4	0.8
Methylprednisolone	PO, IV	4	5	0
Dexamethasone	PO, IV	0.75	30	0
Fludrocortisone	PO	—	10	125

The most common side effects of systemic corticosteroids include behavior disturbances, insomnia, weight gain, and **Cushing's syndrome** (moon face, buffalo hump, hirsutism, obesity, and easy bruising). Other reactions related to the dose and duration of corticosteroid treatment include hyperglycemia, fluid retention, HTN, electrolyte imbalances, osteoporosis, activation of herpes and tuberculosis, and peptic ulcers.

Once remission is achieved, aminosalicylates (such as mesalamine or sulfasalazine) are primarily used to maintain remission.

Case Conclusion   This is MP's initial diagnosis of IBD. She presents with severe symptoms of UC and is therefore started on high doses of IV methylprednisolone to induce remission. After 2 days, MP's stool frequency and pain are decreased. IV methylprednisolone is then converted to oral prednisone. When remission is attained, MP will start a steroid taper and begin mesalamine for maintenance.

Thumbnail: Corticosteroids

Prototypical agent: Prednisone

Clinical use: To induce remission of moderate to severe IBD. Once clinical remission is induced, steroids must be tapered. Other uses: acute asthma exacerbations, arthritis, collagen diseases, immunosuppression for organ transplantation.

MOA: Inhibits release of inflammatory cytokines, interleukin-1 (IL-1), IL-2; reduces adherence and chemotaxis of inflammatory mediators.

Pharmacokinetics

Absorption: Good bioavailability (77% to 99%).

Metabolism: Prednisone is converted to prednisolone (active form) in the liver.

Elimination: Excreted unchanged in the urine.

Adverse reactions: Insomnia, behavioral disturbances, depression, increased appetite, fluid retention, HTN, acne, hyperglycemia, adrenal insufficiency, hirsutism, moon face, osteoporosis.

Questions

1. A patient with a history of UC is experiencing a "flare-up." She has been having six to seven episodes of diarrhea per day and has a loss of appetite. She is currently taking mesalamine for maintenance and loperamide to help minimize bouts of diarrhea. Her labs are significant for an elevated serum sodium of 147 mEq/L and low serum potassium of 3.1 mEq/L. Which corticosteroid would be the most appropriate to start for induction of remission?

   A. Fludrocortisone
   B. Methylprednisolone
   C. Prednisone
   D. Hydrocortisone
   E. Prednisolone

2. JR is a 35-year-old man with an acute exacerbation of his UC, having three stools per day. His disease is limited to the rectum and distal colon. On last admission, he received IV methylprednisolone that made him "crazy." In addition, he experienced weeks of insomnia with his oral steroid taper. Which corticosteroid is the most appropriate for his current situation?

   A. Fludrocortisone
   B. Methylprednisolone
   C. Prednisone
   D. Hydrocortisone
   E. Dexamethasone

HPI: KM is a 57-year-old man who presents with severe pain in his right great toe. He states that the pain was first noticeable 2 days ago. This was several days after he stubbed his toe on the leg of the dining room table. He awoke at 3 A.M. with excruciating pain. His toe is swollen, red, and tender to the touch. He states that the pain is constant and does not go away. This is KM's second attack, the first attack occurring 7 months ago, which was successfully treated. The fluid aspirated from the joint is positive for urate crystals. PMH: HTN, asthma, family history of gout. Medications: Hydrochlorothiazide, beclomethasone inhaler, albuterol inhaler.

PE: Vitals: T 37°C, BP 130/85 mm Hg, HR 90 beats/min, RR 21 breaths/min.

Labs: Serum uric acid 11 mg/dL. All other labs within normal limits.

Thought Questions

- Which NSAID would be a reasonable choice to treat this acute gout attack?

- What is the role of colchicine in the treatment of an acute gout attack?

- What is the role of corticosteroids in the management of gout attacks?

- Which uric acid lowering agent would be reasonable choice for this patient and how would you make that decision?

- What is the impact of hydrochlorothiazide in patients with gout attacks?

Basic Science Review and Discussion

Uric acid, an end product of protein catabolism, was identified as the cause of gout in the middle of the 19th century. Patients with primary **hyperuricemia** have elevated serum uric acid levels because of increased production of uric acid or impaired renal excretion of uric acid.

Overproduction of uric acid can occur due to excessive de novo purine synthesis, excessive dietary purines, or the conversion of tissue nucleic acid to purine nucleotides. When these purines are metabolized, the by-products are converted to uric acid by the enzyme **xanthine oxidase**. Increased levels of uric acid result if the overproduction exceeds excretion. Underexcretion of uric acid can be due to defects in the renal tubular mechanisms that regulate uric acid levels in the body, causing decreased filtration, decreased secretion, or increased reabsorption.

Acute attacks of gout are a result of urate crystal deposits in the synovium of joints. Crystal formation is dependent on a constellation of factors, including the degree of hyperuricemia, physical state of the joint, and presence of synovial fluid. Urate crystals present in the joint space can trigger an acute inflammatory response. **Prostaglandins** play a key role in this inflammatory response, causing vasodilation, increased vascular permeability, and the release of chemotactic substances that attract **polymorphonuclear (PMN) leukocytes**.

Acute gout attacks usually occur between the fourth and sixth decades of life, occurring more often in men than in women. These attacks can occur in younger patients, but it is important to evaluate other possible etiologies of elevated uric acid levels, such as some renal impairment or medications.

One acute gouty attack or isolated hyperuricemia does not make a definitive diagnosis of gout. The gold standard for the diagnosis of gout is the aspiration of joint fluid that is positive for urate crystals. The American College of Rheumatology has set forth criteria for the epidemiologic diagnosis of gout. When aspiration of the joint is not possible, a patient must have 6 of the 11 following criteria to meet the definition of gout: more than one attack of arthritis, exquisite pain involving a joint, joint inflammation maximal within 1 day, oligoarthritis, erythema over involved joints, podagra (first metatarsophalangeal joint), unilateral podagra, tophi, hyperuricemia, asymmetric swelling within a joint on radiologic examination, and complete termination of acute attack.

Elevated levels of uric acid should be treated to decrease the body stores of urate in an attempt to prevent the deposition of urate in joints, thus precipitating an acute gout attack.

The current drug options for treating acute gout attacks include NSAIDs, colchicine, and corticosteroids.

Nonsteroidal Anti-Inflammatory Drugs NSAIDs have now become the drugs of choice over colchicine because of the severe gastrointestinal side effects associated with colchicine and its lack of efficacy to resolve the gouty pain unless used within 24 hours after the occurrence of the initial attack. NSAIDs such as indomethacin, naproxen, and ibuprofen are effective because they have a short T½, a rapid onset of action, and are better tolerated by patients.

Colchicine Colchicine would be a reasonable choice for patients with contraindications or who are intolerant to NSAIDs. The gastrointestinal side effects of colchicine (including severe diarrhea) may make it difficult for patients who are having difficulty accessing the bathroom quickly.

Corticosteroids Corticosteroids are an option for patients who are intolerant to NSAIDs and colchicine. Side effects associated with this regimen may include glucose intolerance, HTN, electrolyte shifts, and increased risk of infection. These regimens are tapered rapidly after 7 to 10 days, but a symptom flare can occur after tapering the therapy.

Prophylaxis Prophylactic treatment of patients with uric acid-lowering agents such as allopurinol or probenecid should not be started until the acute attack resolves. This is because these agents cause mobilization of urate crystals and may prolong the acute attack. Patients may need long-term therapy with these agents to prevent acute gout attacks.

Agents used to treat acute gout attacks as well as to prevent recurrent attacks should be used with caution in patients with **hypertension** and **renal impairment**. Doses may need to be adjusted in patients with decreased renal function. Probenecid is usually recommended for patients who are under 60 years of age, who have normal renal function, are diagnosed as an underexcreter, and have no history of kidney stones. Probenecid causes a marked increase of uric acid in the urine, and decreased renal elimination places the patient at risk for stone formation. Allopurinol is a good choice for patients with uric acid stones or renal insufficiency, as well as for those who are known to be overproducers of uric acid.

Hydrochlorothiazide and loop diuretics may decrease the clearance of uric acid and should be avoided in patients with a history of gout.

Case Conclusion In addition to having urate crystals present in the joint fluid aspirate, KM has met several criteria to support the diagnosis of gout. This acute gout attack is treated with high-dose ibuprofen, which is tapered over 7 days. Once the attack is resolved, maintenance therapy with allopurinol is initiated to lower uric acid levels and prevent future acute gout attacks.

Questions

1. A 55-year-old man presents with complaints of an acute gouty arthritis attack. His left big toe is red, swollen, and tender to the touch. This is his first attack. He has no history of peptic ulcer disease. His uric acid level is 8 mg/dL. Which of the following agents would you recommend for treatment?

   A. Prednisone
   B. Colchicine
   C. Allopurinol
   D. Indomethacin
   E. Probenecid

2. A 65-year-old woman has had several acute gout attacks and now needs to be placed on prophylactic therapy. She has a CrCl rate of 45 mL/min and a uric acid level of 12 mg/dL. The patient refuses to undergo a joint fluid aspiration procedure, but she has 6 of the 11 criteria for epidemiologic diagnosis for gout. Which agent is the best choice for this patient?

   A. Probenecid
   B. Colchicine
   C. Allopurinol
   D. Ibuprofen
   E. Indomethacin

Thumbnail: Agents Used to Treat/Prevent Acute Gout

	NSAIDs	Colchicine	Corticosteroids	Urocosuric agents	Xanthine oxidase inhibitors
Prototype agents	Indomethacin Ibuprofen Naproxen	Colchicine	Prednisone	Probenecid	Allopurinol
Clinical uses	Anti-inflammatory, analgesic, antipyretic	Anti-inflammatory for acute gout attack	Anti-inflammatory for acute gout attack	Prevent acute gouty arthritis; hyperuricemia	Prevent acute gouty arthritis; hyper-uricemia
MOA	Inhibit prostaglandin synthesis by decreasing activity of cyclo-oxygenase	Decreases the deposition of urate crystals in joints by decreasing leukocyte motility	Decreases the motility of PMN leukocytes	Competitive inhibition of uric acid reabsorption at the proximal tubule	Inhibits xanthine oxidase, thus preventing uric acid production
Pharmacokinetics					
Absorption/ distribution	Well absorbed orally; mostly protein bound; crosses the placenta; appears in breast milk	Rapid oral absorption concentrates in leukocytes, kidney, liver, and spleen	Well absorbed orally and highly protein bound	Rapid and complete oral absorption; highly protein bound	Well absorbed orally; distributes into breast milk
Metabolism/ elimination	Hepatically metabolized	Partial metabolism in liver; primary excretion in feces	Metabolism primarily in liver and excreted as inactive metabolites in urine	Metabolized by liver; metabolites excreted in urine	Metabolized in liver to active metabolites (mainly oxypurinol) which is eliminated in urine
Adverse reactions	Nausea, abdominal pain, GI bleeding, ulcers, heartburn, rash, dizziness	Nausea, vomiting, severe diarrhea, abdominal pain	Short-term use: insomnia, nervousness, GI upset, increased appetite	Headache, nausea, vomiting, anorexia	Most common is skin rash
Drug interactions	May decrease anti-hypertensive effects of ACE inhibitors, angiotensin II antagonists. May decrease anti-hypertensive and diuretic effects of thiazide and loop diuretics	May decrease absorption of vitamin B_{12}	Effects decreased by barbiturates, phenytoin, and rifampin; decreases effect of salicylates and vaccines	Decreases clearance of beta-lactams	Risk for hypersensitivity increased in patients who are on thiazides or ACE inhibitors and allopurinol
Warning/ precautions or contraindications	Patients should take medication with food, milk, or antacids. Avoid in patients with active GI bleed or ulcer disease.	Use with caution in elderly patients and patients with severe GI, renal, or liver disease.	Patients should take medication with food or milk to prevent GI upset.	Can precipitate an acute gout attack; should avoid use in patients with CrCl of < 50 mL/min.	Severe skin rashes such as Stevens-Johnson syndrome have been reported.

> **HPI:** KC is a 200-pound 65-year-old woman who has been complaining of pain in her left knee for the past 9 months. Now she is experiencing deep aching pain. Her knee is stiff in the morning, which resolves in about 30 minutes. After periods of inactivity during the day she experiences stiffness in her knee. She states that the pain in her left knee is noticeably worse when she walks. PMH: Obesity and a family history of osteoarthritis.

Thought Questions

- What are the risk factors for **osteoarthritis (OA)**?

- What are the nonpharmacologic options for the treatment of OA?

- What are the pharmacologic options for the treatment of OA?

- What are the toxicities associated with NSAIDs?

Basic Science Review and Discussion

Osteoarthritis is the most common form of arthritis in the United States. This disease affects men and women equally, but symptoms occur earlier and are more severe in women. Risk factors associated with the development of OA include age greater than 50 years, obesity (weight-bearing joints), injury to joints, joint overuse due to prolonged occupational or sports stress, and family history.

There are cellular, mechanical, and biochemical processes that continually remodel and repair healthy joint cartilage. When these processes are altered, as in OA, the disruption leads to degenerative changes of the joint and abnormal repair responses. Inflammation may be present in OA but it is usually mild. Unlike **rheumatoid arthritis,** OA only involves the joints.

Improved function and quality of life are the primary goals of treatment. Nonpharmacologic therapy options for patients with OA are the mainstay of treatment. These measures, in addition to the pharmacologic options, are needed to provide patients with sufficient symptom relief and adequate function. The nonpharmacologic measures include patient education, exercise programs, weight loss if overweight, assistive devices if needed, and support group programs.

Pharmacologic options include **acetaminophen** and **NSAIDs.** Acetaminophen has long been considered the drug of first choice in patients with OA. It provides effective pain relief for a number of patients and is safe to use in a wide range of patients. For patients in whom acetaminophen is not providing adequate pain control, an NSAID should be used. There are many NSAIDs that can be used, and the choice should be based on dosing regimen, cost, tolerance, comorbid diseases, concurrent medications, and patient preferences. The treatment of OA with **COX-2 inhibitors** is still being explored. These agents can be considered as an alternative for patients at risk for adverse GI effects from NSAIDs.

> **Case Conclusion** Treatment plans for patients with OA must be individualized to address the degree of pain and functionality of the patient. Because this patient is elderly, a trial of acetaminophen would be reasonable since it is considered the first-line agent owing to its efficacy, safety profile, and cost. The patient also should be informed of the nonpharmacologic therapy choices, such as a weight loss program and exercise program.

Thumbnail: Agents Used for Osteoarthritis

Drug class	Acetaminophen	NSAIDs	COX-2 inhibitors
Prototypical agent(s)		Indomethacin Ibuprofen Naproxen	Celecoxib Rofecoxib
Clinical uses	Anti-inflammatory; analgesic, antipyretic	Anti-inflammatory; analgesic, antipyretic	Anti-inflammatory; analgesic
MOA	Analgesic	Inhibit prostaglandin synthesis by decreasing activity of cyclo-oxygenase	Decrease prostaglandin synthesis by decreasing activity of cyclooxygenase-2
Pharmacokinetics			
Absorption/ distribution	Well absorbed orally	Well absorbed orally; mostly protein bound; crosses the placenta; appears in breast milk	Good oral absorption; highly protein bound
Metabolism/ elimination	Hepatically metabolized	Hepatically metabolized	Hepatically metabolized
Adverse reactions	Nausea, abdominal pain; liver toxicity with overdosage	Nausea, abdominal pain, GI bleeding, ulcers, heartburn, rash, dizziness, kidney damage	Headache, dyspepsia, diarrhea, abdominal pain, nausea, upper respiratory tract infection
Drug interactions		May decrease antihypertensive effects of ACE inhibitors and angiotensin II antagonists; decrease of antihypertensive and diuretic effects of thiazides and loop diuretics	Agents are CYP2C9 substrates; may decrease effects of ACE inhibitors, thiazides, and loop diuretics; fluconazole increases levels of celecoxib; may increase INR when added to warfarin
Warning/ precautions or contraindications	Avoid excessive concurrent use of alcohol.	Patients should take medication with food, milk, or antacids. Avoid in patients with active GI bleed or ulcer disease. Use with caution in elderly patients. Patients allergic to aspirin may experience cross-reactivity.	Patients should take medication with food, milk, or antacids. Avoid in patients with active GI bleed or ulcer disease. Use with caution in elderly patients. Avoid in patients with severe sulfa allergy.

Questions

1. A 45-year-old man has been diagnosed with OA in his right knee. He has retired from his career as a professional soccer player due to frequent injuries. He has taken maximum doses of acetaminophen with no relief. What agent would be best for this patient?

   A. Aspirin
   B. Celecoxib
   C. Rofecoxib
   D. Indomethacin
   E. Naproxen

2. A 70-year-old woman has left knee and hip pain for over a year. You give the diagnosis of OA and want to begin treatment. She has mild renal insufficiency and a history of GI bleeding. Which agent is the best choice for this patient?

   A. Acetaminophen
   B. Celecoxib
   C. Aspirin
   D. Ibuprofen
   E. Indomethacin

> **HPI:** SM is a 35-year-old woman with a diagnosis of rheumatoid arthritis (RA). She suffers from morning stiffness, fatigue, and generalized muscle and joint pain. She has had to limit her physical activity and is unable to wear her rings because of finger swelling. Her current treatment plan includes education and physical therapy.

Thought Questions

- What are the primary goals of treatment for RA?

- What are the pharmacological options for the treatment of RA?

- What are the pharmacological differences between NSAIDs and disease-modifying antirheumatic drugs (DMARDs)?

- What are the toxicities associated with NSAIDs and DMARDs?

Basic Science Review and Discussion

Rheumatoid arthritis is a chronic, inflammatory, **autoimmune** disease of unknown etiology that if left untreated results in progressive joint destruction, deformity, disability, and premature death. Theories of possible etiologies include genetic, hormonal, viral, autoimmune, and environmental factors. The disease peaks between the fourth through sixth decades of life and is two to three times more common in women than in men. Differences in prevalence rates between ethnic groups are small.

The pathogenesis of RA is a combination of cellular (e.g., macrophages, lymphocytes), biochemical (e.g., prostaglandins, cytotoxins) and mechanical factors that promote the inflammatory condition of the synovial lining. The normal anatomy of joints is altered in RA by immunologically mediated changes in bone, cartilage, supporting tissues, and synovial tissue and fluid.

The primary goals of therapy are to improve or maintain the patient's ability to function and carry out daily living activities, minimize symptoms, and diminish the progression of joint disease. Patient education, rest, exercise, proper diet, and **NSAIDs** are the foundation of RA therapy. NSAIDs are used to reduce joint swelling and pain. Onset effect is within a few days to a week, with peak effects in 1 to 4 weeks. The analgesic and anti-inflammatory effects of these agents do not alter the course of the disease. All NSAIDs are equally efficacious. Factors to be considered when choosing an anti-inflammatory agent are ease of dosing administration, tolerance, cost, patient's age, presence of comorbid diseases, concurrent drugs, and patient preferences.

Disease-modifying antirheumatic drugs are second-line therapy when despite maximum doses of NSAIDs, a patient has ongoing **joint pain,** significant morning stiffness or fatigue, active synovitis, or persistent elevation of the erythrocyte sedimentation rate (ESR) or C-reactive protein (CRP) level. DMARDs have the potential to reduce or prevent joint damage and preserve joint integrity and function. The exact mechanism of action of how this group of drugs works is not known. The drugs in this class are relatively slow acting, with a delay of 1 to 6 months before a clinical response is evident. It is recommended to consider a **rheumatology** consultation when deciding which agent to use.

Case Conclusion There is no known cure for RA or means of preventing it. SM should be started on a course of NSAIDs in addition to her nonpharmacologic interventions. SM should be assessed on a routine basis for disease progression, drug toxicity, and quality of life. If an adequate response is not achieved with NSAIDs alone, DMARDs should be considered with a consultation from a rheumatologist.

Thumbnail: Agents Used for Rheumatoid Arthritis

	Drug class	
	NSAIDs	**DMARDs**
Prototypical agents	Indomethacin Piroxicam Ibuprofen Ketoprofen Naproxen Aspirin	Hydroxychloroquine (HCQ) Methotrexate (MTX) Azathioprine (AZA) Sulfasalazine (SSZ)
Clinical uses	Anti-inflammatory; analgesic, antipyretic	Second-line agents for RA; other clinical uses vary by specific agent
MOA	Inhibit prostaglandin synthesis by decreasing activity of cyclooxygenase.	Exact mechanisms are unknown. All agents interfere with cellular metabolism; possess immunosuppressive properties.
Pharmacokinetics		
Absorption/ distribution	Well absorbed orally; mostly protein bound; cross the placenta; appear in breast milk	Oral absorption complete for HCQ, MTX, AZA SSZ: 10%–15% absorbed MTX and AZA cross placenta
Metabolism/ elimination	Hepatically metabolized	Metabolized in liver; elimination primarily in the urine
Adverse reactions	Nausea, abdominal pain, GI bleeding, ulcers, heartburn, rash, dizziness, kidney damage	All DMARDs can cause nausea, vomiting, diarrhea, leukopenia, thrombocytopenia, liver toxicity, renal toxicity, rash; MTX can cause stomatitis and alopecia
Drug interactions	May decrease antihypertensive effects of ACE inhibitors and angiotensin II antagonists; decrease of antihypertensive and diuretic effects of hydrochlorothiazide and furosemide; concomitant use with other NSAIDs may increase GI adverse effects.	HCQ: cimetidine increases serum levels; absorption decreased when taken with kaolin and magnesium trisilicate MTX: decreases effect of phenytoin; concomitant use with other hepatotoxic drugs can increase risk of hepatotoxicity. NSAIDs can increase half-life and prolong excretion of MTX; however, low doses of MTX with NSAIDs for RA are allowed with close monitoring. AZA: serum levels increased by allopurinol. SSZ: decreases effects of iron, digoxin, folic acid; increases effects of oral anticoagulants, MTX, and oral sulfonylureas.
Warning/ precautions or contraindications	Take medication with food, milk, or antacids. Avoid in patients with active GI bleed or ulcer disease. Use with caution in elderly patients.	Use with caution in patients with renal or liver disease. Avoid SSZ in patients with **G-6-PD deficiency.** Monitor hematologic function closely.

Questions

1. Which agent is most appropriate for a 38-year-old woman with a diagnosis of RA? This is in addition to other nonpharmacologic interventions.

   A. Aspirin
   B. Celecoxib
   C. Rofecoxib
   D. Sulfasalazine
   E. Naproxen

2. A 50-year-old woman has not had an adequate response to NSAIDs. In consultation with a rheumatologist, it is decided to initiate a DMARD agent. The patient has an allergy to "sulfa" drugs. Which agent is the best choice for this patient?

   A. Ibuprofen
   B. Sulfasalazine
   C. Hydroxychloroquine
   D. Injectable gold
   E. Methotrexate

> **HPI:** OF is a 42-year-old white man who presents to the acute care clinic with severe mid-epigastric pain. OF has been working long hours and is under a great deal of stress at work. OF drinks one to two beers per night, and has smoked one pack of cigarettes per day for the past 10 years. He has lost 10 pounds in the past 2 months.
>
> **PE:** Endoscopy reveals a 4-cm gastric ulcer (antral), which tests positive for *Helicobacter pylori*.

Thought Questions

- What are the risk factors for gastroduodenal ulcers?

- What treatment options are available for gastric ulcers?

- What are the pharmacologic differences between each treatment approach?

- What side effects are associated with the use of *H. pylori* treatment regimens?

Basic Science Review and Discussion

Dyspepsia is a chronic or recurrent discomfort/pain in the upper abdomen. The causes for dyspepsia involve gastroduodenal ulcer, atypical gastroesophageal reflux, and gastric cancer. Classic symptoms related to gastroduodenal ulcers, such as postprandial epigastric pain or pain relieved by eating, are common. More importantly, dyspepsia may be associated with certain alarm features such as recurrent vomiting, weight loss, dysphagia, bleeding, or anemia.

Helicobacter pylori is a gram-negative spiral bacterium that has been implicated in the pathogenesis of gastroduodenal ulcers. *H. pylori* has been found in nearly 90% of patients with duodenal ulcers and nearly 70% of patients with gastric ulcers. Eradication of *H. pylori* has been shown to decrease the recurrence rate and accelerate the ulcer healing process.

In cases of *H. pylori*-positive dyspepsia, treatment is aimed at eradicating bacteria as well as alleviating symptoms. In cases of *H. pylori*-negative dyspepsia, empiric antisecretory drugs or prokinetic agents are often initiated. If treatment with these agents fails, the patient should be referred for endoscopy to rule out chronic ulceration or other causes.

Patients with documented *H. pylori* cultures and active ulceration should be treated with **antisecretory agents** and combination antibiotics. Treatment regimens are individualized and may include one, two, or three of the following antimicrobials: amoxicillin, clarithromycin, metronidazole, tetracycline, and bismuth subsalicylate. Treatment regimens for *H. pylori* can be taken together at the same time, without regard to meals or drug interactions among the regimens. This is because systemic blood levels are not necessary; rather, the goal of therapy is local gastrointestinal antimicrobial activity.

Case Conclusion OF began combination antisecretory and antimicrobial therapy for his *H. pylori*-positive gastric ulcer. He has completed a 2-week course of therapy with a four-drug regimen without side effects or other complications. He reports no gastric pain or other symptoms associated with gastric ulcers. OF has also begun a smoking cessation program because smoking has been shown to decrease ulcer healing.

Thumbnail: H₂-Receptor Antagonists

Available agents: Cimetidine, ranitidine, nizatidine, famotidine.

Clinical use: Treatment of dyspepsia, gastroduodenal ulcers, gastroesophageal reflux disease (GERD), and Zollinger-Ellison syndrome.

MOA: Competitively and selectively inhibit the action of histamine on H_2 receptors of the parietal cells.

Pharmacokinetics: All oral H_2-receptor antagonists are rapidly absorbed within 1 to 3 hours. Oral bioavailability is lower for ranitidine, cimetidine, and famotidine than for nizatidine. This is because ranitidine, cimetidine, and famotidine are incompletely absorbed and undergo first-pass hepatic metabolism. All of the H_2-receptor antagonists are eliminated via renal filtration and secretion. For this reason, the H_2-receptor antagonist T½ may be increased in patients with renal dysfunction.

Adverse reactions: All H_2-receptor antagonists are generally well tolerated with few adverse effects. The most common H_2-receptor antagonist adverse effects include confusion, dizziness, headache, constipation, and diarrhea. Rarely, reversible thrombocytopenia has been reported with the H_2-receptor antagonist class. High doses of cimetidine for prolonged periods may lead to dose-dependent elevation in serum prolactin activity and possible alterations in estrogen metabolism. These changes have led to reversible gynecomastia and breast tenderness in males. Famotidine and ranitidine have been associated with headache and CNS changes, specifically in patients with decreased renal function.

Drug interactions: Cimetidine is a CYP450 inhibitor and can inhibit the metabolism of phenytoin, warfarin, and theophylline. Famotidine, nizatidine, and ranitidine are unlikely to cause clinically significant drug interactions. All H_2 antagonists have the potential to interact with other drugs that require gastric acid for absorption (e.g., ketoconazole, itraconazole).

Questions

1. CT is a 47-year-old man who is about to be started on combination therapy for his *H. pylori*-positive ulcer with antibiotics and either a proton pump inhibitor or an H_2-receptor antagonist. Although proton pump inhibitors and H_2-receptor antagonists are well tolerated, which of the following drug side effect combinations is most likely to occur during therapy?

   A. Famotidine/headache
   B. Omeprazole/insomnia
   C. Lansoprazole/rash
   D. Cimetidine/seizure

2. CT is started on omeprazole plus two antimicrobial agents. Which of the following antimicrobial agents has activity against *H. pylori*?

   A. Doxycycline
   B. Ampicillin
   C. Tetracycline
   D. Miconazole

HPI: ST is a 60-year-old man who presents to the clinic with increasing daytime heartburn, episodes of postprandial heartburn, and regurgitation. ST has been using over-the-counter H_2-receptor antagonists and antacids with no relief. He reports a bitter taste in his mouth and mild chest pain. ST recently sustained a compound fracture of his left knee from a motor vehicle accident. He has been immobile for 2 months and has been working long hours on his computer from home. ST drinks occasional alcohol on the weekends, and smokes half a pack of cigarettes per week. He has gained 15 pounds in the past 2 months.

Thought Questions

- What are the risk factors for gastroesophageal reflux disease (GERD)?

- What treatment options are available for GERD?

- What side effects are associated with the use of GERD treatment regimens?

Basic Science Review and Discussion

Gastroesophageal reflux disease results from an imbalance between aggressive factors (acid and pepsin) and defensive factors (antireflux barriers, esophageal clearance, and mucosal resistance). Specifically, GERD causes the reflux of acidic gastric contents into the esophagus. The hallmark symptoms of GERD involve esophagitis and can lead to esophageal complications (esophageal stricture, hemorrhage, Barrett's esophagus, and, rarely, esophageal cancer). Unfortunately the frequency or severity of GERD is not predictive of esophageal damage.

The **lower esophageal sphincter** (LES) is the major barrier to reflux. Spontaneous and transient relaxation of the LES can occur in healthy adults. Patients with GERD experience more frequent relaxation of the LES, resulting in GERD symptoms. Other protective mechanisms, including gravity, saliva, and peristalsis, help to reduce the contact time of gastric acid with the esophagus. These mechanisms, however, may not be active in patients who are supine or lying down.

Treatment of GERD is aimed at relieving symptoms, promoting healing, preventing recurrence, and reducing complications. The most important treatment approach is to incorporate diet and lifestyle changes. The staged approach to GERD facilitates treatment; however, an individualized approach to therapy is preferred. Stage I GERD consists of intermittent heartburn, which typically resolves with lifestyle modification, antacids, and over-the-counter H_2-receptor antagonists. Stage I GERD is classified as mild or infrequent heartburn occurring less than two to three times per week. Stage II GERD involves frequent or consistent episodes of heartburn unrelieved by antacids or H_2-receptor antagonists. This stage of disease requires proton pump inhibitors (PPIs); if no response is observed, the use of promotility agents may be considered. Stage III GERD commonly involves warning symptoms or erosive GERD (cough, dysphagia, odynophagia, weight loss, laryngitis, hematemesis, anemia). Patients with these symptoms should undergo upper endoscopy to identify morphologic or histologic changes in the esophagus (ulceration, erosive esophagitis, cancer, Barrett's esophagus). These patients will typically require long-term therapy with PPIs.

PPIs are considered the drugs of choice for patients with stage II or III GERD. PPIs accelerate esophageal healing and are effective in relieving symptoms. In some patients with chronic symptoms, long-term maintenance therapy with PPIs (3 to 6 months) can help control symptoms and prevent complications. Patients with severe symptoms or atypical GERD (stage III) will require high-dose PPIs along with promotility agents. Promotility agents facilitate gastric emptying by increasing LES pressure and therefore decrease the chance of regurgitation.

Case Conclusion ST was started on a PPI for the treatment of his stage II moderate to severe GERD symptoms. He will need treatment for at least 4 to 8 weeks. ST's recent immobility has led to his weight gain and possibly his worsening symptoms. ST was also counseled on nondrug therapies to help relieve his GERD symptoms.

Thumbnail: Agents for Gastroesophageal Reflux Disease

	PPIs	Prokinetic agents
Available agents	Omeprazole Lansoprazole Pantoprazole Rabeprazole Esomeprazole	Metoclopramide Cisapride
Clinical use	Short-term treatment of gastroduodenal disorders, GERD, and for pathologic secretory conditions such as Zollinger-Ellison syndrome. The PPIs are superior to H_2-receptor antagonists in patients with stage III erosive GERD.	Used in patients with severe symptoms or in those with atypical GERD symptoms. Typically reserved for patients who fail high-dose PPIs. Desired most in patients who also report nausea, constipation, or other related symptoms.
MOA	PPIs are substituted benzimidazoles that irreversibly inhibit gastric parietal cell release of acid. PPIs are prodrugs that must be activated in the acidic environment of the secretory canaliculus located in the parietal cell. PPIs inhibit the H^+/K^+ ATPase pump and can inhibit nearly 100% of the gastric acid secretion.	Promotility agents increase LES tone and accelerate gastric emptying.
Pharmacokinetics	All oral PPIs are rapidly absorbed and undergo hepatic metabolism. The bioavailability of the oral PPIs ranges from 30% to 85%. All of the PPIs have a short elimination $T\frac{1}{2}$ (< 2 hr), but this has minimal effect on the duration of antisecretory action due to irreversible binding to the proton pump.	Both cisapride and metoclopramide have a rapid onset of action, < 1 hr. Both agents have a similar oral bioavailability: 50%–80% and are extensively metabolized by the liver to inactive metabolites.
Adverse reactions	PPIs are very well tolerated. Rarely, headache, diarrhea, constipation, nausea, and pruritus have been observed.	Metoclopramide is associated with CNS side effects, especially in the elderly or in those with decreased renal function. Metoclopramide also leads to drowsiness, diarrhea, abdominal cramps, and **extrapyramidal reactions.** Cisapride, at high doses, is associated with QT segment prolongation. When used at the recommended doses in patients with normal renal and hepatic function, cardiac effects are rare.
Drug interactions	The PPIs differ in their ability to inhibit CYP450. Omeprazole may inhibit the metabolism of diazepam, phenytoin, and warfarin. All PPIs have the potential to interact with other drugs that require gastric acid for absorption (e.g., ketoconazole, itraconazole).	Fatal cardiac arrhythmias have been reported when cisapride was combined with drugs that are metabolized by the CYP450 system. Most of the interactions involved antifungal and antimicrobial agents. For this reason, cisapride is available on a limited access basis in the United States.
Comments	PPIs are most effective when taken 30 min before a meal. PPIs should not be taken with H_2-receptor antagonists since this puts the parietal cell in a resting state. Because consistent gastric acid suppression is desired for healing, the PPIs should not be used for GERD on an as-needed basis.	Cisapride is effective in providing both symptomatic relief and in promoting healing.

Questions

1. SL is a 56-year-old man who was recently diagnosed with stage II GERD. In addition to lifestyle modification, SL is started on a PPI. SL should be counseled to take his PPI:

   A. 30 minutes before breakfast
   B. Together with an H_2 antagonist
   C. With food to decrease stomach upset
   D. On an as-needed basis
   E. All of the above

2. MJ is a 45-year-old man diagnosed with stage III GERD by endoscopy. He is started on a PPI and a promotility agent, cisapride. Cisapride can cause which of the following side effects?

   A. Dry cough
   B. Excessive nausea
   C. Microcytic anemia
   D. Severe constipation
   E. Cardiac arrhythmias

> **HPI:** BL, a 28-year-old woman with a recent diagnosis of acute lymphocytic leukemia (ALL), is admitted for induction chemotherapy with the regimen DVP (daunorubicin, vincristine, prednisone) in hopes of eventually undergoing autologous hematopoietic transplantation as a curative treatment. On day 1 of chemotherapy, BL experiences severe nausea with dry heaves and emesis four times.

Thought Questions

- What are the treatment options for chemotherapy-induced emesis?

- How does treatment vary with different onset times of nausea and vomiting?

- What side effects may be expected with antiemetic treatment?

Basic Science Review and Discussion

Vomiting results from the activation and release of neurotransmitters such as dopamine, histamine, acetycholine, and serotonin. These act in the emetogenic pathway to stimulate the chemoreceptor trigger zone, which in turn sends afferent input to the vomiting center of the brain, located in the medulla. The resulting efferent impulses induce nausea, retching, and vomiting. The major antiemetics serotonin antagonists, dopamine antagonists, anticholinergics, and antihistamines target the specific neurotransmitters through receptor antagonism.

The **emetogenic potential** of individual chemotherapeutic agents is an important factor in the onset and severity of emesis. Acute nausea and vomiting occurs within 24 hours of chemotherapy administration. Delayed nausea and vomiting occurs greater than 24 hours after chemotherapy administration and may occur up to 96 hours postchemotherapy. Anticipatory nausea and vomiting is a psychogenic, conditioned response, occurring before chemotherapy is administered.

The advent of **serotonin antagonists** specific to the 5-hydroxytryptamine-3 receptor ($5-HT_3$) has lead to significant improvements in the treatment of nausea and vomiting and elucidated the role of serotonin in emesis. Interestingly, metoclopramide was thought primarily to be a dopamine antagonist. However, at the high doses used for nausea, it also acts as a serotonin antagonist. Hence, it is believed that cancer chemotherapy triggers the release of both dopamine and serotonin. Unfortunately, at high doses, dopamine antagonist can cause **dystonic reactions** or **extrapyramidal symptoms**. The most effective chemotherapeutic antiemetic is a $5-HT_3$ antagonist in combination with a corticosteroid, usually dexamethasone or methylprednisolone. Although the mechanism is not fully understood in emesis, corticosteroids act synergistically and augment the response to antiemetics when used in combination.

$5-HT_3$ antagonists are effective for acute nausea, but are not effective for anticipatory nausea, and efficacy is low for delayed nausea. Lorazepam is very effective for anticipatory nausea. Other agents used in chemotherapy-induced emesis are dopamine antagonists, scopolamine, and dronabinol. Antihistamines are generally less effective for chemotherapy-induced nausea and vomiting.

Case Conclusion Because BL is experiencing acute nausea and vomiting, she received ondansetron in combination with dexamethasone on a scheduled basis with prompt resolution of her nausea and vomiting.

Thumbnail: Antiemetics

	5-HT$_3$ antagonists	Dopamine antagonists
Agents	Ondansetron Granisetron Dolasetron	Prochlorperazine Droperidol Metoclopramide Promethazine
Clinical use	Prevention of nausea and vomiting, especially that associated with chemotherapy, surgical procedures, and radiotherapy.	Prevention of nausea and vomiting, especially that associated with chemotherapy, surgical procedures, and radiotherapy.
MOA	Antagonism of the 5-HT$_3$ receptor prevents stimulation of the chemoreceptor trigger zone and triggering of the vomiting center.	Central dopaminergic blockade prevents stimulation of the chemoreceptor trigger zone and triggering of the vomit center
Pharmacokinetics		
Absorption	Oral ondansetron is 60% bioavailable	Well absorbed; onset of action in 0.5–1 hr
Distribution	Widely distributed throughout the body	Widely distributed throughout the body
Metabolism	Hepatic metabolism	Hepatic metabolism
Adverse reactions	Well tolerated with few side effects. Headache, especially at higher doses, is the most common adverse effect. Others include dizziness, fatigue, constipation, GI upset, and elevations in hepatic transaminases.	Metoclopramide and prochlorperazine may cause dystonic reactions or EPS at high doses. High doses of droperidol may cause QT$_C$ prolongation. Others include sedation, dizziness, and dry mouth.
Drug interactions	5-HT$_3$ antagonists are CYP450 substrates. Enzyme inducers (i.e., rifampin, phenytoin) may increase 5-HT$_3$ antagonist clearance, and enzyme inhibitors (i.e., cimetidine, allopurinol) may increase toxicity.	Metoclopramide and promethazine are CYP450 substrates. Drug clearance may be altered with concomitant use of enzyme inducers and inhibitors.
Comments	Few side effects. Very effective in combination with corticosteroids.	Phenothiazine antiemetics and metoclopramide may lower the seizure threshold.

Questions

1. A 46-year-old woman with hepatic carcinoma is undergoing weekly infusions of 5-fluorouracil (5-FU). During her third clinic visit, her husband reports that she becomes very nauseated the morning her chemotherapy infusions are due and is unable to eat or drink anything. He has done some research and has found that 5-FU is not a highly emetogenic agent. What is the most appropriate treatment?

   A. Granisetron
   B. Metoclopramide
   C. Dexamethasone with ondansetron
   D. Droperidol
   E. Lorazepam

2. A 66-year-old former smoker is receiving a chemotherapy regimen consisting of cisplatin, vincristine, doxorubicin, and etoposide for small cell lung cancer. Two days after receiving the chemotherapy infusion, he complains of intractable nausea and vomiting. He has been using ondansetron on an as-needed basis, but has experienced no relief. What antiemetic regimen should be offered next?

   A. Schedule ondansetron three times daily (tid).
   B. Dose lorazepam a few hours prior to the next chemotherapy dose.
   C. Give a combination of metoclopramide and dexamethasone.
   D. Give a combination of granisetron and dexamethasone.
   E. Give high-dose metoclopramide with diphenhydramine to counteract EPS effects.

HPI: LE is a 25-year-old woman 4 days s/p C1–C4 laminectomy. She was placed on a morphine patient-controlled analgesia (PCA) immediately postoperatively for 24 hours and is now using oxycodone/acetaminophen every 4 hours for pain control. LE reports stomach discomfort that began 1 day ago. Further questioning reveals that she had not had a bowel movement prior to the procedure and has not had one since the operation, despite regular oral administration of docusate sodium and senna.

PE: Vitals: T 36.9°C, BP 112/69 mm Hg, HR 75 beats/min, RR 18 breaths/min, minimal bowel sounds, and abdomen distended.

Thought Questions

- What are appropriate indications for each type of laxative?
- What are the differences between laxatives?
- What are common adverse effects of laxative use?

Basic Science Review and Discussion

Pharmacologic treatments of constipation are classified by mechanism of action as **stimulants** and **irritants, stool softeners,** or **bulk-forming agents.** Stimulants and irritants generally work in the colon to stimulate peristalsis. Long-term use is not recommended because chronic stimulation of the colon is thought to lead to chronic colon distention. Bulk-forming laxatives are perceived as natural laxatives because their mechanism of action is similar to that of fiber and bran. Bulking laxatives form gels within the large intestine and retain water in the stool to distend the intestine and stimulate peristalsis. Stool softeners become emulsified with the stool and serve to soften it and make passage easier. Stool softeners such as docusate sodium and bulk formers are the only laxatives that should be used prophylactically. Lactulose, an osmotic laxative, also may be used routinely if constipation is refractory to other treatments. Adverse effects associated with long-term use of stimulants and hyperosmotics preclude their chronic use.

The most prominent side effect of laxative use is excessive bowel activity, resulting in diarrhea, nausea, vomiting, and stomach cramping. Obstruction of the esophagus, stomach, small intestine, and rectum has occurred with accumulation of mucilaginous components of bulk laxatives. Large doses or continuous usage of mineral oil may cause anal seepage, leading to local pruritis and irritation. Other side effects include dizziness due to dehydration, gastrointestinal discomfort, bloating, flatulence, and perianal irritation.

Case Conclusion LE has postsurgical and opiate-induced constipation that has been refractory to stool softeners and stimulant/irritants. If distention is not relieved, patients may become nauseated. To mechanically stimulate the sigmoid colon, LE is given a bisacodyl suppository twice. This is not effective, and LE is subsequently given a sodium biphosphate enema, successfully producing a large bowel movement.

Thumbnail: Pharmacologic Actions of Laxatives

Laxative	Onset of action (hr)	MOA	Comments
Saline Sodium biphosphate Magnesium citrate Dibasic sodium Phosphate enemas	0.5–3	Nonabsorbable cations and anions increase osmotic gradient in the gut, drawing in water, causing distention that stimulates peristalsis.	Oral phosphate salts contain ~96.5 mEq of Na^+. Use with caution in Na^+-restricted patients. Use only for acute bowel evacuation.
Stimulants/irritants Cascara Bisacodyl Senna Bisacodyl suppository	6–10 0.25–1	Direct stimulant effect on colon, increasing peristalsis, alters water and electrolyte secretion.	Not for long-term use. Limit to 1 week.
Bulk producing Psyllium Methyl cellulose	12–72	Adsorbs water in the gut; increases stool bulk and moisture, stimulates peristalsis and bowel evacuation	Appropriate for long-term, preventative therapy
Emollient Mineral oil	6–8	Lubricates intestine, retards colonic absorption of fecal water; softens stool	Not indicated for routine use. Impairs absorption of fat-soluble vitamins (ADEK).
Stool softener Docusate sodium	12–72	Acts as detergent in the intestine, reducing surface tension of interfacing liquids and promotes incorporation of fat and liquid, softening stool.	Appropriate for long-term, prophylactic use. Little effect in treating long-standing constipation.
Hyperosmotic Lactulose Glycerin	Glycerin suppository/lactulose enema: 0.25–1 Lactulose oral: 24–48	Osmotic effect retains fluid in the colon and increases colonic peristalsis.	Use when not responsive to stool softeners or stimulants. Titrate to number of stools per day.
Other Castor oil	2–6	Metabolized to ricinoleic acid, which stimulates the intestine, promoting peristalsis and gut motility.	Not for long-term use. Limit to 1 week.

Questions

1. A 45-year-old woman comes into the clinic reporting constipation for the past 2 weeks. She recently started calcium carbonate supplementation per her doctor's advice for the prevention of osteoporosis. She would like to start one of the "natural" laxatives. Which of the following is a bulk-forming agent?

   A. Cascara sagrada
   B. Sodium biphosphate
   C. Polycarbophil
   D. Sennosides
   E. Docusate sodium

2. A 72-year-old man has started taking lactulose for chronic constipation not relieved by stool softeners. He takes 30 mL tid and over the past couple of days he has had two or three loose bowel movements a day. Which of the following would be the appropriate next step?

   A. Discontinue the lactulose as it is not indicated for chronic use.
   B. The lactulose is a hyperosmotic and is too potent. Discontinue the lactulose and start oral senna instead.
   C. Switch to mineral oil as it is more mild.
   D. Hold the lactulose and continue at a lower dose once the diarrhea resolves.
   E. Use the lactulose only on an as-needed basis.

> **HPI:** JB is a 21-year-old man who presents to the ED with a 3-day history of worsening pain, redness, and swelling on his right leg which occurred after falling off his mountain bike.
>
> **PE:** Vitals: T 39.2°C, BP 112/69 mm Hg, HR 80 beats/min, RR 24 breaths/min. He has NKDA. Examination reveals a swollen, warm, and extremely tender leg. JB appears quite ill.

Thought Questions

- Which organisms cause cellulitis?

- Which antibiotics are appropriate for the treatment of cellulitis?

- What is the mechanism of resistance to penicillins?

Basic Science Review and Discussion

Cellulitis results when the integrity of the skin is broken due to an abrasion, ulceration, skin puncture, or surgical wound. Moderate to severe infections can progress to more serious infections such as **osteomyelitis** if not adequately treated. Cellulitis is most commonly caused by group A beta-hemolytic streptococci (*Streptococcus pyogenes*) and *Staphylococcus aureus*. Wound cultures have a very low yield and rarely identify the causative pathogen. Thus, cultures are rarely done and therapy is usually presumptive.

Nafcillin, an antistaphylococcal penicillin, is an appropriate IV antibiotic for the treatment of cellulitis requiring hospitalization. Appropriate alternatives include cefazolin or clindamycin. Second- and third-generation cephalosporins offer no advantage over the listed regimens since they are broader in spectrum and more expensive. While gram-negative organisms such as *Escherichia coli, Pseudomonas aeruginosa,* and *Klebsiella pneumoniae* can cause cellulitis; they should only be considered in patients who either fail first-line regimens or in patients who are immunocompromised. For those patients with severe penicillin allergies, alternative regimens include clindamycin or vancomycin.

Penicillins are classified into several groups depending on their chemical structure: **penicillins,** extended-spectrum penicillins or **aminopenicillins,** and **antistaphylococcal penicillins.** Penicillins inhibit bacterial cell wall synthesis by attaching to **penicillin-binding proteins** (PBP), thereby inhibiting bacterial growth. Although penicillin and ampicillin have activity against *Streptococcus pyogenes,* they lack activity against *Staphylococcus aureus. Staphylococcus aureus* produces an enzyme, **penicillinase,** which breaks down penicillin and ampicillin, rendering them ineffective. Nafcillin is unique because it is stable in the presence of penicillinase. Another common mechanism of resistance to penicillins is through modification of PBPs. Penicillin-resistant *Streptococcus pneumoniae* is an example of an organism that produces modified PBPs.

In general, penicillins are very well tolerated. The most common adverse effects are **hypersensitivity reactions.** While skin rash is the most common manifestation, **anaphylaxis** rarely can occur. In those patients who have experienced an anaphylactic reaction to penicillin, a non-beta-lactam antibiotic should be used.

> **Case Conclusion** The patient is admitted to the hospital and diagnosed with cellulitis. No cultures are done and nafcillin is prescribed. After 3 days of nafcillin, JB was switched to oral dicloxacillin and discharged home to complete his course of therapy.

Thumbnail: Penicillins

	Antibiotic		
	Penicillins	**Aminopenicillins**	**Antistaphylococcal penicillins**
Available agents	Penicillin (IV/IM/PO)	Ampicillin (IV) Amoxicillin (PO)	Dicloxacillin (PO) Nafcillin (IV) Oxacillin (PO/IV)
Clinical usage	Drug of choice for the treatment of infections caused by streptococci, meningococci, penicillin-susceptible pneumococci, and for the treatment of syphilis. The oral form of penicillin is indicated for minor infections only.	Ampicillin is primarily indicated for the treatment of infections due to enterococcus and streptococcal species. Amoxicillin is primarily used for the treatment of upper and lower respiratory tract infections due to streptococcal species or non-beta-lactamase-producing *H. influenzae*.	These agents are primarily used for the treatment of infections caused by beta-lactamase-producing staphylococci. Antistaphylococcal pencillins also are active against penicillin-susceptible strains of streptococci.
Activity	Primarily gram-positive organisms: streptococcal species, enterococcus, penicillin-susceptible pneumococci, *Treponema pallidum*. Few gram-negative anaerobic organisms and *Clostridium* species.	Primarily gram-positive organisms such as streptococcal species, enterococcus, penicillin-susceptible pneumococci, *Treponema pallidum*. Compared with penicillin, aminopenicillins have greater gram-negative activity including *H. influenzae* (non-beta-lactamase producing).	Methicillin-susceptible staphylococci, penicillin-susceptible strains of streptococci and pneumococci.
Pharmacokinetics			
Absorption	Oral penicillin has poor bioavailability.	Amoxicillin has very good bioavailability.	Dicloxacillin has good bioavailability.
Distribution	Penicillins are widely distributed throughout the body. Penicillins penetrate poorly into CSF. However, in the presence of inflamed meninges, CSF concentrations are adequate to treat bacterial meningitis due to susceptible organisms.		
Elimination	Penicillin and ampicillin are excreted by the kidneys into the urine. Dose adjustments are required in the setting of renal dysfunction.	Penicillin and ampicillin are excreted by the kidneys into the urine. Dose adjustments are required in the setting of renal dysfunction.	Nafcillin is primarily cleared by biliary excretion while dicloxacillin is eliminated by both kidney and biliary excretion. No dose adjustments are needed in the setting of renal or hepatic dysfunction.
Adverse reactions	Overall, the penicillins are well tolerated. The most common adverse effects are due to hypersensitivity reactions. Hypersensitivity reactions can be simply categorized as immediate reactions (type 1) or late reactions. Type 1 reactions are IgE mediated and are often associated with systemic manifestations such as diffuse erythema, pruritus, urticaria, angioedema, and bronchospasm. The most severe yet rare IgE-mediated side effect is anaphylaxis (0.05%). Type 1 reactions usually occur within 72 hr of administration. Late reactions usually occur 72 hr after drug administration. The most common late reactions include skin rashes characterized as maculopapular or morbilliform rashes. Rarely, nafcillin may cause **neutropenia**. Seizures in high doses, vaginal moniliasis, and *Clostridium difficile* infection also can occur with all penicillins		
Drug interactions	In general, there are no clinically significant drug interactions associated with the penicillins. Dicloxacillin may increase the effects of warfarin.		

Questions

1. A 42-year-old woman presents to her primary care provider with a 3-day history of redness, swelling, and increasing pain of her right arm after falling off her ladder while washing her windows. The area is warm to the touch with a defined erythematous border. She has NKDA. She has a temperature of 38.5°C. The presumptive diagnosis is cellulitis. What would be an appropriate empiric outpatient regimen?

   A. Clarithromycin
   B. Nafcillin
   C. Penicillin
   D. Cephalexin
   E. Ciprofloxacin

2. A 32-year-old woman is admitted to the hospital with cellulitis after being bitten by a spider 5 days ago. She is empirically started on nafcillin; however, 10 hours later the patient develops hives and difficulty breathing. What alternatives should be considered?

   A. Cefazolin
   B. Ampicillin
   C. Ceftriaxone
   D. Clindamycin
   E. Gentamicin

HPI: MN is a 55-year-old man who is diagnosed with small cell lung cancer. Three days after induction chemotherapy, MN develops a fever to 39.9°C and chills. There was a miscommunication among the medical staff, and ampicillin/sulbactam was started instead of piperacillin/tazobactam.

Labs: Absolute neutrophil count (ANC) 300/μL, hemoglobin (Hgb) 13 g/dL, Hct 42%, platelets 75,000/mm³. MN has NKDA.

Thought Questions

■ Which gram-negative organisms need to be covered in patients with febrile neutropenia?

■ What are the differences in activity among the beta-lactam/beta-lactamase inhibitors?

■ What are the differences in activity among the three available carbapenems?

Basic Science Discussion and Review

Neutropenia is defined as a reduction in the number of circulating granulocytes or neutrophils that predisposes the host to infection. The degree of neutropenia is expressed as the **absolute neutrophil count.** The ANC is defined as the total number of granulocytes (polymorphonuclear leukocytes and band forms) present in the circulating pool of WBCs. Usually the risk of infection is low when the ANC is greater than 1000/μL. As the ANC decreases below 500/μL, the risk for infection increases significantly. Patients with prolonged neutropenia such as those receiving chemotherapy are at high risk for developing serious infections.

Risk factors for infection in the neutropenic host include chemotherapy-induced mucosal damage, invasive medical procedures, in-dwelling medical devices, and altered mucociliary activity. Common infections can be bacterial (gram positive and gram negative), fungal (*Candida* species, *Aspergillus* species), or viral (herpes, cytomegalovirus). The clinical presentation of infection in neutropenic patients varies markedly from patients with normal immune response. The lack of neutrophils results in an absence of many classic signs and symptoms of infection, such as increased WBC or fever. The most common sites of infection are the mouth and pharynx, respiratory tract, skin and soft tissue (IV catheters), perineum, and urinary tract.

The treatment of patients with febrile neutropenia is highly variable, yet empiric antibacterial agents are usually targeted toward gram-negative organisms such as *Pseudomonas aeruginosa* and *Escherichia coli*. Other organisms such as gram-positive bacteria, viruses, and fungi are also considered possible pathogens in the neutropenic host.

Case Conclusion After 2 days of ampicillin/sulbactam therapy, MN continues to spike fevers to 39.5°C. Blood cultures are positive for *Pseudomonas aeruginosa*. Ampicillin/sulbactam is discontinued and MN is started on meropenem and tobramycin. MN is also treated with filgrastim (GCSF) to increase his ANC. He defervesces within 2 days and fully recovers.

Thumbnail: Beta-Lactamase Inhibitors and Carbapenems

	Carbapenems	Beta-lactam/beta-lactamase inhibitors
Agents	Imipenem Meropenem Ertapenem	Piperacillin/tazobactam (PT) Ticarcillin/clavulanic acid (TC) Ampicillin/sulbactam (AS) Amoxicillin/clavulanic acid (AC)
Clinical usage	Used to treat wide range of infections, including septicemia, lower respiratory tract, bone and joint, skin/skin structure, urinary tract, gynecologic and intra-abdominal infections. Carbapenems are reserved for clinical situations associated with highly resistant organisms in which there are few other options.	
MOA	Beta-lactam antibiotics covalently bind to penicillin-binding proteins (PBPs) involved in the biosynthesis of bacterial cell walls.	
Activity	Very broad spectrum of activity. Good activity against gram-positive organisms such as streptococci and staphylococci, but have no activity against methicillin-resistant organisms. All three carbapenems appear to have excellent activity against most strains of clinically significant anaerobes such as *Bacteroides fragilis*. Excellent activity against gram-negative organisms, such as: *Haemophilus influenzae* *Moraxella catarrhalis* *Escherichia coli* *Klebsiella* species *Proteus* species *Morganella morganii* *Pseudomonas aeruginosa* *Enterobacter* species *Acinetobacter* species *Serratia* species *Citrobacter* species Unlike meropenem and imipenem, ertapenem is not active against *Pseudomonas aeruginosa*, *Acinetobacter* species, or *Enterococcus faecalis*.	Broad spectrum activity. All have good activity against gram-positive organisms such as streptococci and staphylococci but have no activity against methicillin-resistant organisms. PT and AS also cover enterococci, unlike TC. TC has activity against *Stenotrophomonas maltophilia* and is considered a second-line agent to trimethoprim/sulfamethoxazole. All beta-lactamase inhibitor combinations have excellent activity against anaerobes. AS and AC gram-negative spectrum: *Haemophilus influenzae* *Moraxella catarrhalis* *Escherichia coli* *Klebsiella* species *Proteus* species *Morganella morganii* *Neisseria gonorrhoeae* In addition to the coverage of AS and AC, PT and TC also have activity against: *Pseudomonas aeruginosa* *Providencia* species *Enterobacter* species *Acinetobacter* species *Serratia* species *Salmonella* species *Citrobacter* species
Mechanism of resistance	Resistance to beta-lactams in clinical isolates is primarily due to the hydrolysis of the antibiotic by beta-lactamases. Mutational events resulting in the modification of PBPs or cellular permeability also can lead to beta-lactam resistance. Beta-lactamase inhibitors such as tazobactam inactivate beta-lactamase.	
Pharmacokinetics		
Absorption	Parenteral: complete bioavailability	PT, TC, and AS are only available parenterally and have complete bioavailability. AC is only available orally and has almost complete absorption.
Distribution	Penetrate well into most body tissues	Penetrate well into most body tissues
Metabolism	Via renal dehydropeptidase Imipenem > meropenem = ertapenem	Minimal—primarily excreted unchanged in the urine
Excretion	Renal	Renal
Adverse reactions	Most common side effects include diarrhea, nausea, vomiting, headache, rash, and infusion-related reactions. Frequency and potential risk of seizures with imipenem appear to be greater in comparison with the other carbapenems and beta-lactam antibiotics. Seizures have occurred most commonly in patients with CNS disorders or bacterial meningitis and/or compromised renal function. May be prevented by dose adjusting for renal insufficiency. Pseudomembranous colitis. Hypersensitivity reaction: in patients with hypersensitivity reactions to penicillins, the incidence of cross-reactivity to carbapenems is 50%.	Most common side effects include nausea, vomiting, diarrhea, pseudomembranous colitis, hypersensitivity reaction, and seizure. Bleeding manifestations have occurred in some patients receiving beta-lactam antibiotics. These reactions have been associated with abnormalities in clotting time, platelet aggregation, and prothrombin time.

Questions

1. OT is a 16-year-old boy who is diagnosed with ALL. Five days after induction chemotherapy, OT develops a fever to 101°F and chills. His ANC is < 500/μL. Overnight, the cross-cover team started piperacillin/tazobactam and imipenem. This regimen is not ideal for which of the following reasons?

   A. Similar adverse event profile
   B. Potential for antagonism
   C. Imipenem is inactivated by tazobactam
   D. Overlapping spectrum of activity
   E. Both are renally excreted

2. JH is a 48-year-old woman with a recent diagnosis of breast cancer and is neutropenic after receiving chemotherapy. She is currently febrile and *Acinetobacter baumannii* is cultured from the blood. Her PMH is significant for chronic renal insufficiency and a history of seizures. Which of the following is considered appropriate therapy for JH?

   A. Imipenem
   B. Piperacillin/tazobactam + imipenem
   C. Ertapenem
   D. Ampicillin/sulbactam + meropenem
   E. Ampicillin/sulbactam
   F. Meropenem

> **HPI:** AL is a 42-year-old febrile and unresponsive man who is brought to the ED by a friend. Over the past several days he was experiencing fever, chills, and a worsening productive cough.
>
> **PE:** He has a temperature of 40.1°C, BP 85/55 mm Hg, RR 25 breaths/min, and HR 115 beats/min. Crackles were heard throughout both lung fields.
>
> **Labs:** Lab tests revealed a WBC count of 22,000/μL (98% PMNs) and Cr 2.0 mg/dL. Results of lumbar puncture showed the following: WBC count 4000/μL, protein 120 mg/dL, and glucose 35 mg/dL. Results of studies on blood, CSF, sputum cultures, and Gram stains are pending. AL has NKDA.

Thought Questions

- What are the most common organisms associated with adult meningitis?

- Which cephalosporins are appropriate for the treatment of meningitis?

- What adverse effects are associated with cephalosporins?

Basic Science Review and Discussion

The etiology of bacterial meningitis is highly dependent on the patient's age and underlying medical conditions. The most common cause of bacterial meningitis in an immunocompetent adult is *Streptococcus pneumoniae* and *Neisseria meningitidis*. In contrast, the most likely causes of bacterial meningitis in a neonate are group B *Streptococcus, Escherichia coli,* and *Listeria monocytogenes*. Bacterial meningitis is a life-threatening infection that necessitates prompt antibiotic administration. Predisposing factors for meningitis in adults include alcohol abuse, splenectomy, chronic obstructive airway disease, and upper respiratory tract infections. The treatment of bacterial meningitis is challenging because antibiotics must cross the blood–brain barrier to reach the CSF. There are a limited number of antibiotics that have adequate penetration into the CSF. Historically, *Neisseria meningitidis* and *Streptococcus pneumoniae* have been susceptible to penicillin G. However, over the past several years in the United States strains of *Streptococcus pneumoniae* demonstrating intermediate and high-level penicillin resistance have emerged, making treatment even more challenging. Third-generation cephalosporins are a mainstay in the management of bacterial meningitis because these agents are active against *Neisseria meningitidis* and *Streptococcus pneumoniae*.

Cephalosporins are divided into four classes: first, second, third and fourth generations. This nomenclature delineates when these agents were developed and, more importantly, their spectrum of activity. In general, the cephalosporins are a heterogeneous group of drugs with differences in spectrum of activity and pharmacokinetics. In general, as the generation increases from first to fourth, the amount of gram-negative coverage increases while gram-positive coverage decreases. More specifically, first-generation cephalosporins are very active against *Staphylococcus aureus* and *Streptococcus* species, whereas gram-negative activity is limited to *Proteus mirabilis, E. coli,* and *Klebsiella pneumoniae,* which can easily be remembered by the pneumonic **PEK.** The second-generation cephalosporins are less active than the first-generation cephalosporins against gram-positive bacteria but have increased gram-negative activity that includes *Haemophilus influenzae* and *N. meningitidis* as well as the **PEK** organisms (**HNPEK**). Among gram-negative bacteria, the third-generation cephalosporins are also active against *Serratia* species; therefore, they cover the **HNPEKS** organisms. Finally the activity of fourth-generation cephalosporins is expanded to include *Enterobacter* species and *Citrobacter* species (**HENPECKS**). Of note, ceftazidime and cefepime are the only two cephalosporins active against *Pseudomonas aeruginosa*. The third- and fourth-generation cephalosporins are active against most staphylococci but less so than the first-generation cephalosporins. However, ceftazidime has very weak antistaphylococcal activity. Cephalosporins are available in both PO and IV formulations. The pharmacologic properties of the cephalosporins are relatively similar, with a few exceptions. The cephalosporins distribute well into most tissues except for the CSF, prostate, and eye. However, the third- and fourth-generation cephalosporins have adequate CSF concentrations in the setting of inflamed meninges. The majority of the cephalosporins are excreted renally via active tubular secretion except for ceftriaxone. Since ceftriaxone has nonrenal elimination, there is no need to adjust the dose in patients with renal insufficiency. The elimination T½ for most of the cephalosporins is 1 to 2 hours, except for cefotetan (3 hours), cefixime (4 hours), and ceftriaxone (8 hours).

Overall, the cephalosporins are remarkably well tolerated. The most common adverse effects are **hypersensitivity** reactions such as skin rashes, fever, and hemolytic anemia.

Cross-reactivity between pencillins and cephalosporins ranges from 5% to 10%. Even though some patients with a history of penicillin allergy may tolerate cephalosporins, patients with a history of anaphylaxis to penicillin should not receive cephalosporins.

Ceftriaxone is associated with biliary sludging or **pseudo-cholithiasis** due to precipitation of the drug in the bile. This occurs when its solubility in bile is exceeded when

used in high doses. Ceftriaxone and cefotaxime are the preferred third-generation cephalosporins for the empiric treatment of bacterial meningitis since these agents are the most active cephalosporins against *Streptococcus pneumoniae*. Cefotetan has a methylthiotetrazole group that may inhibit vitamin K synthesis and cause **hypoprothrombinemia** and bleeding disorders. In addition, **disulfiram-like reactions** can occur if coadministered with alcohol-containing medications.

Case Conclusion Because the etiology of bacterial meningitis in AL is most likely attributable to *S. pneumoniae* and *N. meningitidis*, ceftriaxone, a third-generation cephalosporin, is started empirically. Ceftriaxone will also treat his potential community-acquired pneumonia. Even though the patient has some degree of renal insufficiency (Cr 2.0 mg/dL), the dose of ceftriaxone does not need to be adjusted since it is hepatically eliminated.

Thumbnail: Cephalosporins

	First generation	Second generation	Third generation	Fourth generation
Available agents	PO: Cephradine Cephalexin Cefadroxil IV: Cefazolin	PO: Cefuroxime axetil Cefprozil IV: Cefuroxime Cefotetan Cefoxitin	PO: Cefixime Cefpodoxime Cefdinir Cefditoren IV/IM: Ceftriaxone Ceftazidime Cefotaxime Ceftizoxime	IV: Cefepime
MOA	Inhibition of bacterial cell wall synthesis. **Bactericidal.**			
Activity	*S. aureus, Streptococcus* species, *P. mirabilis, E. coli, K. pneumoniae.*	*S. aureus, Streptococcus* species, *H. influenzae* (including beta-lactamase producing), *N. gonorrhoeae, P. mirabilis, E. coli, K. pneumoniae.* Cefoxitin and cefotetan have good activity against *Bacteroides fragilis.*	*S. aureus* (not as active compared to 1st generation), *Streptococcus* species, *H. influenzae* (including beta-lactamase producing), *N. gonorrhoeae, P. mirabilis, E. coli, K. pneumoniae, S. marcescans. P. aeruginosa* (ceftazadime only).	*S. aureus, Streptococcus* species, *H. influenzae* (including beta-lactamase producing), *Enterobacter* species, *N. gonorrheae, P. mirabilis, E. coli, Citrobacter* species, *K. pneumoniae, S. marcescans, Acinetobacter* species, *Pseudomonas aeruginosa*
Bioavailability	All oral cephalosporins have good absorption.			
Distribution	Widely distributed, except to the prostate, CSF, and eye. In the presence of inflamed meninges, adequate CSF concentrations are achieved by the third- and fourth-generation cephalosporins.			
Elimination	Renally eliminated (> 70%) via active tubular secretion and glomerular filtration, except ceftriaxone, which has nonrenal clearance (biliary). All renally eliminated cephalosporins require dosage adjustment in renal insufficiency.			
Adverse effects	**Hypersensitivity reactions:** Incidence is 5%–10% in patients with history of penicillin allergy vs. 1%–2.5% patients with no penicillin allergy history. Diarrhea: most common with ceftriaxone and oral agents. Pseudomembranous colitis can occur with any cephalosporin. Pseudocholelithiasis (biliary sludging) can occur with ceftriaxone in high doses. Cefotetan can cause hypoprothrombinemia and, if coadministered with alcohol, disulfiram reactions.			
Drug interactions	No clinically significant drug interactions			

Questions

1. JK is a 32-year-old man who was diagnosed with cellulitis. A detailed medication history done by the medical student reveals that JK experienced anaphylaxis after receiving amoxicillin about a year ago. Which of the following antibiotics would you avoid prescribing in JK?

   A. Cefuroxime
   B. Clarithromcyin
   C. Penicillin
   D. Clindamycin
   E. A and C

2. MN is a 54-year-old man who was diagnosed with an intra-abdominal abscess after sustaining a stab wound. He is started on a 21-day course of cefotetan. His social history includes drinking two beers per night. His PMH is significant for peptic ulcer disease, HTN, and seasonal allergies. His medications include omeprazole, enalapril, and cetirizine. Which of the following statements are correct?

   A. While on cefotetan, MN will have to increase his omeprazole dose.
   B. While on cefotetan, MN will have to increase his enalapril dose.
   C. While on cefotetan, MN will have to stop drinking alcohol.
   D. While on cefotetan, MN may resume his current medications and lifestyle.
   E. None of the above.

HPI: MT is a 63-year-old man who presents to the clinic complaining of sudden onset of fever, headache, malaise, and a sore throat. He says he has been feeling ill since taking care of his sick granddaughter, who had group A streptococcal pharyngitis. He has a history of atrial fibrillation and is currently being treated with digoxin and warfarin. He has a history of an allergic reaction to penicillin, which resulted in laryngeal edema, and he has a 30-pack per year tobacco history. A chest radiograph done in the clinic is clear. A rapid antigen detection test is positive for group A streptococcus.

PE: Vitals: T 39.1°C, BP 120/60 mm Hg, HR 130 beats/min (irreg), RR 24 breaths/min.

Thought Questions

- What is the spectrum of activity of the macrolides?

- Which macrolide has poor *Haemophilus influenzae* coverage?

- What is the MOA of macrolides?

- Which macrolide (erythromycin, clarithromycin, or azithromycin) may cause drug interactions with his current medications?

- Which of the three macrolides is most likely to cause GI upset?

Basic Science Review and Discussion

Macrolides are appropriate antibiotics for the management of respiratory tract infections because they are active against *Streptococcus pneumoniae, Streptococcus pyogenes* (group A streptococci), and atypical organisms such as *Legionella pneumophila, Mycoplasma pneumoniae,* and *Chlamydia pneumoniae.* The newer generation macrolides such as clar-ithromycin and the **azalide** azithromycin also have reliable coverage against *Haemophilus influenzae,* unlike erythromycin. However, macrolide-resistant *Streptococcus* is becoming an increasingly important issue in the outpatient treatment of respiratory tract infections such as community-acquired pneumonia. Thus, selection of appropriate antibiotics should be based on local resistance patterns.

Erythromycin inhibits RNA-dependent protein synthesis by binding to the bacterial 50S ribosomal RNA, by blocking aminoacyl translocation reactions, and by blocking formation of the initiation complex. It is also a strong inhibitor of hepatic **cytochrome P450** (CYP450), and will increase the serum concentration of warfarin, prolonging the INR. Erythromycin increases the bioavailability of digoxin, also leading to increased serum concentrations. Clarithromycin, although not as strong an inhibitor against CYP450, may still increase digoxin and warfarin levels. Azithromycin does not inhibit CYP450 and will be least likely to cause drug-drug interactions in this patient. Erythromycin is a **motilin** receptor agonist, and can cause abdominal cramping and diarrhea. Incidentally, erythromycin is often used in patients with diabetic gastroparesis to stimulate GI motility.

Case Conclusion The treatment of choice for group A streptococcal pharyngitis is penicillin. However, due to MT's hypersensitivity reaction to penicillins, macrolides are an appropriate alternative choice. Because erythromycin may increase digoxin and warfarin levels, azithromycin is started for MT's pharyngitis.

Thumbnail: Macrolides

Prototypical agent: Erythromycin. Clarithromycin and azithromycin developed to overcome limitations of erythromycin: poor bioavailability, poor GI tolerability, need for frequent dosing (short T½) and limited *H. influenzae* coverage.

Clinical usage: Primarily as an antibacterial agent for the treatment of respiratory tract infections and sexually transmitted diseases. Also used for treatment of peptic ulcer disease in combination with other agents. Erythromycin is considered the drug of choice for whooping cough.

MOA: Block protein synthesis at 50S ribosomal subunit. The antibacterial action of the macrolides is bacteriostatic.

Activity: Macrolides are active against gram-positive organisms, particularly pneumococci, streptococci, and staphylococci. Some gram-negative organisms, such as *Neisseria* species and *Bordetella pertussis* (whooping cough), are also covered. Other organisms covered include some *Mycobacterium, Legionella, Mycoplasma,* and *Chlamydia* species. Although azithromycin and clarithromycin are active against *H. influenzae* and *Moraxella catarrhalis,* erythromycin is less active. Clarithromycin also has activity against *Helicobacter pylori.*

Pharmacokinetics

Absorption: Erythromycin is poorly absorbed orally and is readily broken down by stomach acid. Thus, erythromycin is enteric coated to increase absorption.

Distribution: Macrolides widely distribute into tissue and obtain high intracellular levels.

Elimination: All macrolides are hepatically eliminated. Clarithromycin is hepatically activated to the 14-OH metabolite. T½: erythromycin < clarithromycin < azithromycin.

Adverse reactions: Erythromycin can cause nausea, vomiting, diarrhea, and abdominal cramping. GI intolerance due to erythromycin is due to direct stimulation of the motilin receptor, leading to increased GI motility. This occurs with both the IV and PO formulation. Although rare, all macrolides can cause hepatotoxicity. The estolate formulation of erythromycin has been associated with cholestatic hepatitis in pregnant women. In high doses, all macrolides can cause **tinnitus.** All macrolides can cause QT$_C$ prolongation and torsade de points

Drug interactions: Erythromycin is a strong inhibitor of CYP450. CYP450 inhibition decreases with the newer macrolides. Thus, clarithromycin is a mild inhibitor, and azithromycin has no effect on CYP450.

Questions

1. CT is a 3-year-old boy brought in by his mother to see the pediatrician for a follow-up appointment. CT was started on high-dose amoxicillin 3 days ago for acute otitis media. CT continues to be febrile with no clinical improvement on amoxicillin. Tympanocentesis reveals gram-negative coccobacilli on Gram stain. What is the most appropriate treatment for CT at this time?

   A. Amoxicillin clavulanic acid
   B. Levofloxacin
   C. Doxycycline
   D. Continue amoxicillin
   E. Erythromycin

2. JC is a 64-year-old man with diabetic gastroparesis. JC has congestive heart failure and atrial fibrillation for which he is taking digoxin and amiodarone. JC's physician would like to prescribe a promotility agent for his gastroparesis. Which of the following is the most appropriate treatment for JC at this time?

   A. Erythromycin
   B. Cisapride
   C. Metoclopramide
   D. Azithromycin
   E. None of the above

HPI: VD, a 23-year-old man about to leave for a Caribbean cruise, complains of mild dysuria with 3 days of painless urethral discharge that started about 2 weeks after his last intercourse. He has been sexually active with his girlfriend for the past 2 to 3 months but admits to being promiscuous. He denies fever.

PE: On examination he has no lymphadenopathy or penile lesions. Examination is remarkable for a white urethral discharge. Gram stain and culture for *Neisseria gonorrhoeae* were negative. A presumptive diagnosis of nongonococcal urethritis (NGU) is made.

Thought Questions

- What is the most common cause of NGU?

- Which tetracycline is preferred for the treatment of NGU?

- What are the adverse effects associated with the tetracyclines?

Basic Science Review and Discussion

Chlamydia trachomatis is the primary cause of nongonococcal urethritis, followed by *Ureaplasma urealyticum*. Doxycycline is the tetracycline of choice for the treatment of nongonococcal urethritis because it has activity against both organisms. There are three tetracyclines that are primarily used for the treatment of infections: tetracycline, doxycycline, and minocycline. Demeclocycline is primarily used for the treatment of chronic syndrome of inappropriate secretion of antidiuretic hormone (SIADH). Doxycycline and minocycline have the advantage of twice daily dosing, whereas tetracycline is dosed four times daily. An alternative to doxycycline for the treatment of NGU is a single 1-g dose of azithromycin. Although azithromycin is an expensive alternative; it may be useful in patients with poor compliance. Both regimens have been shown to be equally effective.

Doxycycline can cause nausea, vomiting, and diarrhea. The bioavailability of doxycycline is reduced if coadministered with multivalent ions such as iron or magnesium. However, unlike tetracycline, it can be administered with food and dairy products. In addition, patients taking tetracyclines may experience **photosensitivity,** especially if they are fair skinned. Patients taking tetracyclines should avoid prolonged exposure to sunlight.

Case Conclusion VD is started on doxycycline for 7 days. The patient is instructed to avoid prolonged exposure to sunlight and to avoid concomitant dosing with antacids or any other medications that may contain multivalent cations.

Thumbnail: Tetracyclines

Available agents: Tetracycline, doxycycline, minocycline.

Clinical usage: Tetracylines are effective for sexually transmitted diseases caused by chlamydia and syphilis. They are also commonly used for the treatment of community-acquired pneumonia, Lyme disease, and Rocky Mountain spotted fever, and in combination with other agents for *Helicobacter pylori*.

MOA: Tetracyclines inhibit protein synthesis by binding with the 30S and 50S ribosomal subunits of bacteria. The antibacterial action of the tetracyclines is **bacteriostatic**.

Activity: Tetracyclines are active against gram-positive organisms, such as pneumococci, *Staphylococcus aureus*, and gram-negative organisms such as *Haemophilus influenzae, Haemophilus ducreyi, Yersinia pestis, Bartonella* species, and *Klebsiella* species. Other organisms covered include *Legionella, Mycoplasma, Chlamydia* species, *Borrelia burgdorferi*, and some mycobacteria.

Pharmacokinetics

Absorption: Tetracyclines are well absorbed after oral administration; however, absorption is impaired by food, by multivalent cations (Ca^{+2}, Mg^{+2}, Fe^{+2} or Al^{+3}), and by dairy products.

Distribution: Tetracyclines widely distribute into tissue and body fluids except CSF.

Elimination: Tetracycline and minocycline are excreted mainly in bile and urine. Doxycycline is eliminated by nonrenal mechanisms. Doxycycline is the tetracycline of choice in patients with renal insufficiency. T½ doxycycline = minocycline > tetracycline.

Rarely, the tetracyclines can cause esophageal ulcers. Patients with esophageal obstruction may be at increased risk. Demeclocycline can cause diabetes insipidus.

Adverse reactions: Tetracyclines can cause nausea, vomiting, and diarrhea. Administering doxycycline with food can minimize these effects. The use of tetracyclines during pregnancy or in children under 8 years of age is contraindicated because it can cause discoloration of teeth and inhibit normal bone growth. The tetracyclines may cause photosensitivity, so patients should avoid prolonged exposure to sunlight. Doxycycline and minocycline can cause dizziness, vertigo, and nausea. Tetracycline and minocycline should be avoided in patients with renal insufficiency because toxic levels may accumulate. *Clostridium difficile* infections and *Monilia* also can occur.

Drug interactions: The bioavailability of tetracyclines is significantly decreased when administered with antacids containing aluminum, calcium, or magnesium, with iron-containing products, or with food. Food or dairy products do not affect the bioavailability of doxycycline or minocycline.

Questions

1. A 32-year-old woman in her first trimester of pregnancy presents with a mucopurulent vaginal discharge and dysuria. She is diagnosed with NGU. Which of the following antibiotics should be avoided?

   A. Azithromycin
   B. Doxycycline
   C. Penicillin
   D. Cefuroxime
   E. Ceftriaxone

2. A 46-year-old woman is prescribed doxycycline for a diagnosis of community-acquired pneumonia. Her PMH is significant for iron-deficiency anemia, peptic ulcer disease, HTN, a recent DVT, and headaches. Her current medications include ferrous sulfate, ibuprofen, enalapril, acetaminophen, famotidine, and warfarin. Which of her following medications is most likely to result in decreased levels of doxycycline?

   A. Acetaminophen
   B. Warfarin
   C. Ferrous sulfate
   D. Famotidine
   E. Ibuprofen

HPI: LD is a 19-year-old female college sophomore who presents to the student health clinic with a 3-day history of dysuria. LD's last menstrual period was 2 weeks ago. She is sexually active, and uses a diaphragm with spermicide for birth control. Her medications include ferrous sulfate and acetaminophen. She has NKDA.

PE: Vitals:T 37.9°, BP 120/78 mm Hg, HR 80 beats/min, RR 15 breaths/min. Mild suprapubic tenderness with no flank pain. No vaginal discharge or lesions were seen.

Labs: A clean-catch mid-stream urine sample shows gram-negative rods on Gram stain.

Thought Questions

- What are the leading organisms that cause urinary tract infections (UTIs)?

- What are some of LD's risk factors for a UTI?

- Which agents achieve high urinary concentrations?

Basic Science Review and Discussion

Urinary tract infections can be classified by anatomic site of involvement into lower and upper urinary tract infections. Lower UTIs include cystitis, urethritis, prostatitis, and epididymitis, whereas upper urinary tract infections include pyelonephritis. UTIs also may be further classified as complicated or uncomplicated. In females with a structurally normal urinary tract, both cystitis and pyelonephritis are considered uncomplicated UTIs. UTIs in men, elderly individuals, pregnant women, or patients with in-dwelling catheters or anatomic or functional abnormalities are considered complicated UTIs.

Escherichia coli is the causative pathogen in 80% of infections. Other organisms that may cause UTIs include *Staphylococcus saprophyticus* and *Enterococcus* species.

The antimicrobial agents most commonly used to treat uncomplicated UTIs include trimethoprim-sulfamethoxazole (TMP-SMX), trimethoprim alone, beta-lactams, fluoroquinolones (Table 51-1), nitrofurantoin, and fosfomycin. These agents are used primarily due to their tolerability, spectrum of activity against the suspected uropathogens, and their favorable pharmacokinetic profiles. All the antimicrobial agents approved for the treatment of UTIs achieve inhibitory urinary concentrations that significantly exceed serum levels. Because most uncomplicated UTIs are treated empirically, therapy should be based on local resistance patterns in the community to ensure that the most appropriate antimicrobial agent is used.

Case Conclusion LD was treated with a 3-day course of TMP-SMX with total resolution of her symptoms.

Table 51-1 Fluorouinolone activity by generation

	First generation	Second generation	Third generation
Agents	Nalidixic acid Cinoxacin Norfloxacin Enoxacin	Ciprofloxacin Ofloxacin	Levofloxacin Moxifloxacin Gatifloxacin
Spectrum of activity	**Gram-negative** *Proteus* species ***Escherichia coli*** *Klebsiella* species *Citrobacter* species *Acinetobacter* species *Pseudomonas aeruginosa* *Enterobacter* species *Serratia marcescens* **Intestinal pathogens** *Shigella* species *Campylobacter jejuni* *Salmonella* species	**Same as first generation** ***Plus:*** **Gram-positive** *S. aureus* *S. epidermidis* **Respiratory pathogens** *H. influenzae* *M. catarrhalis* *Legionella* species **Genital pathogens** *N. gonorrhoeae* *Chlamydia trachomatis*	**Same as first and second generation** ***Plus:*** **Gram-positive** *Streptococcus pneumoniae* **Atypicals** *Chlamydia pneumoniae* *Mycoplasma pneumoniae* *Mycobacterium* species **Anaerobes** *B. fragilis* (moxifloxacin)

Thumbnail: Fluoroquinolones and Trimethoprim-Sulfamethoxazole

	Fluoroquinolones	TMP-SMX
Clinical usage	Quinolones are divided into "generations" based on their spectrum of activity. The higher the generation, the broader the spectrum of activity. First generation: UTIs Second and third generations: UTIs, prostatitis, respiratory tract infections, sinusitis, infectious diarrhea, uncomplicated skin and skin structure infections, traveler's diarrhea	UTIs Prostatitis Acute otitis media Exacerbations of chronic bronchitis Treatment and prophylaxis of *Pneumocystis carinii* infections Traveler's diarrhea
MOA	Inhibition of topoisomerase II (DNA-gyrase) and topoisomerase IV. Inhibition of topoisomerases disrupts DNA replication and transcription resulting in bacterial cell death.	SMX interferes with bacterial folic acid syntheses via inhibition of dihydrofolic acid formation from para-aminobenzoic acid. TMP inhibits dihydrofolic acid reduction to tetrahydrofolate, resulting in sequential inhibition of enzymes of the folic acid pathway. TMP and SMX are synergistic when used together.
Activity	Bactericidal with varying activity against gram-positive, gram-negative, and anaerobic organisms based on generation. Excellent activity against Enterobacteriaceae (such as *E. coli*). Moderate activity against *Enterococcus* species for systemic infections, but the high urinary concentrations are adequate to successfully eradicate the organism in UTIs. Moxifloxacin and gatifloxacin have expanded spectrums of activity that include improved gram-positive (*S. pneumoniae*) and anaerobic activity (*Bacteroides fragilis*).	Gram-positive organisms, particularly *Staphylococcus aureus* Gram-negative organisms: *Haemophilus influenzae*, *E. coli*, *Listeria monocytogenes*, *Moraxella catarrhalis*, and *Salmonella* species Other organisms: *Pneumocystis carinii*, *Toxoplasma gondii*, *Nocardia* species, and *Stenotrophomonas maltophilia*
Pharmacokinetics		
Absorption	High Ciprofloxacin < levofloxacin = gatifloxacin = moxifloxacin	High (PO dose equivalent to IV)
Distribution	Wide distribution into body fluids and tissues including the prostate	
Metabolism	Hepatic Ciprofloxacin = moxifloxacin > levofloxacin = gatifloxacin	Hepatic
Elimination	Renal Gatifloxacin = levofloxacin > ciprofloxacin > moxifloxacin	Renal elimination as metabolites and unchanged drug
Adverse effects	Well tolerated Common adverse effects: CNS side effects (dizziness, headache, insomnia), rash, nausea, vomiting, photosensitivity, elevated transaminases, and tremor. Rare side effects: cartilage toxicity, tendon rupture, and QT_c prolongation. An increase in QT_c prolongation and torsade de pointes has been associated with the use of fluoroquinolones, particularly the newer generations.	Well tolerated Common adverse effects: rash, nausea, vomiting, and photosensitivity. Rare: hepatotoxicity (increased transaminases), anemia, leukopenia, and Stevens-Johnson syndrome. TMP-SMX should be used with caution in patients with G6PD deficiency since this can cause hemolytic anemia.
Drug interactions	Cytochrome interactions: CYP450 inhibitors Norfloxacin > ciprofloxacin > moxifloxacin > levofloxacin = gatifloxacin. Warfarin: The exact warfarin-quinolone drug interaction is unknown. Reduction of intestinal flora responsible for vitamin K production by antibiotics is probable, as are decreased metabolism and clearance of warfarin due to CYP450 inhibition by the quinolones. Multivalent cations such as aluminum, magnesium, calcium, iron, zinc, and multivitamins with minerals may chelate with fluoroquinolones and decrease the oral absorption if administered concurrently.	TMP-SMX is a known inhibitor of CYP450 and can substantially increase warfarin plasma concentrations and hypopro-thrombinemic response.

Questions

1. HG is a 65-year-old man diagnosed with acute prostatitis. He has an allergy to sulfa drugs, which gives him urticaria. Which of the following agents would be the most appropriate option for treatment of his prostatitis?
   A. Cephalexin
   B. TMP-SMX
   C. Ciprofloxacin
   D. Amoxicillin
   E. Nitrofurantoin

2. JP is a 35-year-old woman who presents with an uncomplicated UTI. She has a history of cardiac arrhythmias for which she takes amiodarone and digoxin. Her allergies include anaphylaxis to sulfa medications. Which of the following medications would be the best choice to treat her UTI?
   A. Gatifloxacin
   B. Moxifloxacin
   C. TMP-SMX
   D. TMP

HPI: After 2 days of treatment for her UTI, LD now returns to the clinic complaining of chills, fever, nausea, flank pain, and increased lower tract symptoms (frequency, dysuria, and urgency).

Thought Questions

■ What are the most likely organisms to be causing LD's pyelonephritis?

■ What are appropriate antibiotics that can be used for the treatment of pyelonephritis?

■ What toxicities are associated with aminoglycosides?

■ What dosing regimens are available for aminoglycosides?

Basic Science Review and Discussion

The infecting organisms causing pyelonephritis are typically similar to the infecting pathogens responsible for lower UTIs. In uncomplicated cases, antibiotics used for treatment of lower tract infections also can be used for the treatment of upper tract infections. These agents typically include fluoroquinolones and TMP-SMX. In more serious cases, pyelonephritis may be accompanied by bacteremia, warranting hospitalization and parenteral therapy.

Aminoglycosides are parenteral antibiotics most widely used in the treatment of infections due to enteric gram-negative bacteria. However, aminoglycosides are often used in combination with cell wall–active agents such as beta-lactams or vancomycin for treatment of endocarditis. Aminoglycosides initially diffuse passively across the bacterial outer membrane and are then actively transported into the cytoplasm. This active transport is inhibited in low pH or anaerobic conditions. Once inside the cytoplasm, aminoglycosides inhibit protein synthesis by binding to the bacterial 30S ribosomal subunit and preventing the formation of the initiation complex and interfering with the accuracy of translation and translocation. Because aminoglycosides are inhibited in acidic or anaerobic conditions, aminoglycosides are not active against anaerobic bacteria or in low pH conditions such as abscesses or necrotic tissue.

Aminoglycosides are most notably associated with **ototoxicity** and **nephrotoxicity** and have a narrow therapeutic window. Risk factors include prolonged therapy, preexisting renal dysfunction, elderly patients, and concurrent use of other ototoxic or nephrotoxic agents. Ototoxicity typically presents as cochlear (tinnitus, high-frequency hearing loss) and, not as commonly, vestibular toxicity (vertigo, ataxia). Nephrotoxicity due to aminoglycosides typically presents as an increase in serum creatinine or a decrease in creatinine clearance. Rarely, in high doses, aminoglycosides can cause neuromuscular paralysis due to a concentration-dependent inhibition of presynaptic release and postsynaptic binding of acetylcholine. This can lead to tingling, muscle paralysis, and apnea.

There are two dosing regimens used for aminoglycosides: once daily and conventional (three times daily). Because aminoglycosides exhibit **concentration-dependent killing,** increasing concentrations kill an increasing proportion of bacteria. In addition, aminoglycosides exhibit a **postantibiotic effect**. Thus, antibacterial activity persists even when the drug falls below levels that are detectable in serum. By dosing aminoglycosides once daily, higher peak concentrations are achieved, leading to a more rapid bactericidal effect and longer postantibiotic effect. The less frequent dosing of once-daily aminoglycosides leads to lower or nondetectable trough concentrations and may lead to less nephrotoxicity.

Case Conclusion LD is admitted to the hospital for treatment of her pyelonephritis. On admission, blood and urine cultures are drawn and LD is empirically started on ampicillin and gentamicin for coverage for *Enterococcus* species and gram-negative organisms pending culture results. Parenteral therapy is used because LD is nauseated and is exhibiting signs of a systemic infection. Two days later, cultures return positive for *Escherichia coli.*

Thumbnail: Aminoglycosides

Available agents: Gentamicin, tobramycin, amikacin, streptomycin, neomycin

MOA: Irreversible protein synthesis inhibitor that binds to the 30S subunit of bacterial ribosomes. Prevents the formation of the initiation complex, interferes with the translational accuracy of the mRNA, and inhibits translocation.

Activity: Aerobic bacteria only. Primary activity is against aerobic gram-negative bacilli. Tobramycin is more active against *Pseudomonas aeruginosa*. Can be used in combination with cell wall-active agents for treatment of infections due to staphylococcal or enterococcal species. Streptomycin is used for infections due to mycobacteria.

Pharmacokinetics

Absorption: Poorly absorbed orally, thus limited to parenteral use. However, neomycin can be used for GI decontamination.

Distribution: Requires aerobic environment for activity. Effectiveness is reduced in low pH or anaerobic environments such as abscess fluid or necrotic tissue. Does not cross the blood-brain barrier. Treatment of CNS infections require intraventricular or intrathecal administration.

Elimination: Renal. Excretion occurs via glomerular filtration and is directly proportional to creatinine clearance. Dose adjustment is needed in renal impairment.

Adverse reactions: Irreversible ototoxicity (cochlear and vestibular) in 0.5% to 5% of patients. High-frequency hearing is affected first and can progress to low-frequency hearing loss. Reversible nephrotoxicity is seen in up to 25% of patients, particularly in patients receiving aminoglycosides for more than 7 days. Rarely, neuromuscular paralysis (curare-like effect) can occur.

Questions

1. KC is a 45-year-old man receiving ampicillin and gentamicin for endocarditis due to *Enterococcus faecalis*. He has a baseline serum Cr of 1.5 mg/dL secondary to uncontrolled diabetes mellitus. His other medications include furosemide, aspirin, and captopril. During his second week of therapy KC complains of ringing in his ears and a sensation of fullness. Risk factors for ototoxicity in KC include:

   A. Age
   B. Preexisting renal dysfunction
   C. Prolonged aminoglycoside therapy
   D. Furosemide
   E. Ampicillin
   F. Captopril
   G. A, B, C
   H. B, C, D
   I. All of the above

2. CJ is a 7-year-old boy with neuroblastoma receiving chemotherapy. He is currently neutropenic and is febrile at 38.2°C. His physicians would like to empirically cover him for *Pseudomonas aeruginosa* with two agents and he is started on cefepime and an aminoglycoside. Which aminoglycoside would be the best choice?

   A. Gentamicin
   B. Streptomycin
   C. Tobramycin
   D. Amikacin
   E. Neomycin

HPI: KS is a 25-year-old woman with ALL who presents to the oncology clinic complaining that she has had fevers and chills for the past day. KM receives chemotherapy via a peripherally inserted central catheter (PICC) inserted in her left antecubital vein, last dose 3 weeks ago.

PE: Vitals: T 39.6°C, BP 100/60 mm Hg, HR 110 beats/min, RR 20 breaths/min; lungs are clear. Her PICC site appears hot and erythematous.

Labs: WBC 3500/mm^3, Hgb 14 gm/dL, Hct 40%, Plt 178,000/mm^3, Cr 0.7 mg/dL, BUN 20 mg/dL.

Thought Questions

- What is the most likely organism to cause a catheter-related infection in KM?

- What are common side effects of vancomycin?

- How is toxicity or efficacy of vancomycin assessed?

Basic Science Review and Discussion

Coagulase-negative staphylococci, such as *Staphylococcus epidermidis,* are the most common causes of catheter-related infections due to their ability to adhere to prosthetic material. *Staphylococcus aureus,* aerobic gram-negative bacilli, and *Candida albicans* are also common causes of catheter-related infections. Depending on local susceptibility patterns, methicillin-resistant *S. aureus* (MRSA) may represent up to 20% of all isolates. In contrast, upward of 80% of *S. epidermidis* are methicillin-resistant (MRSE).

In the past, side effects attributed to vancomycin were most likely due to impurities in the earlier preparations. Today, the majority of side effects due to vancomycin are minor and include "**red man**" or "**red neck**" syndrome, rash, or chemical **phlebitis** at the infusion site. The poten-

tial for vancomycin to cause **nephrotoxocity** and **ototoxicity** remains controversial. Early reports of vancomycin-induced nephrotoxocity and ototoxicity may be exaggerated. In patients who receive vancomycin alone, nephrotoxicity and ototoxicity appears to be rare. However, nephro-toxocity can be enhanced when given in combination with an agent known to cause nephrotoxocity such as an aminoglycoside. Similarly, ototoxicity can occur when vancomycin is given in combination with a known ototoxic agent such as erythromycin or an aminoglycoside. When given for prolonged periods, vancomycin can cause **neu-tropenia** in rare cases.

Serum monitoring of vancomycin levels should be done in patients receiving prolonged courses of vancomycin, partic-ularly in the setting of preexisting renal insufficiency. However, elevated trough levels have been poorly corre-lated with the development of nephrotoxocity. Similarly, a relationship between vancomycin levels and ototoxocitiy has not been well established. Trough levels are typically used to evaluate efficacy, because vancomycin exhibits **time-dependent killing.** Therapeutic trough levels range from 5 to 15 μg/mL. Higher trough levels may be indicated in the setting of meningitis, due to poor penetration across the blood-brain barrier. In general, peak concentrations are not routinely measured.

Case Conclusion KM is admitted to the hospital and two sets of blood cultures are drawn. Vancomycin is started empirically. The next day, the 2/2 blood cultures return positive for MRSE. KS is continued on vancomycin for 10 days.

Thumbnail: Vancomycin

Clinical usage: Intravenous vancomycin is primarily indicated for the treatment of infections such as sepsis and endocarditis, due to methicillin-resistant staphylococci and meningitis secondary to penicillin-resistant *Streptococcus pneumoniae*. Vancomycin is also indicated in patients with hypersensitivity reactions to beta-lactams. Oral vancomycin is used for the treatment of antibiotic-associated colitis secondary to *Clostridium difficile*.

MOA: Glycopeptide antibiotic that inhibits cell wall synthesis by binding to the D-Ala-D-Ala terminus of the peptidoglycan pentapeptide. This prevents elongation and cross-linking of the cell wall, leading to the inability to form a rigid cell wall, and ultimately, cell lysis. Vancomycin exhibits time-dependent killing.

Activity: Vancomycin is bactericidal against most gram-positive organisms such as streptococci and staphylococci (including those that are methicillin resistant). Vancomycin is bacteriostatic against *Enterococcus* species, and is usually given in combination with an aminoglycoside to achieve a bactericidal effect. Other bacteria include gram-positive bacilli such as *Bacillus* species, corynebacteria, and *Lactobacillus,* and most *Clostridium* species, including *Clostridium difficile*.

Pharmacokinetics

Absorption: Vancomycin is poorly absorbed orally; thus, oral vancomycin is used only for the treatment of antibiotic-associated enterocolitis due to *Clostridium difficile*.

Distribution: Vancomycin is widely distributed. Vancomycin penetrates poorly into CSF. However, in the presence of inflamed meninges, CSF vancomycin concentrations range from 7% to 21% of simultaneous serum concentrations.

Elimination: 85% to 90% of vancomycin is excreted unchanged in the urine. Dose adjustments are necessary in the setting of renal dysfunction. The T½ of vancomycin ranges from 5 to 10 hours, and is prolonged in patients with renal insufficiency. In patients with end-stage renal disease, the T½ can approach 7 days.

Therapeutic range: Recommended trough concentrations range from 5 to 15 µg/mL. Recommended peak concentrations range from 20 to 50 µg/mL, although it is not routinely recommended to check peak levels.

Adverse reactions: Although long thought to be nephrotoxic and ototoxic, the incidence of nephrotoxicity and ototoxicity secondary to vancomycin is rare, yet may occur when given in combination with other nephrotoxic or ototoxic agents. Peak levels of greater than 60 to 80 µg/mL may be associated with an increased risk of ototoxicity. Flushing, rash, and hypotension (i.e., red man syndrome), may occur during IV infusion and is mediated by histamine.

Questions

1. TM is a 56-year-old man who is dialysis dependent secondary to diabetes mellitus. Upon arrival for his thrice-weekly hemodialysis, TM is found to be febrile to 39°C. TM has NKDA. Which of the following is the best course of treatment for TM?

   A. Draw two sets of blood cultures and wait for culture results.
   B. Draw two sets of blood cultures and start nafcillin IV.
   C. Draw two sets of blood cultures and start vancomycin IV.
   D. Start vancomycin PO.
   E. Start vancomycin IV.
   F. A and C.
   G. A and D.

2. TM is given a single dose of vancomycin. Ten minutes into the infusion, TM's blood pressure suddenly drops to 80/60 mm Hg, and he feels "hot and flushed." What is the best course of action for TM's "red man syndrome"?

   A. Discontinue the infusion, start nafcillin.
   B. Discontinue the infusion, give vancomycin PO.
   C. Slow down the rate of infusion.
   D. Give diphenhydramine.
   E. Give epinephrine.
   F. C and D.
   G. D and E.

HPI: While on duty, FD, a 42-year-old policeman, sustains a gunshot wound to the stomach and colon. He is admitted to the hospital and within 1 hour he undergoes an emergency laparotomy. During surgery there is spillage of gastrointestinal contents into his peritoneal cavity.

PE: Vitals: BP 90/65 mm Hg, HR 100 beats/min, T 39.7°C, WBC 20,000/mm³. Allergy: anaphylaxis to penicillin.

Thought Questions

- Which bacteria should be considered as potential pathogens in intra-abdominal infections?

- What are the common adverse effects associated with metronidazole and clindamycin?

Basic Science Review and Discussion

Normal GI flora sparsely populate the stomach, whereas the large bowel contains a high bacterial inoculum of *Bacteroides* species, particularly *Bacteroides fragilis* and gram-negative organisms such as *Escherichia coli, Klebsiella,* and *Enterobacter* species. Since the colon has significantly more bacteria than the stomach, it is much more likely to be associated with infections if ruptured. Thus, *B. fragilis* is the most common anaerobe isolated, and *E. coli, Klebsiella,* and *Enterobacter* are the most common gram-negative bacteria associated with intra-abdominal infections.

Metronidazole and clindamycin are **protein synthesis inhibitors** that inhibit bacteria by interacting with the DNA to cause a loss of helical DNA structure and strand breakage. This results in inhibition of protein synthesis and cell death. Metronidazole and clindamycin are commonly used in the treatment of intra-abdominal infections. Metronidazole has excellent activity against gram-negative anaerobes, whereas clindamycin has activity against both gram-positive and gram-negative anaerobes. The expression, "clindamycin for above the belt and metronidazole for below the belt" highlights the fact that metronidazole does not have good activity against gram-positive anaerobes found in the mouth, whereas clindamycin does. Metronidazole is also an antiprotozoan drug, and is the treatment of choice for amebiasis, giardiasis, and trichomoniasis. The most troublesome side effect associated with metronidazole is GI intolerance. Metronidazole can cause a **disulfiram-like** reaction in patients who consume ethanol, due to inhibition of aldehyde dehydrogenase.

The most notable adverse effect associated with clindamycin is **antibiotic-associated colitis** secondary to toxigenic *Clostridium difficile*. This organism usually overgrows in the GI tract in the presence of antibiotics due to the inhibition of normal GI flora. Ironically, the drug of choice for the treatment of antibiotic-associated colitis is metronidazole. Clindamycin also can cause diarrhea that is not related to *C. difficile*.

Case Conclusion Because the etiology of intra-abdominal infections is most often polymicrobial (gram-negative and anaerobic bacteria) and the patient has an allergy to penicillin, FD can be treated empirically with tobramycin and metronidazole or clindamycin. This regimen provides adequate empiric coverage of the most noteworthy pathogens associated with intra-abdominal infections.

Thumbnail: Antianaerobic Agents

	Metronidazole	Clindamycin
MOA	Inhibits bacteria by interacting with the DNA to cause a loss of helical DNA structure and strand breakage, resulting in inhibition of protein synthesis and cell death	Reversibly binds to 50S ribosomal subunits, thereby inhibiting bacterial protein synthesis
Activity	*Bacteroides* species, *Clostridium difficile*, *Clostridium perfringens*, *Gardnerella vaginalis* (a common cause of bacterial vaginosis in women), *Trichomonas vaginalis*, *Entamoeba histolytica*, *Giardia lamblia*, *Helicobacter pylori*	*Bacteroides* species, *Streptococcus* species, *Staphylococcus aureus* (not MRSA), anaerobic streptococci (i.e., peptostreptococcus), *Clostridium perfringens*. Other noteworthy pathogens: *Pneumocystis carinii*, *Toxoplasma gondii*.
Pharmacokinetics		
Bioavailability	High	Moderate absorption (70%)
Distribution	Widely distributed. Readily crosses the blood-brain barrier	Widely distributed. Minimal levels achieved in CSF
Elimination	Hepatic	Hepatic
Adverse effects	Metallic taste, anorexia, nausea, vomiting (administering with food or milk can reduce GI side effects). Neurologic: vertigo, headache. Dark urine due to azo metabolite in some patients.	Diarrhea, nausea and vomiting (2%–20%). Pseudomembranous colitis (0.1%–10%) is a result of *C. difficile* overgrowth in the stool.
Drug interactions	Can cause a disulfiram-like reaction in patients who concomitantly consume ethanol due to inhibition of aldehyde dehydrogenase. Metronidazole prolongs the prothrombin time in patients taking warfarin.	No clinically significant drug interactions

Questions

1. MB is a 39-year-old man who is diagnosed with cellulitis. Since he has an allergy to penicillins (urticarial rash), he is prescribed clindamycin for 10 days. Nine days into therapy he develops diarrhea. A stool culture detects *C. difficile* toxin. What is the best treatment for MB's diarrhea?

   A. Cefotetan
   B. Metronidazole
   C. No treatment necessary
   D. Oral vancomycin
   E. Penicillin

2. GQ is 33-year-old alcoholic who is placed on metronidazole, clarithromycin, and omeprazole for a recently diagnosed peptic ulcer. A urease breath test is positive for *H. pylori*. His other medications include ibuprofen, lisinopril, and meclizine. Which of the following is most likely to interact with GQ's metronidazole?

   A. Omeprazole
   B. Ibuprofen
   C. Alcohol
   D. Meclizine
   E. None of the above

HPI: BB is a 21-year-old female nursing student who presents to her primary care physician with a 24-hour history of fever to 102°F, headache, myalgia, and sore throat. She notes that her roommate has had "flu-like" symptoms for the past 2 days and she thinks she is coming down with the same symptoms. BB states she has finals next week and cannot afford to get sick at this time. Her PMH is significant for mild asthma and seizures. Her medications include phenytoin, albuterol inhaler, ibuprofen, and birth control pills.

Note: Influenza surveillance this year in the area shows a predominance of influenza B virus.

Thought Questions

- What is the best means for preventing influenza?

- Which agents are active against influenza B virus?

- When is the ideal time for therapy to be initiated?

- How do amantadine and rimantadine differ with regard to renal elimination and potential for CNS toxicity?

Basic Science Review and Discussion

Influenza is characterized by the abrupt onset of constitutional and respiratory signs and symptoms such as fever, myalgia, headache, severe malaise, nonproductive cough, sore throat, and rhinitis. In the United States, influenza is responsible for approximately 20,000 deaths annually.

Immunoprophylaxis with inactivated vaccine remains the principal means for reducing influenza-related morbidity and death. Although the vaccine provides the best protection against influenza, there are four antiviral agents that are used to prevent or treat influenza: amantadine, rimantadine, zanamivir, and oseltamivir. To shorten the duration of influenza symptoms, all agents should be initiated within 2 days of onset of symptoms.

Amantadine and rimantadine are chemically related antiviral drugs active against influenza A but not influenza B viruses. Amantadine differs from rimantadine because it is primarily renally eliminated and is associated with more CNS side effects and can potentially lower the seizure threshold.

Zanamivir and oseltamivir are **neuraminidase inhibitors** that are active against influenza A and B viruses.

Case Conclusion   BB was started on oseltamivir since the neuraminidase inhibitors also have activity against influenza B, unlike amantadine and rimantadine. Also, with her seizure history, amantadine would not be an option because it may lower the seizure threshold. Her symptoms resolve 2 days sooner than her roommate's, and her finals go smoothly.

Thumbnail: Agents for Influenza

	Available agents			
	Amantadine	Rimantadine	Neuraminidase inhibitors	
			Zanamivir	Oseltamivir
Clinical usage	Prophylaxis or symptomatic treatment of influenza A Parkinson's disease Drug-induced extrapyramidal reactions		Prophylaxis or symptomatic treatment of influenza A and B	
Route of administration	Oral	Oral	Oral inhalation	Oral
MOA	Antiviral: Mechanism not fully understood—appears to block the viral uncoating of influenza. Antiparkinson: Mechanism not fully understood—appears to increase dopamine release, block dopamine reuptake, and stimulate dopamine receptors.		Antiviral: Neuraminidase inhibitors are analogues of sialic acid. Proposed mechanism of action is to block the active site of neuraminidase to produce uncleaved sialic acid residues. This results in viral aggregation at the host cell surface and a reduction in the amount of virus that is released from the infected cell.	
Activity	Influenza A virus	Influenza A virus	Influenza A and B viruses	Influenza A and B viruses
Pharmacokinetics				
Absorption	Well absorbed from the GI tract		4%–17% inhaled dose absorbed systemically	75% oral dose absorbed systemically
Distribution	Wide distribution throughout the body and crosses the blood–brain barrier		Wide distribution	Wide distribution
Metabolism	Minimal	Extensive hepatic	None	Converted to oseltamivir carboxylate by hepatic esterases
Elimination	90% renal Dose adjust for renal dysfunction	< 25% excreted in urine	All systemically absorbed drug renally eliminated	renal
Adverse reactions	CNS: dizziness, irritability, insomnia, fatigue, headache Increased seizure activity with amantadine GI: dry mouth, abdominal pain CV: orthostatic hypotension, peripheral edema, heart failure		Zanamivir: diarrhea, nausea, sinusitis, nasal signs and symptoms, bronchitis, cough	Oseltamivir: nausea, vomiting, diarrhea
Comments	Amantadine requires dose adjustment in **renal insufficiency** but rimantadine does not. Amantadine has increased **CNS toxicity** in the elderly compared to rimantadine.			

Questions

1. AK is an 80-year-old woman who presents to her physician after a 36-hour history of fever, chills, and myalgias. She is diagnosed with influenza B. Her PMH is significant for chronic renal insufficiency (CrCl ~15 mL/min) and hypertension. Which of the following would be considered the most appropriate therapy for her symptoms?

    A. Amantadine
    B. Rimantadine
    C. No agent can be used since it needs to be started within 24 hours
    D. Oseltamivir
    E. Influenza vaccine

2. CD is a 70-year-old man who resides in a nursing home. His PMH is significant for Parkinson's disease and COPD. His medications include carbidopa/levodopa, and amantadine, as well as ipratropium, albuterol, and triamcinolone inhalers. One of the residents is diagnosed with influenza A and all the residents now require prophylaxis for influenza A with rimantadine. Which of the following would be the most appropriate therapy for prevention of influenza A in CD?

    A. Continue amantadine
    B. Discontinue amantadine, add rimantadine
    C. Start zanamivir
    D. Start rimantadine
    E. A and C
    F. A and D

HPI: SL is a 35-year-old female lawyer who is complaining of itching and burning in her genital area. She states that she has had these symptoms in the past, particularly when she is under a lot of stress.

Thought Questions

- What is the difference between primary herpes and recurrent herpes?

- When should therapy for genital herpes be started?

- What is the MOA of acyclovir?

- Which of the antiviral agents are active against herpes simplex virus (HSV)?

Basic Sciences Review and Discussion

Herpes simplex virus is divided into HSV-1 and HSV-2. Genital herpes is usually caused by HSV-2, whereas oral herpes is caused by HSV-1. **Primary herpes** refers to the first outbreak of infection, whereas **recurrent herpes** refers to subsequent infections. With each outbreak, patients typically experience symptoms 2 to 10 days after the initial infection. Symptoms may include a "prodrome" of burning or itching, followed by the appearance of blisters and open sores within a few days. Other symptoms such as fever, headache, muscle aches, painful urination, or vaginal discharge are also common. In general, recurrent outbreaks are usually mild and shorter in duration.

Because viral replication occurs prior to the onset of symptoms, initiation of early therapy is imperative for optimum clinical efficacy. Thus, treatment must be initiated at the first signs and symptoms of infection, typically during the prodrome period.

Acyclovir is an acyclic guanosine derivative that requires three phosphorylation steps for activation. Conversion to the monophosphate is carried out by the virus thymidine kinase, and conversion to the di- and triphosphate is carried out by host kineases. The active nucleotide triphosphate inhibits viral replication by competing with the viral deoxy-GTP for the viral DNA polymerase. Thus, acyclovir triphosphate is inserted into the growing viral DNA, leading to irreversible chain termination. Reduced susceptibility to acyclovir is due to altered viral thymidine kinase. Because the MOA of ganciclovir is similar to that of acyclovir, HSV that is resistant to acyclovir is also resistant to ganciclovir.

Although acyclovir is considered the drug of choice for the treatment of HSV infection, ganciclovir, foscarnet, and cidofovir also have in vitro activity against HSV, but these agents are most commonly used for the treatment of infections due to cytomegalovirus (CMV). Valacyclovir is the L-valyl ester of acyclovir and was developed to overcome the poor bioavailability of acyclovir. Famciclovir is the ester prodrug of penciclovir, an acyclovir analogue. Although the serum $T\frac{1}{2}$ of penciclovir is similar to that of acyclovir, the intracellular $T\frac{1}{2}$ of penciclovir is extended. Penciclovir is not available as an oral agent, but only as a cream.

Case Conclusion   SL is experiencing a recurrent genital herpes outbreak. The treatment of choice is either acyclovir or one of the acyclovir analogues. The duration of symptoms may be shortened because SL was able to identify and seek treatment for her outbreak early.

Thumbnail: Antiviral Agents for Herpes Viruses

	Acyclovir	Ganciclovir	Foscarnet	Cidofovir
MOA	Monophosphorylation by viral kinases and di- and triphosphorylation via host kinases; inhibition of viral DNA polymerase; insertion into forming DNA, leading to chain termination.		Inorganic pyrophosphate compound that inhibits viral DNA and RNA polymerase. Does not require phosphorylation for activity.	Cystosine nucleotide analogue diphosphorylated by cellular kinases; inhibition of viral DNA polymerase, insertion into forming DNA, leading to chain termination.
Activity	HSV-1, HSV-2, varicella zoster virus (VZV). Weak activity against Epstein-Barr virus (EBV), CMV.	HSV-1, HSV-2, VZV, CMV, EBV, human herpes virus (HHV)-8.	HSV-1, HSV-2, VZV, CMV, EBV, HHV-6, HHV-8. May be used for treatment of resistant HSV or CMV.	
Pharmacokinetics				
Absorption	Poor oral absorption (10%–30%)	Poor oral absorption (5%)	IV only	IV and intravitreal
Distribution	All medications distribute widely, including CSF			
Elimination	Renal, via glomerular filtration and tubular secretion. Dose adjustment needed in renal insufficiency.			
T½	3–4 hr	2–4 hr	6–8 hr	2 hr; intracellular T½ 17–60 hr
Adverse reactions	Thrombophlebitis from IV administration, headache, crystal nephropathy, concentration-dependent neurotoxicity (lethargy, coma, seizure, tremor, hallucinations).	Bone marrow suppression: neutropenia (40%), thrombocytopenia, anemia, GI symptoms with oral formulation, teratogenic, carcinogenic.	Thrombophlebitis, nephro-toxicity (acute tubular necrosis, crystalluria, interstitial nephritis), anemia, electrolyte disturbances ($\downarrow Ca^{2+}$, $\downarrow Mg^{2+}$, $\uparrow/\downarrow PO_4^{3-}$), neurotoxicity.	Nephrotoxicity, teratogenic, carcinogenic. With intraocular adminis-tration: hypotony, iritis, vitritis.
Comments	Valacyclovir, famciclovir formulated to improve bioavailability. Penciclovir only available topically.	Oral valganciclovir formulated to improve bioavailability.	Risk factors for nephrotoxicity include dehydration, high doses, rapid infusion.	IV prehydration and administration with probenicid necessary to prevent nephrotoxicity.

Questions

1. SL is a 34-year-old HIV positive man with CMV who is receiving his second week of induction therapy with ganciclovir. His current labs are Cr 1.8 mg/dL (previously 1.0 mg/dL), WBC 800/mm³, platelets 89,000/mm³. How would you treat SL?

   A. Decrease the dose of ganciclovir
   B. Administer filgrastim
   C. Discontinue ganciclovir and switch to cidofovir
   D. Discontinue ganciclovir and switch to foscarnet
   E. A and B
   F. B and C
   G. C and D

2. LY is a 32-year-old woman s/p liver transplantation who is started on foscarnet for treatment of ganciclovir-resistant CMV. Side effects of foscarnet include:

   A. Hypocalcemia
   B. Hyperphosphatemia
   C. Hypophosphatemia
   D. Thrombophlebitis
   E. Acute tubular necrosis
   F. All of the above

HPI: CJ is a 32-year-old man with acquired immunodeficiency syndrome (AIDS) (CD4$^+$ cell count 160 cells/mm^3, viral load 35,000 copies/mL) who presents to the clinic with altered taste sensation and difficulty swallowing. CJ is noted to have white plaques on the tongue and upper oral pharynx that are easily scraped off with a tongue depressor. PMH is significant for renal insufficiency secondary to his HIV. His antiretroviral regimen includes stavudine, lamivudine, and lopinavir/ritonavir and he is receiving TMP-SMX for *Pneumocystis carinii* pneumonia (PCP) prophylaxis. He has NKDA.

Labs: Cr 2.0 mg/dL, BUN 43 mg/dL.

Thought Questions

■ What are risk factors for developing candidal infections?

■ What are options for the treatment of CJ's esophageal candidiasis?

■ What are the pharmacologic differences among the azole antifungals?

■ What are the toxicities associated with amphotericin B?

Basic Science Review and Discussion

Candida organisms are common inhabitants of the GI tract, skin, and female genital tract. Patients at risk for invasive candidal infections include those who are immunocompromised or diabetic. Iatrogenic risk factors, such as prolonged hospitalization, use of in-dwelling catheters, parenteral nutrition, and antibiotics have all been identified as risk factors for developing candidiasis. In patients infected with HIV, the rate of candidal infections increases as the CD4$^+$ lymphocyte count decreases. Since the introduction of highly active antiretroviral therapy (HAART), the incidence of opportunistic infections in patients with HIV has significantly declined.

The two main classes of systemic antifungals that are used in the treatment of candidiasis are **azoles** and **amphotericin**

B. Azole antifungals include systemic agents such as ketoconazole, fluconazole, itraconazole, and voriconazole. Topical agents used for the treatment of vaginal candidiasis and thrush include miconazole and clotrimazole. The pharmacologic properties of the systemic azoles differ considerably. Ketoconazole, the first oral azole developed, has poor bioavailability and requires an acidic environment for enhanced absorption. Thus, initial studies required ketoconazole to be administered with a cola to increase bioavailability. Fluconazole, unlike itraconazole and ketoconazole, is hydrophillic and has increased penetration across the blood-brain barrier. Fluconazole is also the only azole that is renally eliminated.

Amphotericin B, sometimes referred to as "amphoterrible," is associated with multiple **infusion-related reactions** and adverse effects on the kidneys. Chills, rigors, fevers, and hypotension are common during amphotericin administration. Thus, patients are typically premedicated with diphenhydramine and acetaminophen or NSAIDs prior to infusion. Meperidine can be given in response to rigors. Renal toxicity is also commonly associated with amphotericin and can be irreversible. Renal toxicity may present as azotemia, renal tubular acidosis, or electrolyte wasting. Almost all patients receiving amphotericin will experience some degree of renal insufficiency.

Case Conclusion   Because esophageal candidiasis is most often attributable to *Candida albicans,* CJ can be given either IV amphotericin or an azole antifungal. However, itraconazole, ketoconazole, and voriconazole are potent CYP450 inhibitors and will thus interact with his protease inhibitors. Amphotericin B is also not a good choice due to his preexisting renal insufficiency. Fluconazole is chosen for treatment of his esophageal candidiasis because it is less likely to interact with his protease inhibitors and will not negatively impact his renal function.

Thumbnail: Antifungal Agents

	Azoles		Amphotericin B
Available agents	Systemic: Ketoconazole Itraconazole Fluconazole Voriconazole	Topical: Butaconazole Clotrimazole Econazole Ketoconazole Miconazole Terconazole	Lipid-based formulations created to attenuate the renal toxicity associated with conventional amphotericin B
MOA	Inhibition of ergosterol synthesis by binding to fungal CYP450. **Fungistatic.**		Binds to ergosterol, altering fungal cell membrane permeability, leading to cell lysis. **Fungicidal.**
Activity	*Candida* species, *Cryptococcus neoformans*, *Blastomyces dermatitidis*, *Coccidioides immitis*, dermatophytes. Itraconazole and voriconazole are the only azoles active against *Aspergillus* species.		*Candida* species (except *C. lusinatia*), *Cryptococcus neoformans*, *Histoplasma capsulatum*, *Blastomyces dermatitidis*, *Coccidioides immitis*. Molds include *Aspergillus* species and mucor.
Pharmacokinetics			
Bioavailability	Ketoconazole: low Itraconazole: low Fluconazole: high Voriconazole: high		Poorly absorbed; IV only
Distribution	Widely distributed. Fluconazole readily crosses the blood–brain barrier.		Widely distributed; minimal levels achieved in CSF.
Elimination	Ketoconazole, itraconazole, voriconazole: hepatic Fluconazole: renal		Minimal excretion in the urine
Adverse reactions	All azoles can cause GI upset and hepatotoxicity. Ketoconazole can cause gynecomastia and oligospermia in men and menstrual irregularities in women due to inhibition of gonadal steroid production. Voriconazole can cause reversible visual disturbances such as blurred vision, photophobia, altered color perception, and enhanced light perception. Most common during 1st month of therapy. Photosensitivity can occur with long-term use.		Renal dysfunction common. Electrolyte wasting, including hypokalemia, hypomagnemesia. Infusion-related toxicities include fever, chills, and rigors and hypotension.
Drug interactions	Ketoconazole and itraconazole absorption decreased with agents that increase gastric pH. All azoles are CYP450 inhibitors and can increase serum levels of drugs metabolized through this pathway. Voriconazole > itraconazole = ketoconazole >> fluconazole.		Increased renal toxicity used in combination with other nephrotoxic agents such as cyclosporine, tacrolimus, or aminoglycosides.

Questions

1. PJ is a 23-year-old man with ALL hospitalized for induction chemotherapy. He is scheduled to receive amphotericin B tonight as part of his prophylactic regimen against opportunistic infections. His premedications for amphotericin should include the following:

   A. Diphenhydramine
   B. Acetaminophen
   C. Meperidine
   D. 1 liter of normal saline
   E. A and B only
   F. A, B, and C
   G. A, B, and D
   H. All of the above

2. GM is a 43-year-old woman with poorly controlled insulin-dependent diabetes mellitus. She is complaining of vaginal itching and a thick, "cottage cheese"-appearing vaginal discharge. Her PMH includes gastroesophageal reflux disease, for which she is taking omeprazole. What is the best treatment for GM's vulvovaginal candidiasis?

   A. Ketoconazole
   B. Clotrimazole
   C. Itraconazole
   D. Amphotericin
   E. No treatment necessary

HPI: KC is a 50-year-old Mexican man who presents to the clinic with upper right quadrant pain and dark-colored urine. KC recently began antitubercular therapy 4 weeks ago for pulmonary *Mycobacterium tuberculosis* (MTB). He has no other significant PMH. Medications: Rifampin, isoniazid, ethambutol, and pyrazinamide.

Labs: AST 450 IU/L, ALT 368 IU/L, total bilirubin 4.1 mg/dL.

Thought Questions

- Which agents are considered first-line therapy for TB?

- Which agents cause clinically significant drug interactions?

- What are the primary side effects of each first-line agent?

Basic Science Discussion and Review

Tuberculosis (TB) may be caused by one of three mycobacterial organisms: MTB, *Mycobacterium bovis,* or *M. africanum.* The vast majority of MTB cases throughout the world are due to *M. tuberculosis.*

The agents most commonly used for the treatment of active MTB are **isoniazid, rifampin, pyrazinamide,** and **ethambutol.** Usually a four-drug regimen consisting of these first-line agents is preferred for the initial empiric treatment of MTB. When drug susceptibilities are known, the regimen should be tailored based on the results. Resistance develops rapidly with monotherapy; thus, multiple agents are used. Many of these drugs have significant drug-drug interactions, so it is always important to take a complete medication history. Rifampin is a potent inducer of CYP450 and isoniazid is an inhibitor of CYP450.

Side effects caused by isoniazid, rifampin, pyrazinamide, and ethambutol are common and can include **hepatotoxicity, peripheral neuropathy, optic neuritis,** and GI side effects. All four agents can potentially be hepatotoxic, but this side effect is most frequently associated with isoniazid and rifampin. Peripheral neuropathy is most commonly associated with isoniazid, whereas optic neuritis is associated with ethambutol. The metabolism of isoniazid is genetically predetermined. Patients of Scandinavian, European, and African descent metabolize isoniazid slower (slow acetylators) and are therefore more predisposed to hepatotoxicity and peripheral neuropathy due to isoniazid. Fast acetylators include people of Asian or American Indian descent and are less predisposed to these adverse effects.

Case Conclusion KC was diagnosed with hepatitis and all his medications were discontinued. After 7 days, his LFTs and bilirubin returned to normal. To determine which one of his medications was causing his hepatotoxicity, each medication was restarted one at a time with close monitoring of his LFTs. On rechallenge with isoniazid, KC experienced a similar increase in LFTs and was diagnosed with isoniazid-induced hepatitis. Because KC's MTB was highly susceptible, KC was successfully treated with a three-drug regimen of pyrazinamide, rifampin, and ethambutol.

Thumbnail: Agents for Tuberculosis

	Isoniazid	Rifampin	Pyrazinamide	Ethambutol
Clinical usage	Active MTB Latent TB infection	Active MTB Latent TB infection Eliminating meningococci from asymptomatic carriers Postexposure prophylaxis of *Haemophilus influenzae* type B Treatment of staphylococcal infections	Active MTB	Active MTB
MOA	Interferes with mycolic acid synthesis, a component of the mycobacterial cell wall Bactericidal	Inhibits bacterial RNA synthesis by binding to the beta subunit of DNA-dependent RNA polymerase Bactericidal	Exact mechanism unknown Converted to pyrazinoic acid in susceptible strains of MTB, which lowers the pH of the environment Requires an acidic pH for activity Bactericidal	Interferes with RNA synthesis and mycolic acid incorporation into the cell wall Bacteriostatic
Activity	MTB *M. bovis* *M. kansasii*	MTB *M. leprae* *Mycobacterium bovis* *M. kansasii* *Haemophilus* species *Neisseria* species *Brucella* species *Legionella pneumophilia* *Rhodococcus* species *S. aureus,* *S. epidermidis,* *S. pneumoniae* (only in combination with a cell wall-active agent)	MTB	MTB *M. avium-intracellulare* *M. bovis* *M. kansasii*
Pharmacokinetics				
Absorption	All well absorbed			
Distribution	All widely distributed, including CSF	All widely distributed		
Metabolism	Hepatic acetylation by *N*-acetyltransferase	Hepatic	Hepatic	Hepatic (20%)
Excretion	Renal	Enterohepatic recirculation Unchanged in feces (60%) Urine (30%)	Renal	Renal (50%) Feces (20%)
Adverse reactions	Nausea Vomiting Hepatotoxicity Peripheral neuropathy Hematologic side effects: agranulocytosis, aplastic anemia, thrombocytopenia	Nausea Vomiting Diarrhea Rash Hepatotoxicity Orange or red discoloration of sweat, tears, and urine	Nausea Vomiting Thrombocytopenia Rash Photosensitivity Hyperuricemia Hepatotoxicity	Nausea Vomiting Headache Peripheral neuropathy Thrombocytopenia Hepatotoxicity Retrobulbar neuritis leading to red-green color blindness and optic neuritis
Drug interactions	Inhibitor of hepatic CYP450	Substrate and potent inducer of hepatic CYP450		

Questions

1. A 62-year-old Chinese man is to be started on rifampin for treatment of his latent TB infection. His PMH is significant for HTN, CAD, and hypercholesterolemia. His current medications include metoprolol, diltiazem, aspirin, pravastatin, and nitroglycerin patches. Which of his current medications will most likely interact with rifampin?

   A. Metoprolol
   B. Pravastatin
   C. Aspirin
   D. Diltiazem
   E. Nitroglycerin

2. A 56-year-old man is currently on rifampin, ethambutol, and isoniazid for MTB for the past 3 weeks. His PMH is significant for diabetes and alcoholism. He is now complaining of a burning sensation in his feet and hands. What would be the most appropriate treatment for this patient's peripheral neuropathy?

   A. Add thiamine to his regimen.
   B. Discontinue rifampin and add another antitubercular agent.
   C. Add pyridoxine to his regimen.
   D. Discontinue ethambutol and add another antitubercular agent.
   E. Discontinue isoniazid and add another antitubercular agent.

HPI: GL is 35-year-old man who presents to the HIV clinic with complaints of rash, nausea, and vomiting. He has been on his current antiretrovirals (ARVs) for 8 months, with immune reconstitution and undetectable viral load. Per the patient report, he missed many of his doses last week since he was on vacation. After he returned from his trip 4 days ago, he restarted taking all his medications. His medications include nelfinavir, lamivudine, abacavir, and TMP-SMX.

Labs: CD4+ cell count 190 cells/mm³ (nadir 60 cells/mm³), viral load < 50 copies/mL, glucose 168 mg/dL (fasting), triglycerides 450 mg/dL (fasting).

Thought Questions

- What are the most common side effects of each class of ARV?

- Which ARVs should not be used in combination?

- Which ARVs may interact with his current medications?

- Which ARVs are associated with hyperlipidemia or glucose intolerance?

Basic Science Review and Discussion

HIV is a human retrovirus that infects lymphocytes and other cells with the CD4 surface protein. Infection eventually leads to lymphopenia and CD4 T-cell depletion. The time from onset of HIV infection to development of AIDS varies from months to years.

There are two enzymes, **reverse transcriptase** (RT) and **protease**, within the HIV life cycle to which therapy is directed

(Figure 59-1). HIV is able to convert its own RNA into DNA for incorporation into the host cell genome. This conversion is catalyzed by the enzyme RT, which is the target of two of the available classes of ARVs. These two classes are the **nucleoside (and nucleotide) reverse transcriptase inhibitors** (NRTIs, NtRTIs) and the **non-nucleoside reverse transcriptase inhibitors** (NNRTIs). After uptake by host cells, NRTIs and NtRTIs are converted to their triphosphate forms by cellular kinases. Phosphorylation by nucleoside kinases is crucial for rendering the drugs active in suppressing viral replication. NNRTIs, on the other hand, do not require phosphorylation or intracellular processing to become activated. They are noncompetitive inhibitors of RT and cause allosteric inhibition of enzyme function by binding at sites distinct from the nucleoside-binding site.

Later in the life cycle during the process of budding, the enzyme HIV protease cleaves the polyproteins in the core, converting the immature viral particles into infectious virions. **Protease inhibitors** (PIs) inhibit the viral protease enzyme to prevent cleavage of the polyproteins so that

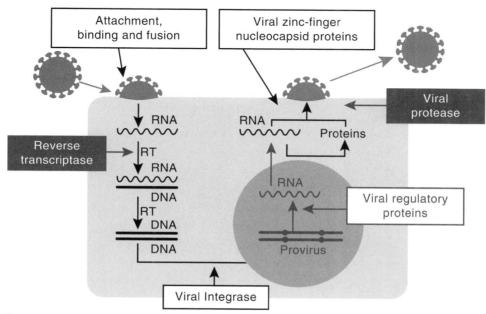

Figure 59-1

the viral particles remain immature and replication defective.

Initial regimens usually consist of two NRTIs plus either a potent PI or NNRTI. Frequent changes in therapy are required over time due to adverse effects, lack of response, or both. As a general rule, NRTIs do not require dose adjustments when combined with other ARVs. However, PIs and NNRTIs tend to have complex metabolisms and in combination affect each other's levels and potency. Drug resistance occurs with all available agents, and resistance to one agent will often confer resistance to the entire class (Table 59-1).

Table 59-1 Overview of available antiretroviral agents

NRTIs and NtRTIs	NNRTIs	Protease inhibitors
Zidovudine	Nevirapine	Saquinavir
Didanosine	Delavirdine	Ritonavir
Zalcitabine	Efavirenz	Indinavir
Stavudine		Nelfinavir
Lamivudine		Amprenavir
Abacavir		Lopinavir + ritonavir (combination)
Tenofovir (NtRTI)		

Case Conclusion Based on GL's history of nonadherence and his symptoms of rash, nausea, and vomiting, **abacavir hypersensitivity** is suspected and the agent is discontinued. The symptoms most commonly associated with abacavir hypersensitivity reaction are fever, rash, GI effects (nausea, vomiting, diarrhea, or abdominal pain), lethargy or malaise, and upper or lower respiratory effects. The majority of symptoms include either fever or rash and laboratory abnormalities may include elevated LFTs, increased creatine phosphokinase or Cr, and lymphopenia. Another nucleoside analogue is started and his symptoms resolve. He is counseled on the importance of adherence, especially when he travels.

Thumbnail: Nucleoside Reverse Transcriptase Inhibitors (NRTIs), Nucleotide Reverse Transcriptase Inhibitors (NtRTIs), NNRTI, PIs

Name	Pharmacokinetics	Side effects/comments
Abacavir (ABC)	Metabolism: hepatic Elimination: 80% renal	Hypersensitivity reaction (~4%): fever, malaise, rash, GI, respiratory. Resolves within 2 days of discontinuation. Do not rechallenge. Rash alone without hypersensitivity
Didanosine (ddI)	Metabolism: unknown Elimination: 40%–60% renal	Peripheral neuropathy Pancreatitis
Lamivudine (3TC)	Metabolism: minor hepatic Elimination: 70% renal	Generally the best tolerated ARV Active against hepatitis B
Stavudine (d4T)	Metabolism: unknown Elimination: 40% renal 60% nonrenal (hepatic)	Peripheral neuropathy Pancreatitis
Zalcitabine (ddC)	Metabolism: minimal hepatic Elimination: 60%–80% renal	Peripheral neuropathy Oral ulcers Rarely used due to toxicity and low potency
Zidovudine (ZDV, AZT)	Metabolism: hepatic Elimination: 15%–25% renal via filtration and tubular secretion	Nausea, headache, fatigue Macrocytic anemia, neutropenia Peripheral neuropathy Myopathy
Tenofovir (TDF)	Metabolism: minimal Elimination: 80% recovered unchanged in the urine from glomerular filtration and secretion	First NtRTI Renal toxicity Active against hepatitis B Avoid in patients with CrCl < 60 mL/min

NRTI Side Effects Class effects of the NRTIs include **lactic acidosis** and **hepatic steatosis.** The "d" drugs such as ddl (didanosine), d4T (stavudine), and ddC (zalcitabine) are associated with an increased risk of **pancreatitis** and **peripheral neuropathy.** Although the PIs are usually associated with lipodystrophy, the NRTIs also have been linked to metabolic abnormalities.

NRTI Drug Interactions The NRTIs are not metabolized by CYP450 and are not usually associated with many drug interactions. The buffered (chewable) form of ddl contains an antacid that can bind or inhibit the absorption of other medications such as fluoroquinolones, itraconazole, or ketoconazole. NRTI combinations that should be avoided include zidovudine with stavudine (antagonistic in vivo) and didanosine with zalcitabine (increased risk for peripheral neuropathy).

NNRTI Side Effects Class effects of the NNRTIs include **rash** and **hepatotoxicity. Sleep disturbances** due to efavirenz can include hallucinations and vivid dreams, most commonly within the first month of therapy.

NNRTI Drug Interactions The NNRTIs are either inducers or inhibitors of CYP450, and these interactions are drug specific. In general, delavirdine is an inhibitor of CYP450, nevirapine an inducer, and efavirenz is a mixed inducer and inhibitor. For example, efavirenz can reduce the serum levels of PIs such as amprenavir, increase serum levels of ethinyl estradiol, and potentially increase or decrease warfarin serum levels.

PI Side Effects The PIs are associated with many varied side effects that are highly patient specific. All PIs can cause GI side effects such as diarrhea and abdominal cramping. Several metabolic adverse effects have been associated with the chronic use of PIs. **Glucose intolerance** and new-onset or exacerbation of previous diabetes mellitus have been noted, as has **hyperlipidemia.** A **lipodystrophy** syndrome with symmetric loss of subcutaneous fat from the face and extremities can be seen after the initiation of PI therapy. Abnormal fat deposits at the posterior base of the neck and in the abdominal viscera, often with elevated serum triglyceride levels, also have been reported.

PI Drug Interactions PIs are extensively metabolized by the hepatic CYP450 enzyme complex. PIs may interfere, to varied degrees, with the hepatic metabolism of other drugs due to their CYP450-inhibiting effects. Although these effects are most prominent with ritonavir, the use of any PI should prompt a careful review of concurrently used medications to avoid potential adverse drug interactions. The metabolism of PIs also can be affected by other CYP450 inducers or inhibitors. Inhibitors of CYP450 (such as ketoconazole) may increase PI levels markedly, whereas inducers (such as rifampin and rifabutin) may decrease levels. Although the PIs can be potent inhibitors of CYP450, this pharmacokinetic property can be exploited therapeutically. For example, ritonavir is rarely used as a sole PI and is used in combination with another PI to "boost" its drug levels and to inhibit metabolism (e.g., ritonavir/lopinavir).

Non-nucleoside reverse transcriptase inhibitors (NNRTIs)

Name	Pharmacokinetics	Side effects/comments
Delavirdine	Metabolism: extensive hepatic via CYP450-3A4 Elimination: 50% renal, 40% feces	Transient rash CYP450 inhibitor
Nevirapine	Metabolism: extensive hepatic via CYP3A4 Elimination: 90% renal	Rash Hepatitis CYP450 inducer
Efavirenz	Metabolism: extensive hepatic via CYP3A4 and -2B6 Elimination: 14%–34% renal, 16%–61% feces	Rash Insomnia or sedation Sleep disturbances Dizziness Hepatitis Contraindicated in pregnancy Mixed CYP450 inducer and inhibitor

Protease inhibitors (PIs)

Name	Pharmacokinetics	Side effects/comments
Amprenavir	Metabolism: hepatic CYP3A4 Elimination: 14% renal, 75% hepatic	Rash Nausea, diarrhea
Indinavir	Metabolism: hepatic CYP3A4 Elimination: < 20% renal	Nephrolithiasis (hydration essential) Nausea, GI
Lopinavir/ritonavir	Metabolism: CYP3A4 Elimination: 10% renal, 83% feces	GI Combination capsule
Nelfinavir	Metabolism: CYP3A4 Elimination: 87% feces	Diarrhea common Nausea
Ritonavir	Metabolism: CYP3A4 and -2D6 Elimination: 86% feces	Nausea Diarrhea Circumoral paresthesia
Saquinavir (soft gel)	Metabolism: CYP3A4 Elimination: 88% feces	Soft gel: improved absorption
Saquinavir (hard gel)	Metabolism: CYP3A4 Elimination: 81% feces	Hard gel: poor bioavailability

Questions

1. KJ is a 45-year-old woman currently on the following medications: nelfinavir, lamivudine, zidovudine, fluconazole (prophylaxis for thrush), and TMP-SMX. Which of the following two agents are most likely to be causing her anemia?

   A. Fluconazole and zidovudine
   B. Zidovudine and TMP-SMX
   C. Lamivudine and zidovudine
   D. Fluconazole and lamivudine
   E. Nelfinavir and TMP-SMX

2. GR is a 55-year-old HIV positive man currently receiving ritonavir/lopinavir, nevirapine, and lamivudine. You would like to start simvastatin to decrease his triglycerides. Which of his ARVs will interact with simvastatin?

   A. Nevirapine only
   B. Lamivudine only
   C. Ritonavir/lopinavir only
   D. Nevirapine and lamivudine
   E. Nevirapine and ritonavir/lopinavir
   F. Ritonavir/lopinavir and lamivudine

HPI: LJ is a 48 year-old man who presents with increasing fatigue. He notes that his skin and eyes have progressively become more yellow. PMH includes chronic hepatitis C virus (HCV) infection and hemorrhoids. Social History: IV drug use 25 years ago; alcohol abuse for 15 years.

Labs: HCV Ab (+), Serum Cr 1.1 mg/dL, HCV RNA (+), Total bilirubin 3.1 mg/dL, WBC 7500/mm^3, ALT 133 IU/L, HCT 38%, AST 103 IU/L, Platelets 125,000/mm^3, INR 1.4. The patient asks if there are any treatment options for the management of his chronic HCV infection.

Thought Questions

■ What treatment modalities are available for the management of chronic HCV infection?

■ What are common side effects of interferon and ribavirin?

■ When should patients be treated with interferon and ribavirin?

■ What is the role of the combination therapy (interferon plus ribavirin) compared with interferon monotherapy?

Basic Science Review and Discussion

Hepatitis C virus infection is a leading cause of chronic liver disease in the United States. It is the leading cause of **cirrhosis,** and is the most common reason for liver transplantation.

HCV transmission is primarily through exposure to infected blood. Most patients do not show symptoms acutely after infection, and approximately 15% will clear the infection. The remaining 85% will be chronically infected. Of those chronically infected, about 20% will develop cirrhosis of the liver. Alcohol consumption, coinfection with hepatitis B and/or HIV, older age at time of infection, and male gender are factors that increase the risk for progressive liver disease. HCV accounts for about one third of **hepatocellular carcinoma** cases in the United States.

The goal of therapy in the management of chronic HCV is to prevent progression of the disease to cirrhosis. Patients with moderate liver histologic changes, persistently abnormal ALT levels, and the presence of HCV RNA in the serum are potential candidates for treatment. Treatment is not indicated in patients with mild histologic findings on liver biopsy (minimal inflammation without fibrosis), persistently normal serum ALT levels, or patients with complications of advanced liver disease (ascites, hepatic encephalopathy, impaired hepatic synthetic function, hepatocellular carcinoma, or variceal hemorrhage).

Interferon-α and the combination of interferon-α plus oral **ribavirin** are the only FDA-approved drugs for the treatment of chronic HCV infection. Multiple forms of interferon-α are available, including **interferon-α_{2a}, interferon-α_{2b},** and interferon-α_{con-1}, as well as **pegylated interferon-α_{2b} and interferon-α_{2b}.** The pegylated form of interferon has a much slower elimination from the body, and thus can be given once a week compared with three times a week with the standard forms of interferon.

Interferon therapy is associated with many adverse effects. Fatigue, **fever,** headache, chills, **myalgia,** dizziness, anorexia, nausea, alopecia, **myelosuppression,** and **depression** are some of the more common side effects. Interferon therapy is contraindicated in patients with a history of autoimmune disorders, and should be used with extreme caution in organ transplant recipients, and those with a history of neuropsychiatric disorders. Common side effects of ribavirin therapy include dose-dependent **hemolytic anemia,** pruritis, and anemia. Because ribavirin is highly **teratogenic** (pregnancy category X), ribavirin is contraindicated in women who are pregnant or in men whose female partners are pregnant.

Interferon and ribavirin are indicated for the treatment of chronic hepatitis C with compensated liver disease. Compensated liver disease typically is defined as no history of hepatic encephalopathy, variceal hemorrhage, ascites, or other signs of decompensation. In addition, laboratory values should be near normal (bilirubin ≤ 2 mg/dL, stable [near normal] albumin, PT < 3 second prolongation, WBC ≥ 3000/mm^3, platelets $\geq 70,000$/mm^3, Cr near normal).

The combination of interferon and ribavirin has a significant benefit on sustained virologic response (the absence of detectable HCV RNA more than 6 months after treatment), biochemical response (normalization of transaminases), and liver histology in patients with hepatitis C compared with interferon by itself. Ribavirin is ineffective by itself and should not be used as monotherapy.

Case Conclusion   The patient is a candidate for interferon and ribavirin as part of the management of his chronic HCV infection to prevent progression of his disease.

Thumbnail: Agents Used for Hepatitis C Infection

	Prototypical Agent	
	Interferon-α	Ribavirin
Clinical use	Chronic hepatitis C and chronic hepatitis B infection; various malignancies (hairy cell leukemia, malignant melanoma, follicular lymphoma, AIDS-related Kaposi's sarcoma); condylomata acuminata	Given orally in combination with interferon for treatment of chronic HCV infection; inhaled ribavirin used in treatment of severe lower respiratory tract infections due to respiratory syncytial virus (RSV)
MOA	Cytokine released in response to viral infections; immunomodulating activity by inhibiting cell proliferation, increasing phagocytic activity and augmenting cytotoxicity of lymphocytes; inhibits viral replication	Oral guanosine analogue with antiviral activity against variety of RNA and DNA viruses. For HCV infections, combination of ribavirin plus interferon improves virologic response compared to interferon monotherapy.
Pharmacokinetics		
Absorption/distribution	Poor oral absorption, should be given SC or IM. Injected intralesionally for condylomata acuminata.	Rapid oral absorption (bioavailability 64%); distributes extensively into red blood cells (RBCs)
Elimination	Elimination T½ of interferon is 2–3 hr. The T½ of pegylated interferon is 40–80 hr.	Long elimination T½ (~298 hr) reflects slow elimination from RBCs. Ribavirin and metabolites are renally eliminated.
Adverse reactions	Flulike symptoms (headache, fever, chills, myalgia, arthralgia), fatigue, bone marrow suppression, nausea, anorexia, diarrhea, depression, parasthesia, dyspnea, pruritis, rash, alopecia	Dose-related hemolytic anemia, dyspnea, pruritis, rash
Precautions	Avoid use in patients with autoimmune disorders. Use caution in patients with neuropsychiatric problems.	Not effective by itself for treatment of HCV infection (must be used in combination with interferon); teratogenic (pregnancy category X).

Questions

1. CW is a 50-year-old woman with a history of chronic HCV infection. She states that she gained approximately 8 kg over the past 2 weeks. On examination she has icteric sclera, spider angiomas, mild asterexis, and a positive abdominal fluid wave. Her ALT level is 141 U/L, total bilirubin 5.5 mg/dL, serum Cr 1.3 mg/dL, INR 1.8, platelet count 95 × 10⁹/L, and a hemoglobin of 13 g/dL. Which of the following drugs or drug regimens can be used to treat this patient's chronic HCV infection?

   A. Interferon-α_{2b}
   B. Ribavirin
   C. Interferon-α_{2b} plus ribavirin
   D. Pegylated interferon-α_{2b}
   E. Pegylated interferon-α_{2b} plus ribavirin
   F. No treatment for chronic HCV infection is warranted at this time.

2. MM is a 48-year-old man with a history of chronic HCV infection. He complains of increasing fatigue and shortness of breath over the past 2 weeks. He started therapy for his chronic HCV infection 4 weeks ago with interferon-α_{2b} and ribavirin. His serum ALT is 80 U/L, serum Cr 1.2 mg/dL, INR 1.1, hematocrit 22%, hemoglobin 7 g/dL, total bilirubin 12 mg/dL, and G6PD within normal limits. Peripheral blood smear reveals hemolysis. Which of the following drugs is the most likely to cause hemolytic anemia?

   A. Interferon-α_{2a}
   B. Pegylated interferon-α_{2a}
   C. Interferon-α_{2b}
   D. Ribavirin
   E. Interferon-α_{con-1}

HPI: DS is a 48-year-old woman recently diagnosed with treatment-induced acute myelogenous leukemia (AML). She was successfully treated for breast cancer 4 years prior after receiving six cycles of AC chemotherapy (doxorubicin [Adriamycin] and cyclophosphamide). Her total cumulative dose of doxorubicin was 360 mg/m^2. Her current oncologist would like to begin induction chemotherapy for her AML with the goal of achieving remission. He recommends a regimen consisting of high-dose cytarabine and daunorubicin. She is otherwise in good health.

Thought Questions

- Describe the pharmacology and major side effects of anthracycline agents.

- What special precautions should be considered when administering anthracyclines?

- What labs might be helpful to evaluate prior to proceeding with anthracycline therapy?

- Is this patient at risk for anthracycline-induced cardiotoxicity? How should she be monitored?

Basic Science Review and Discussion

The **anthracyclines** (doxorubicin, daunorubicin, idarubicin, epirubicin) are antineoplastic antibiotics with a broad range of clinical uses. Doxorubicin has activity against a number of solid tumors (such as sarcomas, adenocarcinomas) and hematologic malignances (leukemia, lymphoma, multiple myeloma). Compared with doxorubicin, daunorubicin and idarubicin are much less active against solid tumors but highly effective against leukemia.

Anthracyclines have several modes of action leading to anticancer activity. They intercalate between base pairs in DNA, interfering with nucleic acid synthesis. Anthracyclines also inhibit DNA topoisomerases I and II, which leads to DNA double-strand breaks. In addition, doxorubicin and daunorubicin may form complexes with metals such as iron. Although these metal-anthracycline complexes result in oxygen free radical formation, which may contribute to antitumor activity, membrane damage incurred from the free radicals is thought to be the mechanism responsible for

cardiotoxicity. Free radical generation may be less prominent with idarubicin compared with other anthracyclines. Anthracyclines can be cytotoxic in all phases of the cell cycle and are not considered to be cell cycle phase specific.

Administration and Metabolism All of the anthracyclines are administered parenterally because oral absorption is poor. Anthracyclines can cause severe tissue damage if **extravasated,** so it is recommended that they be administered via central venous catheters or as a short IV push over 1 to 2 minutes. Anthracyclines are primarily eliminated via hepatic metabolism. Patients with **cholestasis** have impaired clearance and experience greater toxicity. It is recommended that patients receiving anthracyclines have LFTs monitored prior to administration, and that dose reductions be considered if total bilirubin is elevated.

Toxicities Anthracyclines have a number of significant toxicities. They may result in **myelosuppression,** which is considered the acute dose-limiting toxicity. Leukopenia has a nadir of approximately 10 to 14 days but recovery is usually quick following the nadir. The most significant delayed adverse effect of anthracyclines is **cardiotoxicity.** It may manifest as acute toxicity (arrhythmias) or delayed cardiomyopathy, which is related to total cumulative lifetime exposure. The cardiomyopathy syndrome classically presents as CHF and it may be irreversible. Patients may be at increased risk for anthracycline-induced cardiomyopathy if they have been exposed to cumulative doses of doxorubicin greater than 550 mg/m^2 (or equivalent for other anthracyclines), prior mediastinal irradiation, are over 70 years of age, or have preexisting cardiovascular disease. It is recommended to obtain baseline cardiac function evaluations prior to commencing anthracycline therapy.

Case Conclusion Given that DS's prior doxorubicin exposure was 360 mg/m^2, and the current regimen will expose her to an additional 180 mg/m^2 of anthracycline, it was decided safe to proceed with treatment. After induction therapy, she will have been exposed to 540 mg/m^2 anthracycline and should be monitored carefully for the potential development of cardiomyopathy.

Thumbnail: Anthracyclines

Prototype drug: Doxorubicin (Adriamycin). Other examples in class: daunorubicin, idarubicin, epirubicin, liposomal doxorubicin, liposomal daunorubicin.

Clinical uses: Leukemia, lymphoma, multiple myeloma, sarcomas, germ cell tumors of ovaries or testes, head and neck cancer, lung cancer, Wilms' tumor, breast cancer, stomach cancer, pancreatic cancer, liver cancer, ovarian cancer, bladder cancer, uterine cancer, neuroblastoma.

MOA: Intercalation into DNA, which leads to blockade of DNA and RNA synthesis; DNA strand breaks; free radical formation.

Pharmacokinetics

Absorption: Poor oral absorption (<50%), given IV.

Distribution: Rapidly distributes into liver, spleen, kidney, lung, and heart. Poor penetration into CNS.

Metabolism/elimination: Triphasic elimination (primarily in liver); adjust dose or withhold use in patients with increased total bilirubin levels.

Adverse reactions: Cardiotoxicity (increased risk when lifetime cumulative dose equivalent to doxorubicin 400–550 mg/m^2 is exceeded), alopecia, vesicant, nausea/vomiting (moderate to high emetogenic potential for doses > 60 mg), mucositis, myelosuppression (primarily leukopenia, nadir 10 to 14 days).

Drug interactions: CYP450 enzyme substrate and inhibitor. Unclear clinical significance.

Questions

1. AR is a 48-year-old woman who was treated for Hodgkin's disease 15 years ago with ABVD (doxorubicin, bleomycin, vinblastine, dacarbazine). She now presents with breast cancer and her oncologist feels that chemotherapy with FAC (fluorouracil, doxorubicin [Adriamycin], and cyclophosphamide) is the most appropriate regimen. Her previous chemotherapy included a total of 300 mg/m^2 doxorubicin exposure. Which of the following agents may be utilized to reduce risk of cardiotoxicity associated with the anthracycline therapy she is about to receive?

   A. Leucovorin
   B. Mesna
   C. Amifostine
   D. Dexrazoxane
   E. *N*-acetylcysteine

2. MT is a 49-year-old man admitted for his first cycle of chemotherapy for multiple myeloma. He is scheduled to receive VAD therapy (vincristine, doxorubicin [Adriamycin] and dexamethasone). Past medical history includes asthma and diabetes. Admission laboratory values include WBC count 3400 mm^3, platelets 9500 mm^3 (low), Cr 1.8 mg/dL (high), bilirubin 2.4 mg/dL (high). Which of the following factors may lead you to consider dose modification of doxorubicin?

   A. Diabetes
   B. Asthma
   C. Platelet count
   D. Cr
   E. Bilirubin

HPI: GH is a 48-year-old woman who presents with stage III epithelial adenocarcinoma of the ovaries. She has received three cycles of cisplatin and paclitaxel, but has now progressed. Her course has been complicated by severe side effects, including numbness of her feet, persistent nausea and vomiting, severe neutropenia, and renal dysfunction (serum Cr 1.5 mg/dL). Her physician is considering switching to an alternative regimen consisting of ifosfamide and etoposide. She is reluctant due to her poor tolerability of her previous therapy.

Thought Questions

- What issues should be considered when selecting an alternative regimen?

- Which agents caused her complications?

- What can be done to minimize toxicities with her alternative regimen?

Basic Science Review and Discussion

Poor response or tolerability are often the rationale for switching chemotherapy regimens. Cisplatin, a platinum **alkylating agent,** and paclitaxel, a **taxane,** are two of the most effective drugs for ovarian cancer. Cisplatin is known to be the most **emetogenic** chemotherapy agent. It is also known to cause **neuropathy, nephrotoxicity, myelosuppression,** electrolyte wasting, and **ototoxicity.** Switching to another platinum alkylating agent, such as carboplatin, may help with nausea, vomiting, nephrotoxicity, and neurotoxicity, but since GH is having a poor response, it may not be the best choice. Paclitaxel may also cause neurotoxicity and myelosuppression, and may have additive toxic effects to the cisplatin (see Case 65 for discussion of taxanes).

Cisplatin acts as an alkylating agent to react with cellular DNA, forming both intrastrand and interstrand cross-links, which results in DNA conformational changes and disruption of DNA replication. Alkylating agents are generally considered to be non-cell cycle specific; however, they exhibit the most activity in cells that are rapidly dividing. Cisplatin metabolites also may react with thiol groups on proteins, and some cisplatin toxicity (ototoxicity, nephrotoxicity, and neurotoxicity) may result from these interactions. **Amifostine** is metabolized to a free thiol product and may be used to bind and detoxify reactive metabolites of cisplatin.

Ifosfamide is an alkylating agent related to cyclophosphamide. It is often used as a second-line agent for ovarian cancer. Its main side effect is **hemorrhagic cystitis.** Hemorrhagic cystitis is caused by the acrolein metabolite, which binds to the bladder and causes irritation and tissue damage. Aggressive hydration and the use of the chemoprotective agent **mesna** are necessary for safe administration. Mesna tends to have a shorter T½ than ifosfamide, so it is imperative that the dose be given for at least 8 to 12 hours after the end of the ifosfamide infusion.

Case Conclusion GH had a measured 24-hour CrCl rate of 55 mL/min. This was considered adequate for her to proceed with the proposed alternative regimen without dose modification. She was given aggressive hydration and mesna with her ifosfamide. She tolerated the etoposide with minimal problems. Compared with her previous regimen, she had less nausea and vomiting, although she still experienced 7 days of neutropenia.

Thumbnail: Alkylating Agents

	Drug class			
	Platinum analogues	Nitrogen mustards	Nitrosoureas	Other
Agents	Cisplatin Carboplatin	Mechlorethamine Cyclophosphamide Ifosfamide	Carmustine Lomustine Streptozocin	Busulfan
Clinical uses	Cancer of the testes, ovaries, bladder, lung, head and neck, cervix, and endometrium; sarcoma	Mechlorethamine: lymphoma Cyclophosphamide: leukemia, lymphoma, cancer of the breast, lung, sarcoma Ifosfamide: ovarian, breast cancers, sarcomas	Carmustine and lomustine: lymphomas, brain tumors Streptozocin: pancreatic, insulinoma	Busulfan: leukemia Dacarbazine: melanoma, Hodgkin's lymphoma, soft tissue sarcoma
MOA	Form intrastrand and interstrand cross-links in DNA, which interferes with DNA replication. Usually considered cell cycle nonspecific, but do work best when cells are rapidly multiplying.			
Pharmacokinetics	Only available as IV injection; predominantly renally excreted.	Mechlorethamine: IV only; undergoes rapid chemical transformation. Cyclophosphamide and ifosfamide: biotransformed by the liver to active compounds. Requires dose adjustment for both hepatic and renal impairment. Usually IV, but can be taken orally.	Carmustine: renally cleared, readily crosses blood-brain barrier. Lomustine: extensive metabolism by the liver to active metabolites; oral only.	Busulfan: may give IV or PO; hepatic metabolism, readily distributes to CNS. Dacarbazine: hepatic metabolism, but prolonged elimination in the presence of renal dysfunction; IV only.
Adverse reactions	Cisplatin: severe nausea/vomiting (N/V), neuropathy, nephrotoxicity, ototoxicity, electrolyte wasting, myelosuppression Carboplatin: thrombocytopenia, leukopenia, less N/V, renal and neurotoxicity than cisplatin	Mechlorethamine: vesicant, myelosuppression, N/V, skin rash Cyclophosphamide and ifosfamide: hemorrhagic cystitis, SIADH, acute and delayed N/V, myelosuppression	Myelosuppression Carmustine: pulmonary fibrosis with high dose	Myelosuppression, N/V Busulfan: pulmonary fibrosis, hepatic dysfunction, hyperpigmentation Dacarbazine: severe N/V, fatigue, hepatic dysfunction, flulike symptoms
Special precautions	Amifostine may be used to reduce cumulative renal toxicity associated with repeated cisplatin therapy	Mesna to prevent hemorrhagic cystitis		

Questions

1. WD is a 24-year-old woman with metastatic melanoma, who is being treated with cisplatin, dacarbazine, IL-2, and interferon-α. What precautions should be taken while she is being treated?

   A. Monitor magnesium and potassium levels.
   B. Premedicate with antiemetics, including a serotonin antagonist.
   C. Monitor pulmonary function tests.
   D. A and B only.
   E. All of the above.

2. GF is a 43-year-old man with Burkitt's lymphoma who is about to receive high-dose cyclophosphamide (4000 mg/m² for one dose) for stem cell mobilization. Which of the following factors should be considered prior to administration?

   A. Prehydration with normal saline (NS)
   B. Use in combination with mesna
   C. Use of a serotonin antagonist for acute nausea and vomiting
   D. Use of antiemetic regimen including dexamethasone for delayed nausea and vomiting
   E. All of the above

> **HPI:** TB is a 46-year-old woman with osteosarcoma who is admitted for treatment with very high dose methotrexate. All of her admit laboratory values were within normal limits. She is given 1000 mL NS IV over 2 hours, then started on D5W with 2 amps (100 mEq) sodium bicarbonate/liter to run at 250 mL/hr. Her urine pH is checked hourly. Once her urine pH is sufficiently alkaline and her urine output is considered adequate, methotrexate is administered IV over 4 hours. Twenty-four hours after the methotrexate infusion, leucovorin "rescue" is begun.

Thought Questions

- What is the pharmacology of methotrexate and what are the main side effects?

- What is the role of hydration in this patient?

- How does leucovorin work in this case and when should it be stopped?

- What other factors should be considered in patients receiving high-dose methotrexate?

- What are other antimetabolites used in cancer treatment and what are their principal side effects?

Basic Science Review and Discussion

Methotexate is an antineoplastic folic acid analogue that blocks the conversion of dihydrofolate (FH_2) to tetrahydro-folate (FH_4) by binding to **dihydrofolate reductase** (DHFR) enzyme. Folate is essential for the normal synthesis of purines and pyrimidines, and therefore DNA and RNA. In order for folate to function as a cofactor, it must be reduced to FH_4 by DHFR. Methotrexate binds to DHFR, prevents the conversion of FH_2 to FH_4, and, consequently, inhibits purine and pyrimidine synthesis. The **antimetabolites** are considered cell cycle specific, with most activity for cells in the S (synthesis) phase. With high-dose methotrexate, **leucovorin** rescue is often used to prevent severe toxicity to normal body tissues. Leucovorin (folinic acid) is a reduced form of folate (similar to FH_4) that does not require the use of DHFR. Leucovorin is transported into healthy cells and is utilized for DNA and RNA synthesis. Tumor cells tend to have impaired transport mechanisms and usually cannot use leucovorin. Leucovorin is usually started within 24 to 36 hours of high-dose methotrexate administration and continues until methotrexate serum levels are below nontoxic levels (0.1 to 0.05 mol/L).

Common side effects seen with methotrexate include **mucositis, leukopenia, thrombocytopenia,** and anemia. At normal doses, methotrexate is primarily excreted unchanged in the urine. Adequate renal function is essential for safe administration of methotrexate. At high doses, methotrexate is partially metabolized to 7-hydroxymethotrexate, which is slightly soluble in acidic environments, so alkalinization of the urine with sodium bicarbonate will help prevent precipitation in the renal tubules. Some drugs (trimethoprim, penicillins, NSAIDs, aspirin, probenecid) may compete with methotrexate for renal elimination, and concurrent use may lead to methotrexate toxicity. Drugs that create an acidic environment in the kidneys also may reduce the rate of methotrexate excretion. Methotrexate is extensively distributed in body water. Patients with fluid accumulations such as **pleural effusions** or **ascites** may have significant difficulty in methotrexate elimination.

Other anitimetabolites used in cancer therapy include pyrimidine analogues and purine analogues. Pyrimidine analogues such as **fluorouracil** are used extensively for gastric and colorectal cancers. Fluorouracil is converted to a monophosphate nucleotide (F-UMP) which is reduced to a deoxynucleotide (F-dUMP). With a folate coenzyme, F-dUMP will bind and inactivate thymidylate synthetase, and therefore inhibit DNA synthesis. Significant side effects include mucositis, **myelosuppression,** and **alopecia.** **Capecitabine** is an oral prodrug which is converted to fluorouracil intracellularly. It is used in the treatment of metastatic breast cancer and has been associated with severe **diarrhea** and **hand-foot syndrome** (chemotherapy-induced acral erythema) as side effects. **Cytarabine** is a pyrimidine analogue used primarily in the treatment of leukemias. In high doses, this agent is associated with myelosuppression, **rash** (which may be severe), chemical conjunctivitis, and cerebellar dysfunction (especially when used in the presence of renal dysfunction).

Purine analogues including **cladribine** and **fludarabine** are used to treat a variety of leukemias. Compared with the pyrimidine analogues, these agents are associated with a lower incidence of significant mucositis; however, **neutropenia** tends to be prolonged (4 weeks compared with 2 weeks).

Case Conclusion   TB tolerated her high-dose methotrexate and leucovorin rescue. She received leucovorin rescue for 4 days before her methotrexate levels became nontoxic. Her neutrophil count dropped around day 6 but she did not become neutropenic (ANC <500). She had no evidence of mucositis.

Thumbnail: Antimetabolites

| | Drug class | | |
	Folate antagonists	Purine analogues	Pyrimidine analogues
Agents	Methotrexate	Thioguanine Cladribine Fludarabine Mercaptopurine	Cytarabine (Ara-C) Fluorouracil (5FU) Capecitabine
Clinical uses	Leukemia, lymphoma, sarcoma, cancers of the lung, breast, ovaries, head and neck	Thioguanine: leukemia Cladribine: hairy cell leukemia Fludarabine: chronic lymphocytic leukemia Mercaptopurine : leukemia	Cytarabine: leukemias Fluorouracil: gastric, colon, bladder, breast, head and neck cancers Capecitabine: metastatic breast cancer
MOA	Inhibits DHFR enzyme, preventing reduction of FH_2 to FH_4; inhibits purine and pyrimidine synthesis necessary for DNA and RNA synthesis. Cell cycle specific (S phase)	Metabolized to a false purine analogue that will act as a competitive inhibitor after incorporation into cellular DNA	Metabolized to a false pyrimidine analogue that will act as a competitive inhibitor after incorporation into cellular DNA
Pharmacokinetics	Predominantly renally excreted (partially metabolized at high doses). Widely distributed into body fluids. At high doses, will penetrate CNS. May be given intrathecally. Oral administration is rapid, but often incomplete.	Thioguanine: oral only, eliminated renally, poor CNS penetration. Cladribine: IV only; rapid plasma clearance. Fludarabine: IV only. Mercaptopurine: oral only, poor absorption.	Cytarabine: extensive hepatic metabolism, but active metabolite is renally cleared. Adequate CNS levels may be achieved with high doses. May be given intrathecally. Not absorbed orally. Fluorouracil: distributes rapidly, and is extensively metabolized. Oral absorption is erratic, but can be given orally as prodrug (capecitabine).
Adverse reactions	Renal dysfunction, myelosuppression, mucositis, hepatotoxicity	Rash, neutropenia, diarrhea	Cytarabine: rash, fever, conjunctivitis, myelosuppression, cerebellar dysfunction if given with renal impairment Fluorouracil: rash, fever, mucositis, alopecia, hyperpigmentation, myelosuppression, neurotoxicity
Special precautions	NSAIDs, penicillins, and other drugs may interfere with methotrexate clearance. Consider leucovorin rescue with high-dose methotrexate.		Steroid eye drops may help prevent conjunctivitis. Increased CNS toxicity with renal impairment. Leucovorin is sometimes added to fluorouracil therapy for added cytotoxic effects.

Questions

1. HG is a 68-year-old man with AML. He is to receive induction chemotherapy consisting of high-dose cytarabine and daunorubicin. Which condition(s) should be evaluated in this patient prior to and during treatment with high-dose cytarabine?

   A. Renal function
   B. Conjunctivitis
   C. Rash
   D. Fever
   E. All of the above

2. PO is a 58-year-old Asian man with colorectal cancer. He is on a regimen consisting of fluorouracil and leucovorin over 1 week, every 28 days. What is the role of leucovorin in this case?

   A. Rescues normal cells like it does for methotrexate toxicity
   B. Enhances the cytotoxicity of fluorouracil
   C. Has antitumor activity on its own
   D. Is an antiemetic agent
   E. Is used to prevent hypersensitivity

HPI: RE is a 26-year-old woman recently diagnosed with ALL. She was admitted for induction therapy consisting of daunorubicin daily for 3 days (on days 1 through 3), vincristine once weekly for four doses (days 1, 8, 15, and 22), prednisone daily for 28 days (days 1 through 28), and asparaginase daily on days 17 through 28. She has no past medical history.

She is currently day 15 and due for her third dose of vincristine. Her main complaints consist of mild numbness in her fingertips and severe constipation (no bowel movement for 4 days).

Labs: Laboratory parameters are generally within normal limits, with the exception of neutropenia (neutrophil count 40/mm³) and elevated bilirubin (1.5 mg/dL).

Thought Questions

- What is the most likely drug that is causing her complaints?

- Describe the pharmacology and major side effects of vinca alkaloids.

- What should be done?

- Could another vinca alkaloid be substituted?

Basic Science Review and Discussion

The patient's symptoms are most likely due to her vincristine therapy. Vinca alkaloids exert antineoplastic effects by binding to tubulin and thereby inhibiting assembly of microtubules. This results in the dissolution of the mitotic spindle apparatus, and cell arrest occurs in the mitosis (M) phase of the cell cycle. Vinca alkaloids are used for a variety of hematologic malignancies and solid tumors, such as lung, testicular, and breast cancers. The most common vinca alkaloids include vincristine, vinblastine, and vinorelbine.

All of the vinca alkaloids exhibit very poor oral absorption and are given parenterally. Vinca alkaloids are predominantly excreted through the **biliary tract** or by hepatic metabolism. Generally, for patients with mild elevations in bilirubin (serum bilirubin 1.5 to 3 mg/dL), the dose of these agents should be reduced. For patients with severely abnormal bilirubin levels (more than 5 mg/dL), the use of vinca alkaloids should be avoided.

Compared with vincristine, vinblastine and vinorelbine are more likely to cause **myelosuppression** (considered to be the dose-limiting toxicity of these agents). In addition, vincristine has very low **emetogenic potential** compared with vinblastine and vinorelbine, which present a more moderate risk.

Vincristine and the vinca alkaloids are known to cause **neuropathy.** Neuropathy may be related to nerve conduction alteration due to microtubule arrest. Although neuropathy is most often seen as finger numbness, it can also manifest as an ileus or **constipation.** Effects are usually reversible, and therapy should be delayed if symptoms are disabling. Use of concomitant drugs that may cause constipation (i.e., opiates) should be avoided if possible, and patients receiving vinca alkaloids should be managed with an aggressive bowel regimen to prevent these complications.

All the vinca alkaloids cause peripheral neuropathy, although a lower incidence of neuropathy is associated with vinorelbine. Vinorelbine, however, does not have an indication for leukemia, and therefore should not be substituted for the vincristine.

Case Conclusion RE was given lactulose to help her constipation, and after three doses she had a bowel movement. Due to her elevated bilirubin, RE's vincristine dose was lowered by 50%. Her finger numbness was slightly better. Her neutrophils remained low until day 23. A repeat bone marrow biopsy performed after recovery demonstrated remission of her ALL.

Thumbnail: Vinca Alkaloids

	Vincristine	Vinblastine	Vinorelbine
Clinical uses	Leukemia, sarcoma, lymphoma	Lymphoma, testicular, bladder, renal cancers	Lung, breast, ovarian cancers, lymphoma
MOA	Inhibit polymerization of tubulin, which is necessary for the formation of mitotic spindles for mitosis. Cell cycle specific for M phase of cell cycle.		
Pharmacokinetics	Poor oral absorption (given IV); predominantly hepatic elimination, slow clearance due to extensive tissue binding		
Adverse reactions	Peripheral neuropathy (may be dose-limiting), ileus, low emetogenic potential, low risk for severe myelosuppression	Peripheral neuropathy, ileus, dose-limiting myelosuppression (neutropenia and thrombocytopenia), moderate emetogenic potential	Peripheral neuropathy, ileus, moderate emetogenic potential, moderate risk for severe myelosuppression
Special precautions	All vinca alkaloids are considered vesicants, and extravasations should be avoided. All vinca alkaloids may be **fatal if given intrathecally.**		

Questions

1. TR is a 24-year-old man with testicular cancer who is about to receive a combination of cisplatin, etoposide, and vinblastine. Which factor(s) should be considered prior to administration of the vinblastine?

   A. LFTs
   B. Bowel movements
   C. WBC counts
   D. Venous access
   E. All of the above

2. LS is a 57-year-old woman with multiple myeloma being treated with VAD chemotherapy, a regimen consisting of a 4-day continuous infusion of vincristine and doxorubicin (Adriamycin) plus oral dexamethasone. Both vincristine and doxorubicin are vesicants. Which of the following precautions should be taken?

   A. Administer via a peripheral line.
   B. Administer via a central line.
   C. Use warm compresses on the skin in the area prior to administration.
   D. Premedicate with hyaluronidase .
   E. All of the above.

HPI: ML is a 57-year-old woman with advanced ovarian cancer. She has recently recovered from debulking surgery and presents to receive her first course of adjuvant chemotherapy with carboplatin and paclitaxel. Past medical history is noncontributory and she has no known drug allergies. She receives an antiemetic (ondansetron) as premedication. Ten minutes into the paclitaxel infusion, ML develops dyspnea and urticaria. The infusion is stopped and supportive care is given.

Thought Questions

- What is the mechanism of action of taxane antineoplastic agents?

- What are some clinical uses for taxanes?

- What precautions should be taken when administering taxanes?

- What pretreatment regimens can be used to minimize adverse reactions to taxanes?

Basic Science Review and Discussion

The taxane antineoplastic agents (paclitaxel and docetaxel) act by promoting formation and stabilization of microtubules. Accumulation of these polymerized microtubules may lead to mitotic arrest and cell death from nonfunctional tubules. They are considered to be cell cycle-specific agents (acting with greatest activity on cells in Gap 2 [G_2] and mitosis [M] phases).

Paclitaxel is indicated for the treatment of various solid malignancies. It is considered first-line therapy (usually in combination with a platinum analogue such as cisplatin) for advanced **ovarian cancer.** It is also useful in breast cancer, non–small cell lung cancer (in combination with cisplatin), and as second-line therapy for AIDS-related Kaposi's sarcoma. Docetaxel is indicated for the treatment of patients with locally advanced or metastatic breast cancer and non–small cell lung cancer.

Both paclitaxel and docetaxel may result in **anaphylactoid** or severe **hypersensitivity** reactions manifested by dyspnea, bronchospasm, angioedema, hypotension (occasionally HTN), and urticarial skin reactions. The reaction may be due to the active drug itself or to the vehicle (Cremophor or polysorbate 80). Additionally, patients receiving docetaxel may experience serious or life-threatening **fluid retention.** This syndrome is characterized by poorly tolerated peripheral or generalized edema, pleural effusion, dyspnea, ascites, and cardiac tamponade.

It is recommended that all patients receiving paclitaxel receive **pretreatment** with corticosteroids (such as dexamethasone) and antihistamines, both H_1 (diphenydramine) and H_2 (cimetidine or ranitidine) antagonists. All patients must be premedicated with corticosteroids prior to receiving each cycle of docetaxel to reduce the incidence and severity of hypersensitivity reactions or fluid retention. Patients who experience severe hypersensitivity reactions should not be rechallenged.

Case Conclusion   ML quickly recovered from her mild hypersensitivity reaction to the paclitaxel. For the remaining cycles of chemotherapy, she was pretreated with steroids and antihistamines and tolerated the paclitaxel without further reaction. After six cycles of chemotherapy, her CA-125 marker level was normal, her abdominal CT scan appeared normal, and she appeared to have a complete clinical response.

Thumbnail: Taxanes

Prototype drug: Paclitaxel

Other examples in class: Docetaxel

Clinical uses: Advanced ovarian carcinoma, node-positive breast cancer (adjuvant), metastatic breast cancer, non–small cell lung cancer, cervical, bladder, head and neck cancer, AIDS-related Kaposi's sarcoma (second line).

MOA: Inhibits mitosis by promoting and maintaining assembly of microtubules. Cell cycle specific (G2 and M phases). May also lead to chromosome breakage by distorting mitotic spindle apparatus.

Pharmacokinetics

Absorption: Administered IV

Distribution: Highly protein bound

Metabolism/elimination: Hepatic metabolism

Adverse reactions: Alopecia, nausea/vomiting/diarrhea, **myelosuppression** (dose-limiting, granulocytopenia, and thrombocytopenia), hepatic toxicity, peripheral neuropathy, hypersensitivity reactions, myalgias/arthralgias, rare cardiovascular events, fluid retention/pulmonary edema (docetaxel).

Precautions: Doses may be modified or therapy delayed for toxicity (myelosuppression). Adjust dose for hepatic impairment. Avoid use of docetaxel in patients with elevated bilirubin. Corticosteroids and antihistamines (i.e., cimetidine and diphenhydramine) are recommended to lessen risk for anaphylactoid reactions with paclitaxel. Pretreatment with steroids is *required* for docetaxel to minimize risk for fluid retention and hypersensitivity.

Questions

1. A 65-year-old man is about to receive his first course of paclitaxel therapy for refractory non–small cell lung cancer. Past medical history includes HTN and depression. He has NKDA. Which of the following pretreatment regimens would you recommend prior to infusing the paclitaxel?

   A. Dexamethasone alone
   B. Diphenhydramine alone
   C. Dexamethasone + diphenhydramine + ranitidine
   D. Dexamethasone + diphenhydramine + omeprazole
   E. Omeprazole alone

2. A 48-year-old woman presents for her third cycle of docetaxel therapy for her metastatic breast cancer. Which of the following laboratory parameters are necessary to evaluate prior to administering the docetaxel?

   A. Absolute neutrophil count
   B. Total bilirubin
   C. AST
   D. Alkaline phosphatase
   E. All of the above

HPI: EN is a 62-year-old white man with a 35-pack per year smoking history who was recently diagnosed with extensive small cell lung cancer. His oncologist is recommending therapy with cisplatin and etoposide. He is anxious to start treatment but is also wondering about other chemotherapy options.

Thought Questions

- What chemotherapy drugs are commonly used as first-line therapy for small cell lung cancer?

- How do topoisomerase inhibitors act as antineoplastic agents?

- What are some clinical indications for the different topoisomerase inhibitors?

- What are the toxicities associated with the use of these agents?

Basic Science Review and Discussion

Several combination chemotherapy regimens are available to treat small cell lung cancer (SCLC), although clear survival advantages have not been demonstrated with one regimen over another. Common regimens include etoposide plus a platinum analogue (cisplatin or carboplatin). Alternatives include a combination of cyclophosphamide plus doxorubicin plus vincristine. Topotecan and paclitaxel are also being investigated as first-line, single-agent therapy.

Etoposide and teniposide act by binding to cellular topoisomerase II (topo II) enzymes and **blocking DNA replication.** They are considered to be cell cycle specific by causing cellular arrest in the late synthesis (S) phase and early growth 2 (G2) phase. Etoposide has a wide variety of clinical uses, including lung cancer, germ cell cancers, gastric cancers, lymphomas (Hodgkin's and non-Hodgkin's), acute leukemias, and some sarcomas. Teniposide is used primarily in pediatric ALL.

Toxicities associated with etoposide include dose-limiting **myelosuppression** (granulocytopenia and thrombocytopenia), mild to moderate nausea/vomiting, dermatologic reactions (alopecia, pruritic rash), and mucositis (which can be severe with high doses). Rapid infusion of high doses may be associated with fever, hypotension, bronchospasm, and metabolic acidosis.

Topotecan and irinotecan both act by inhibiting topoisomerase I (topo I) enzymes, thereby inhibiting DNA replication. They are cell cycle-specific agents with most activity for cells in the S phase. Topotecan is used for treatment of refractory metastatic ovarian carcinoma and small cell lung cancer. It also may be useful in the treatment of head and neck cancer. Irinotecan is indicated for the treatment of metastatic carcinoma of the colon or rectum.

Topotecan is associated with bone marrow suppression (dose-limiting **neutropenia**). Other side effects include mild to moderate nausea/vomiting, alopecia, and abdominal complaints. Irinotecan has been associated with both acute (within 24 hours) and delayed (3 to 11 days posttherapy) **diarrhea.** The diarrhea may be severe or prolonged and may lead to fluid and electrolyte imbalances. The early diarrhea may be mediated by cholinergic mechanisms and can sometimes be ameliorated by administration of atropine.

Case Conclusion EN decides to proceed with the cisplatin/etoposide therapy as originally recommended. He tolerated 6 months of therapy with a complete response and minimal complications (moderate nausea/vomiting and alopecia).

Thumbnail: Topoisomerase Inhibitors

	Topoisomerase I inhibitors	Topoisomerase II inhibitors
Prototype drugs	Topotecan Irinotecan	Etoposide (VP16)
Clinical uses	Topotecan: ovarian cancer, small cell and non–small cell lung cancer Irinotecan: metastatic colon and rectal carcinoma	Small cell and non–small cell lung cancer, gastric cancer, germ cell cancers, leukemias and lymphomas.
MOA	Inhibits topoisomerase I enzyme; blocks effective replication and transcription.	Forms complex with topoisomerase II enzyme, which blocks DNA replication; results in DNA strand breakage.
Pharmacokinetics		
Absorption/distribution	Topotecan and irinotecan available IV only	Etoposide available IV and PO (50% bioavailable)
Metabolism/elimination	Topotecan: primarily renal clearance Irinotecan: converted to active metabolite in the liver	Renal and nonrenal clearance
Adverse reactions	Topotecan: myelosuppression (universal and dose limiting), mild nausea/vomiting, alopecia, diarrhea, fever, headache, fatigue Irinotecan: diarrhea, neutropenia and anemia, nausea/vomiting, alopecia, fever	Myelosuppression (dose-limiting neutropenia), nausea/vomiting, alopecia, stomatitis, skin changes, infusion-related reactions (hypotension)

Questions

1. A 60-year-old woman is being treated for metastatic colon cancer with her first course of irinotecan combined with fluorouracil (5-FU) and leucovorin. One hour after completing the irinotecan infusion, she complains of diaphoresis, crampy abdominal pain, and diarrhea. Which of the following measures would you consider as the most appropriate intervention at this time?

   A. Atropine
   B. Docusate sodium
   C. Metoclopramide
   D. Ondansetron
   E. Loperamide

2. A 51-year-old woman is being treated with topotecan for refractory ovarian cancer that failed to respond to initial therapy. She wishes to be as aggressive as possible with her therapy and would like you to explain why the recommended dose of topotecan cannot be exceeded. What is the dose-limiting toxicity of topotecan?

   A. Alopecia
   B. Nausea/vomiting
   C. Paresthesia
   D. Diarrhea
   E. Neutropenia

HPI: BB is a 76-year-old man with metastatic prostate cancer. He was diagnosed 4 years ago and underwent a radical prostatectomy but elected to delay other treatment because he was asymptomatic. Today he presents to evaluate treatment options because he is experiencing bone pain from his metastases. He is very opposed to orchiectomy, but is willing to try hormonal therapy to control his disease. He is in otherwise good health.

Thought Questions

- What hormonal agents are available for treatment of metastatic prostate cancer?

- What other types of cancer can be treated with hormonal manipulation?

- What are the main actions and side effects associated with hormonal agents used to treat malignancies?

Basic Science Review and Discussion

Alterations in hormonal balance may be used to treat a variety of neoplastic conditions. Since the sex hormones are involved in the stimulation and function of certain tissues, appropriate modification of hormone levels may inhibit growth of cancers arising from these tissues. The agents used to modify sex hormone levels or function can be separated into broad categories based on their general activities. With continued exposure, the **luteinizing hormone releasing hormone (LHRH) agonists** will suppress gonadal steroidogenesis (decrease estrogen in females, decrease testosterone in males). Estrogenic compounds and antiandrogens may be used to treat prostate cancer. The aromatase inhibitors and estrogen receptor antagonists result in antiestrogenic properties and are useful in the treatment of breast cancer. The adrenal corticosteroids (particularly glucocorticoid analogues such as prednisone) may be useful in the treatment of acute leukemia, lymphomas, multiple myeloma, and other hematologic malignancies.

The LHRH agonists (leuprolide and goserelin) are synthetic peptide analogues of naturally occurring LHRH (also referred to as gonadotropin-releasing hormone). They function with paradoxic effects on the pituitary when given continuously. They initially result in stimulation followed by inhibition of release of **follicle stimulating hormone (FSH)** and **luteinizing hormone (LH).** Inhibition of FSH and LH results in reduced production of **testosterone** and **estrogen** in the gonads. They are used in the treatment of prostate cancer, and low doses are approved for use in endometriosis. These agents are destroyed in the GI tract and not absorbed orally. They are administered as daily SC injections or long-acting depot preparations. During the initial few weeks of treatment, patients may experience a flare of

symptoms. This can often be avoided by starting antiandrogen therapy concurrently with initiation of the LHRH agonist.

The **antiandrogen** agents (flutamide, bicalutamide, and nilutamide) are used in combination with surgical castration or LHRH agonists in the treatment of metastatic prostate cancer. They act by inhibiting androgen uptake and/or inhibiting nuclear binding of androgen in target tissues. Side effects include **sexual dysfunction** (loss of libido, impotence), hot flashes, **gynecomastia,** and rare but potentially serious **hepatotoxicity.**

Estrogenic agents (diethylstilbestrol [DES] and estramustine) can be effective in the treatment of metastatic prostate cancer; however, concerns about potential **thromboembolic** events and other side effects (painful gynecomastia) have limited their use.

Most hormone-sensitive cancers will express hormone receptors that can be assayed on biopsy specimens. This allows the clinician to predict whether an individual patient is likely to benefit from hormonal therapy. For example, it is now standard to measure **estrogen receptor (ER)** and progesterone receptor (PR) content in breast cancer tissue. Patients with ER- or PR-positive tumors are more likely to respond to antiestrogen therapy compared with patients who lack these hormone receptors.

The antiestrogens tamoxifen and toremifene have been used to treat patients with ER-positive breast cancer. Tamoxifen also has been used as a chemopreventative agent in women with very high risk of developing breast cancer. Tamoxifen functions as a competitive partial agonist-inhibitor by binding to estrogen receptors of estrogen-sensitive tissues and tumors and inducing a conformational change. These agents are generally well tolerated but may cause **menopausal symptoms** (hot flashes, vaginal dryness) in premenopausal women. An initial flare of tumor or bone pain may arise when therapy is started, but these effects usually dissipate with continued treatment.

Aminoglutethimide is a nonsteroidal inhibitor of corticosteroid biosynthesis. It results in decreased production of endogenous estrogens, androgens, and cortisol. It has been used to treat patients with breast cancer, and off-label uses include treatment of prostate cancer. Because this is a relatively nonselective inhibitor, corticosteroid supplementation must be used concurrently to prevent symptoms of **adrenal insufficiency**. Anastrozole and letrozole are nonsteroidal specific inhibitors of the **aromatase** enzyme. By inhibiting this enzyme, they reduce conversion of androgens to estrogens without affecting adrenal steroid synthesis. Aromatization may occur in adipose tissue, and these agents are useful to decrease extragonadal estrogen synthesis in postmenopausal women with breast cancer (ER positive or unknown status).

Due to potentially serious adverse effects on the fetus, all the hormonal agents that affect sex hormones must be avoided during pregnancy.

Case Conclusion BB began treatment with flutamide and leuprolide (intramuscular depot). For the first few days he noted increased bone pain, which was manageable with analgesics. After 2 weeks of therapy, his bone pain was much improved compared with baseline. Upon questioning, he admits to some loss of libido but is otherwise tolerating the medications.

Thumbnail: Hormonal Agents Used in Cancer Therapy

	Drug class			
	Aromatase inhibitors	Antiestrogens	Antiandrogens	LHRH agonists
Prototype agent	Anastrozole	Tamoxifen	Flutamide	Leuprolide
Other agents in class	Letrozole Exemestane Aminoglutethimide	Toremifene	Bicalutamide Nilutamide	Goserelin
Clinical uses	Breast cancer in post-menopausal women (ER positive or unknown)	Breast cancer (ER positive or unknown)	Prostate cancer	Prostate cancer, palliative treatment of advanced breast cancer (goserelin), endometriosis (low dose)
MOA	Nonsteroidal inhibitors of aromatase enzyme; decrease conversion of androgens to estrogens	Competitively block estrogen receptors	Inhibit androgen uptake or inhibit androgen binding in target tissues	Suppress production of LH and FSH, resulting in decreased testosterone and estrogen levels
Pharmacokinetics				
Absorption/ distribution	Good oral absorption	Good oral absorption	Good oral absorption	Not absorbed orally; give SC or long-acting IM depot
Metabolism/ elimination	Hepatic metabolism (85%); T½ 50 hr	Hepatic metabolism, T½ 7 days	Extensive metabolism with metabolites eliminated in urine; T½ 5–6 hr	Metabolism and elimination not well defined
Adverse reactions	Hot flashes, mild nausea, anorexia, edema, headache, diarrhea	Hot flashes, mild nausea, vaginal dryness, transient thrombocytopenia, bone/ tumor pain, thromboembolic events, hepatotoxicity, fluid retention	Hot flashes, loss of libido, impotence, diarrhea, nausea, anorexia, gyneco-mastia, edema, rare hepatotoxicity	Depression, hot flashes, nausea, weight gain, edema, gynecomastia
Precautions	Aminoglutethimide administered with adrenal replacement doses of hydrocortisone.	Hypercalcemia may occur in patients with bone metastases.	Use in combination with LHRH agonist.	

Questions

1. A 37-year-old premenopausal woman with breast cancer (ER and PR positive) is being started on hormonal therapy after a modified radical mastectomy. She is still interested in having children in the future, if possible. Which of the following regimens is most appropriate for her?

   A. Ethinyl estradiol
   B. Letrozole
   C. Tamoxifen
   D. Flutamide
   E. Nilutamide

2. A 62-year-old postmenopausal woman with metastatic breast cancer is starting treatment with anastrozole. Which potential side effect(s) do you anticipate and monitor?

   A. Severe myelosuppression
   B. Hot flashes
   C. Adrenal insufficiency
   D. Hepatotoxicity
   E. All of the above

HPI: PS is a 65-year-old man with follicular B-cell non-Hodgkin's lymphoma (NHL). He had undergone treatment with standard chemotherapy last year but now has relapsed. Past medical history includes diabetes mellitus and depression. He is willing to undergo further treatment for his NHL but refuses to have any chemotherapy that would require him to be admitted to a hospital. He wonders what treatment options are available for him.

Thought Questions

- How are monoclonal antibodies (MoAbs) used to treat cancer?

- What MoAbs are currently available for treating cancer?

- What are some adverse effects of MoAb treatment?

- What precautions may be taken to avoid some of these side effects?

Basic Science Review and Discussion

Monoclonal antibodies may be used as passive immunotherapy to treat malignancies. They react with specific antigens present on the surface of tumor cells and result in cell destruction. Rituximab was the first MoAb approved in the United States for the treatment of cancer. It is a chimeric MoAb directed against cluster differentiation 20 (CD20) markers, which are expressed on over 90% of B-cell NHL tumors. Rituximab is thought to result in B-cell depletion by a number of mechanisms, including complement-mediated and antibody-dependent cell lysis and induction of apoptosis.

Additional MoAbs used in treating cancer are listed in Table 68-1. The mechanism of action is generally thought to be similar, although the unique cellular targets differentiate the agents. Of the four MoAbs available, only gemtuzumab ozogamicin incorporates a toxin (calicheamicin) that is covalently linked to the MoAb. After the MoAb binds to the CD33 antigen, the entire complex is internalized into the cell where the calicheamicin is released and results in cellular toxicity due to double-strand DNA breaks.

In general, the MoAbs used in treating cancer are relatively well tolerated compared with conventional cytotoxic chemotherapy. The main adverse effect associated with rituximab use is infusion-related or **hypersensitivity** reactions. Patients may experience fever, rigors, dyspnea, hypotension, and rarely anaphylactoid reactions. Premedication with acetaminophen, diphenhydramine, and corticosteroids can reduce these reactions. Patients with significant tumor burden at the time of first treatment with rituximab may experience **tumor lysis syndrome,** and appropriate measures should be implemented to prevent this complication in these patients.

Trastuzumab also may cause infusion-related or hypersensitivity reactions (particularly with the first infusion). However, a more concerning possible side effect is **cardiac dysfunction** (including CHF). Although patients may develop cardiac dysfunction with trastuzumab alone, the incidence is significantly increased in patients who receive trastuzumab in combination with paclitaxel or in those patients with previous use of anthracyclines.

Alemtuzumab has been associated with significant infusion-related reactions (almost 90% of patients will experience fever and rigors during the infusion) and premedication is recommended. In addition, patients treated with this agent may become profoundly immunocompromised and are at

Table 68-1 Monoclonal antibodies used in treatment of malignancies

MoAb	Target antigen and cells expressing antigen	Clinical indications	Adverse reactions
Rituximab	CD20 Normal and malignant B-lymphocytes	B-cell NHL	Hypersensitivity and infusion-related reactions
Trastuzumab	Her2/neu Overexpressed in 25%–30% of primary breast cancer	Metastatic breast cancer (overexpressing Her2/neu)	Hypersensitivity; cardiac dysfunction
Alemtuzumab	CD52 Normal and malignant B-lymphocytes, T cells, NK cells, monocytes, macrophages, platelets (not hematopoietic stem cells)	Chronic lymphocytic leukemia	Hypersensitivity and infusion related reactions, profound immunosuppression
Gemtuzumab ozogamicin	CD33 Immature myeloid cells and leukemic cells (not normal hematopoietic stem cells)	AML	Hypersensitivity and profound neutropenia and thrombocytopenia

high risk for developing **opportunistic infections** such as PCP and herpes virus infections. All patients receiving alemtuzumab should be appropriately prophylaxed against these infections, and the drug is absolutely contraindicated in patients with active infections.

Gemtuzumab ozogamicin is almost universally associated with profound **neutropenia** and **thrombocytopenia.** These effects may last weeks after the therapy is completed, and patients must be monitored closely for infections and bleeding complications.

Case Conclusion   PS agrees to treatment with rituximab for his NHL, which can easily be administered weekly in the outpatient clinic. He was appropriately premedicated prior to each infusion and tolerated the regimen well.

Thumbnail: Monoclonal Antibodies for Cancer

Prototype drug: Rituximab

Clinical uses: Relapsed or refractory low-grade or follicular B-cell NHL, which expresses CD20.

MOA: Chimeric monoclonal antibody directed against CD20 surface antigen expressed on B-lymphocytes. Results in cell death by complement-mediated and antibody-dependent cell lysis and induction of apoptosis.

Pharmacokinetics

Absorption: Administered IV only.

Adverse reactions: Infusion-related and hypersensitivity reactions, occasional nausea/vomiting, headache, rare cardiac arrhythmias, leukopenia, thrombocytopenia.

Precautions: Consider premedication with diphenhydramine, acetaminophen with or without corticosteroids to minimize infusion-related and hypersensitivity reactions.

Questions

1. GL is a 56-year-old man with refractory chronic lymphocytic leukemia. He has failed prior therapy with fludarabine and chlorambucil. His oncologist wishes to start treatment with alemtuzumab. Which of the following precautions should be undertaken prior to starting this therapy?

   A. Rule out any current active infections.
   B. Premedication with acetaminophen, antihistamine, and corticosteroids prior to each infusion.
   C. Begin patient on daily doses of TMP-SMX.
   D. Start prophylactic doses of acyclovir.
   E. A and B only.
   F. A and C only.
   G. B, C, and D only.
   H. All of the above.

2. A 68-year-old man with relapsed AML presents to the clinic to evaluate further treatment options. He received high-dose chemotherapy (cytarabine and daunorubicin) earlier this year with complications of cardiotoxicity due to the daunorubicin and neurotoxicity from the cytarabine. He has relapsed after a brief remission. Which of the following MoAbs may be considered for use in this patient?

   A. Rituximab
   B. Trastuzumab
   C. Alemtuzumab
   D. Gemtuzumab ozogamicin
   E. Daclizumab

> **HPI:** CC is a 55-year-old woman with chronic myelogenous leukemia (CML) in chronic phase. She was diagnosed with CML 2 years ago. Due to her age, she is deemed not a candidate for allogeneic bone marrow transplantation. She had been maintained on interferon-α therapy for the past year but has not achieved cytogenetic remission and complains that she "hates the way the interferon makes me feel." She is in otherwise good health.

Thought Questions

- What treatment options are available for chronic phase CML?

- What is the Philadelphia chromosome? How does its presence lead to CML?

- What is the MOA of imatinib mesylate?

- What are the major adverse reactions associated with imatinib and how are they managed?

Basic Science Review and Discussion

Chronic myelogenous leukemia may progress through several clinical phases. Most patients are diagnosed with CML in **chronic phase**. CML may then progress to **accelerated phase** and finally to **blast crisis** (either lymphoid or myeloid), which resembles acute leukemia and may be difficult to treat.

Hydroxyurea and busulfan are oral chemotherapy agents that have been used to stabilize and maintain blood counts; however, they do not prevent disease evolution. For patients in chronic phase, the only known curative option is **allogeneic bone marrow transplantation**. However, this procedure requires patients to have a suitable sibling donor or a matched unrelated donor and carries a high mortality rate due to complications. Patients who are not candidates for allogeneic transplantation (due to age, underlying medical conditions, inability to find a suitable donor) may be maintained on interferon-α therapy (with or without cytarabine) with the goal of remaining in chronic phase. This therapy is generally not considered curative.

Chronic myelogenous leukemia results from a reciprocal translocation between chromosomes 9 and 22, which forms the **Philadelphia chromosome** (Ph+). This chromosomal abnormality leads to the constitutive production of an **abnormal tyrosine kinase (Bcr-Abl)**, which in turn signals growth of leukemic cells.

Imatinib mesylate is a new tyrosine kinase inhibitor designed for the treatment of CML. It inhibits the Bcr-Abl tyrosine kinase leading to inhibition of proliferation and induction of apoptosis in Bcr-Abl-positive cells. Imatinib is indicated for treatment of CML in blast crisis, accelerated phase, or chronic phase in patients who have failed interferon therapy. Response rates have been evaluated in terms of hematologic and cytogenetic (decrease or disappearance of Philadelphia chromosome) responses.

Response rates vary depending on the phase of CML. Hematologic and cytogenetic responses are best in patients treated while in chronic phase. Note that while imatinib is promising and results in favorable hematologic and cytogenetic response rates compared with existing therapies, there are currently no available randomized studies to demonstrate clinical benefit (such as survival) compared with existing therapies. It also has activity in gastrointestinal stromal tumors (GISTs) and is indicated for treatment of patients with unresectable or metastatic GISTs.

Imatinib is relatively well tolerated, but it has some significant adverse effects. Some of the most common side effects include nausea, vomiting, diarrhea, **edema**, muscle cramps, and rash. The edema is usually characterized by periorbital swelling or lower limb edema but may manifest as pleural effusions, ascites, and pulmonary edema. The fluid retention is often managed with dose reduction, diuretics and other supportive care measures. Imatinib also may be associated with **cytopenias** (primarily neutropenia and thrombocytopenia). These effects are thought to be dose related and are more common in patients with accelerated phase or blast crisis compared with chronic phase CML. Dose reduction or interruption in imatinib therapy may be considered to manage the cytopenias.

> **Case Conclusion** CC's oncologist decides to stop the interferon therapy and initiate a trial of imatinib mesylate. She tolerated the imatinib well, with minimal complaints of lower extremity edema for which she was prescribed furosemide. Six weeks after starting imatinib, CC's peripheral blood smear appeared normal (hematologic response) and cytogenetic evaluation of her bone marrow revealed disappearance of the Philadelphia chromosome.

Thumbnail: Imatinib Mesylate

Clinical uses: CML—patients in blast crisis, accelerated phase, or chronic phase after failure of interferon therapy; unresectable or metastatic GISTs.

MOA: Inhibits abnormal Bcr-Abl tyrosine kinase resulting from Philadelphia chromosome; inhibits proliferation and induces apoptosis of Bcr-Abl-positive cells.

Pharmacokinetics

Absorption: Excellent oral absorption (98%). No IV formulation.

Metabolism/elimination: Hepatically metabolized (primarily by CYP3A4) to active metabolite. Metabolites are eliminated in the feces.

Adverse reactions: Gastrointestinal (nausea, diarrhea, vomiting), fluid retention and edema, cytopenias (neutropenia and thrombocytopenia), hepatotoxicity, rash, muscle cramps.

Drug interactions: CYP3A4 enzyme substrate and inhibitor. Use caution when coadministering imatinib with CYP3A4 inhibitors (increased exposure and toxicity due to imatinib). Imatinib may inhibit clearance of other CYP3A4 substrates (such as HMG CoA reductase inhibitors, warfarin, etc.).

Questions

1. A 66-year-old man with CML in accelerated phase is being evaluated prior to initiation of imatinib mesylate therapy. PMH includes hypertension. Vital signs are within normal limits. Weight is 71 kg. Labs: WBC 11,500/mm^3, ANC 3200/mm^3, platelets 9800/mm^3, Cr 1.2 mg/dL, electrolytes normal, total bilirubin 0.8 mg/dL, AST 46 IU/L, ALT 55 IU/L. Which of the following is (are) important baseline parameters to obtain prior to initiating therapy with imatinib?

   A. Weight
   B. ANC
   C. Platelets
   D. Total bilirubin
   E. All of the above

2. A 47-year-old woman was started on imatinib for chronic phase CML 3 weeks ago. She returns to clinic for follow-up but states that she has been tolerating the new drug very poorly. She complains of periorbital edema and moderately severe GI upset (nausea, diarrhea). Her oncologist checks the dose and verifies that she has been taking the proper amount. PMH includes HTN (on furosemide and atenolol), asthma (albuterol inhaler), diabetes (controlled with glipizide), and fungal pneumonia being treated with itraconazole oral solution. Which of the following medications may be contributing to this patient's imatinib toxicity?

   A. Furosemide
   B. Atenolol
   C. Albuterol
   D. Glipizide
   E. Itraconazole

HPI: AH is a 57-year-old man who just received an orthotopic liver transplant for hepatitis C cirrhosis. PMH includes hepatitis C cirrhosis, ascites, and hepatic encephalopathy.

Labs: Serum Cr 1.2 mg/dL, BUN 12 mg/dL, K 4.5 mEq/L, Na 140 mEq/L, WBC 6700/mm³, HCT 39%, Platelets 8900/mm³, ALT 50 IU/L, INR 1.2, Total bilirubin 1.2 mg/dL. AH will receive prednisone, mycophenolate mofetil, and tacrolimus to prevent allograft rejection.

Thought Questions

- Why are immunosuppressive drugs necessary following solid organ transplantation?

- What immunosuppressive drugs are used to *prevent* allograft rejection in solid organ transplantation?

- What immunosuppressive drugs can be used to *treat* allograft rejection?

- What are some potential complications as a result of immunosuppression?

Basic Science Review and Discussion

Organ transplantation can be a life-saving procedure or can be used to improve the quality of life. Heart, kidney, liver, lung, pancreas, and small bowel are the organs most commonly transplanted in clinical practice.

Immunosuppressive drugs are necessary following transplantation to prevent **acute rejection** of the grafted organ. Acute rejection is a normal alloresponse because the grafted organ is recognized as foreign by the recipient's immune system. Antigens from the donor organ are presented by macrophages to lymphocytes. The lymphocytes in turn are activated and begin to proliferate. Cytotoxic lymphocytes attack the allograft, causing organ damage. Immunosuppressive drugs are used to block this alloresponse to prevent rejection. Acute rejection is a predictor for chronic rejection. Chronic rejection is a common cause of graft loss in kidney transplant recipients.

Immunosuppressive drugs can be divided into five basic categories. **Corticosteroids** such as **methylprednisolone** and **prednisone** are a part of virtually all immunosuppressive drug regimens. Corticosteroids block the production of IL-1 and have potent anti-inflammatory effects. **Calcineurin inhibitors** such as **cyclosporine** and **tacrolimus** are also used in a majority of immunosuppressive drug regimens. Calcineurin inhibitors inhibit the production and secretion of IL-2. IL-2 is involved with T-lymphocyte activation and proliferation. **Antiproliferative agents** such as **azathioprine, mycophenolate mofetil,** and **sirolimus** block T-lymphocyte proliferation by a variety of mechanisms. **The IL-2 receptor antagonists** such as **basiliximab** and **daclizumab** are monoclonal antibodies that competitively block the IL-2 receptor, preventing IL-2 from binding to it. **Antithymocyte globulin** and **muromonab CD3** are collectively called the **antilymphocyte antibodies**. These antibodies bind to lymphocytes that express certain surface markers such as CD2, CD3, CD4, CD8, CD25, etc., inactivate them, and remove them from circulation.

Immunosuppressive drugs of different classes are used in combination to maximize immunosuppression while minimizing side effects. The choice of a particular agent or combination may be specific to the organ(s) transplanted, reason for transplantation, concomitant medical conditions, and transplant center. The most common combination is a triple regimen that consists of a corticosteroid (prednisone), a calcineurin inhibitor (cyclosporine or tacrolimus), and an antiproliferative drug (mycophenolate, sirolimus, or azathioprine). The goal of immunosuppression is to decrease the patient's immune response to the allograft while avoiding side effects, **opportunistic infections,** and malignancies.

Complications can be medication related or the result of overimmunosuppression. Common medication-related side effects are reviewed in the Thumbnail section. Common side effects of corticosteroids include insomnia, psychosis, **hyperglycemia,** HTN, and adrenal suppression. Treatment with calcineurin inhibitors may result in **HTN, nephrotoxicity,** neurotoxicity, and electrolyte imbalances. The antiproliferative agents may cause bone marrow suppression and gastrointestinal upset. Adverse effects associated with the antilymphocyte antibodies include infusion-related reactions (including **anaphylactoid** reactions), flulike symptoms, opportunistic infections, and malignancies. Overimmunosuppression may predispose the patient to opportunistic infections such as PCP, **viral infections** (herpes virus, cytomegalovirus), and **fungal infections** (Candida and Aspergillus species). In addition, patients on long-term immunosuppression may be prone to develop malignancies such as lymphomas and skin cancers (squamous cell, basal cell carcinoma).

The calcineurin inhibitors (cyclosporine and tacrolimus) and sirolimus are metabolized in the liver and gut by **CYP450-**

3A4. There are many drugs that can interact with CYP450-3A4. Caution must be used when choosing drug therapy in a patient taking one of these immunosuppressive drugs to avoid potentially serious **drug-drug interactions**. Target concentrations may vary depending on organ(s) transplanted and transplant center-specific protocols. In general, concentrations of cyclosporine between 200 and 300 ng/mL are considered therapeutic. Similarly, concentrations of both tacrolimus and sirolimus should be maintained between 5 and 15 ng/mL.

Case Conclusion   AH recovered uneventfully from his liver transplantation. He continues to tolerate his immunosuppressive regimen relatively well with mild complications of hyperglycemia (controlled with insulin) and HTN (for which amlodipine was prescribed).

Thumbnail: Immunosuppressants

	Drug class				
	Corticosteroid	Calcineurin inhibitor	Antiproliferative	Antilymphocyte antibody	IL-2 receptor antagonist
Prototype agent(s)	Prednisone and methylprednisolone	Cyclosporine (CSA) and tacrolimus	Azathioprine, mycophenolate mofetil, sirolimus	Muromonab CD3, antithymocyte globulin (ATG)	Basiliximab and daclizumab
MOA	Inhibition of IL-1; anti-inflammatory	Inhibit of T-lymphocyte activation and proliferation by blocking production of IL-2	Purine antagonist (azathioprine); inhibit purine biosynthesis (mycophenolate); sirolimus inhibits IL-2-driven cell cycle progression	Anti-CD3 antibody (muromonab CD3); deplete T-lymphocytes (ATG)	MoAb that blocks IL-2 receptor
Pharmacokinetics					
Absorption	Well absorbed; available IV and PO	Variable oral absorption; both are available IV and PO	Azathioprine IV and PO; mycophenolate IV and PO; sirolimus has rapid oral absorption (PO only)	Not absorbed orally; IV only	Not absorbed orally, IV only
Elimination	Hepatic; T½ 3 hr	Hepatic (CYP 3A4); T½ 8–12 hr	Renal (azathioprine T½ 3 hr and mycophenolate T½ 18 hr); sirolimus is hepatic (CYP3A4), T½ 60 hr	N/A; muromomab T½ 18 hr; ATG T½ 72 hr	N/A; T½ 14–20 days
Adverse reactions	Psychosis, insomnia, edema, weight gain, HTN, hyperglycemia, osteoporosis, adrenal suppression, impaired wound healing, infection	Nephrotoxicity, neurotoxicity, HTN, tremors, headache, hyperglycemia, hyperkalemia, nausea, diarrhea (tacrolimus), hirsutism (CSA)	Leukopenia, thrombocytopenia, nausea, diarrhea, gastritis (mycophenolate), stomatitis (azathioprine), sirolimus also may cause hyperlipidemia and hypertension	Flulike symptoms, pulmonary edema, anaphylactoid reactions, infection, malignancies, aseptic meningitis (muromonab), bone marrow suppression (ATG)	Infusion reactions

Questions

1. AH is a 58-year-old man who received a liver transplant for hepatitis C cirrhosis. His ALT is 40 IU/L, INR 1.1, serum Cr 1.2 mg/dL, WBC 1900/mm^3, platelets 88/mm^3. Which drug can cause AH's leukopenia and thrombocytopenia?

   A. Tacrolimus
   B. Mycophenolate mofetil
   C. Prednisone
   D. Basiliximab
   E. Cyclosporine

2. CW is a 45-year-old woman who received a cadaveric renal transplant for diabetic nephropathy 2 months ago. A recent renal biopsy reveals acute cellular rejection. Her immunosuppressive medications include cyclosporine modified, mycophenolate mofetil, and prednisone. What immunosuppressive drugs can be used for the treatment of acute rejection?

   A. Basiliximab
   B. Sirolimus
   C. Azathioprine
   D. Daclizumab
   E. Antithymocyte globulin

Answer Key

Case 1
1. B
2. G

Case 2
1. D
2. E

Case 3
1. E
2. E

Case 4
1. A
2. D

Case 5
1. C
2. B

Case 6
1. B
2. E

Case 7
1. B
2. A

Case 8
1. B
2. C

Case 9
1. C
2. D

Case 10
1. B
2. B

Case 11
1. E
2. B

Case 12
1. A
2. E

Case 13
1. D
2. A

Case 14
1. C
2. E

Case 15
1. B
2. E

Case 16
1. D
2. B

Case 17
1. E
2. A

Case 18
1. B
2. C

Case 19
1. E
2. F

Case 20
1. A
2. C

Case 21
1. B
2. C

Case 22
1. C
2. B

Case 23
1. B
2. D

Case 24
1. A
2. B

Case 25
1. D
2. C

Case 26
1. D
2. E

Case 27
1. B
2. A

Case 28
1. E
2. F

Case 29
1. A
2. D

Case 30
1. C
2. E

Case 31
1. B
2. E

Case 32
1. E
2. D

Case 33
1. B
2. E

Case 34
1. E
2. B

Case 35
1. C
2. E

Case 36
1. A
2. E

Case 37
1. A
2. C

Case 38
1. B
2. D

Case 39
1. D
2. C

Case 40
1. E
2. A

Case 41
1. E
2. C

Case 42
1. A
2. C

Case 43
1. A
2. E

Case 44
1. E
2. C

Case 45
1. C
2. D

Case 46
1. D
2. D

Case 47
1. B
2. F

Case 48
1. E
2. C

Case 49
1. A
2. C

Case 50
1. B
2. C

Case 51
1. C
2. D

Case 52
1. H
2. C

Case 53
1. C
2. F

Case 54
1. B
2. C

Case 55
1. D
2. A

Case 56
1. E
2. F

Case 57
1. G
2. B

Case 58
1. D
2. C

Case 59
1. B
2. E

Case 60
1. F
2. D

Case 61

1. D
2. E

Case 62

1. D
2. E

Case 63

1. E
2. B

Case 64

1. E
2. B

Case 65

1. C
2. E

Case 66

1. A
2. E

Case 67

1. C
2. B

Case 68

1. H
2. D

Case 69

1. E
2. E

Case 70

1. B
2. E

Answers

Case 1

1. B Amiodarone reduces the clearance of digoxin by half, and the digoxin levels double approximately 1 to 2 weeks following the initiation of amiodarone therapy. Although hypokalemia increases the potential for any digoxin level to produce toxicity (pharmacodynamic effect), hypokalemia does not change either the absorption, distribution, or metabolism/elimination of digoxin. With a digoxin T½ of 4 days, the digoxin concentration should decrease to 1.8 µg/L (3.6/2) after 4 days, and an additional 4 days (8 days total) would be required for the digoxin level to decline to about 0.9 µg/L (1.8/2). Digoxin is normally 20% metabolized and 80% renally eliminated. Even if the patient had half the normal renal function and the 80% were reduced in half, the remaining 40% would still be the majority of the route by which digoxin is cleared from the body. Benazepril does not change the pharmacokinetics of digoxin. It does have the potential to increase serum potassium.

2. G Given the patient's, age, weight, sex, and serum Cr, his calculated CrCl rate is 20 mL/min:

$$\text{CrCl for males (mL/min)} = \frac{(140 - \text{age})(\text{weight})}{(72)(\text{Cr})}$$

$$= \frac{(140 - 80 \text{ yr})(72 \text{ kg})}{(72)(3 \text{ mg/dL})}$$

$$= 20 \text{ mL/min}$$

That would indicate that the recommended dose of cefepime is 0.5 to 1 g every 24 hours. Because the CrCl rate is in the middle of the recommended range, either dose would be reasonable. If only the serum Cr were used to approximate renal function, the serum Cr of 3 is three times higher than the usual value of 1 mg/dL, indicating a one-third normal value or about 33 mL/min. Thus, only using the serum creatinine to estimate a patient's renal function overestimates the actual value when patients weigh significantly less than 70 kg or are of advanced age.

Case 2

1. D The prolonged administration of procainamide often leads to the development of a positive ANA test result, with or without symptoms of a lupus erythematous-like syndrome. The common symptoms of lupus erythematous-like syndrome are arthralgia, malaise, rash, fever, chills, and arthritis, which may occur more often in slow acetylators because they do not metabolize procainamide as well. If a positive ANA titer develops, assess the benefit/risk ratio related to continued procainamide therapy.

2. E All of the above. Disopyramide is poorly tolerated in the elderly due to anticholinergic side effects and should be avoided in patients with CHF due to negative inotropic effects. Flecainide should be avoided in patients with underlying cardiac disease because these patients are more prone to experience cardiac

arrhythmias and sudden death with this drug. Procainamide is not the best choice in this patient due to his underlying renal dysfunction. Procainamide's active metabolite (NAPA) is renally eliminated, and accumulation of NAPA has been associated with toxicity such as torsade de pointes.

Case 3

1. E Congestive heart failure. Lidocaine is cleared by liver metabolism. Any condition that decreases liver metabolism or liver blood flow may increase lidocaine levels. If a patient has CHF, advanced age, shock, or liver cirrhosis, a lower infusion rate should be considered. Diabetes, atrial flutter, tachycardia, and sodium levels are unlikely to affect hepatic blood flow or lidocaine clearance.

2. E All of the above. At high lidocaine levels of 6 to 10 µg/mL, patients may start to experience confusion, agitation, psychosis, seizures, and coma. The active metabolite of lidocaine, GX, is responsible for most of the CNS toxicities. Since the active metabolite is renally cleared, caution should be taken in patients with renal insufficiency.

Case 4

1. A Sotalol has nonselective beta-blocking properties that may cause bronchospasm in patients with asthma and COPD. Although amiodarone has beta-blocking activity, this effect is specific to the heart and therefore is not contraindicated in patients with asthma. Also, the patient has not taken amiodarone for a long enough period to develop pulmonary fibrosis. Procainamide, quinidine, and lidocaine are unlikely to cause bronchospasm.

2. D Amiodarone is the best option. Disopyramide, quinidine, and sotalol all have negative inotropic effects, which may exacerbate his CHF. Lidocaine may be given in patients with CHF, but it is only administered IV due to its low bioavailability and is not suitable for long-term maintenance.

Case 5

1. C Methylxanthines such as theophylline are adenosine receptor antagonists. In the presence of methylxanthines, larger doses of adenosine may be required or some patients may be refractory to adenosine. The other drugs are not likely to interfere with adenosine's efficacy.

2. B Because this patient has asthma and is wheezing, calcium channel blockers are the drug class of choice. Unlike beta-blockers and adenosine, they do not cause bronchospasm. Beta-blockers and adenosine should be used cautiously in patients with obstructive lung disease, and use should be avoided in patients with asthma. Digoxin is not contraindicated, but it is not the drug of choice due to its slow onset. Amiodarone is indicated for ventricular arrhythmias, but not PSVT.

Case 6

1. B Hypokalemia. Electrolyte imbalances, such as hypokalemia, hypomagnesemia, and hypercalcimia are risk factors for digoxin toxicity. This 55-year-old man with a serum Cr of 0.8 mg/dL appears to have normal renal clearance; therefore, it should not contribute to digoxin toxicity. Hyperkalemia also can put a patient at risk for toxicity by inhibiting digoxin effects on the Na^+/K^+ ATPase pump. However, amphotericin B is known to cause a decrease in potassium and magnesium levels; therefore, hypokalemia is the best choice.

2. E Digoxin-immune Fab (digoxin antibodies). Lidocaine is useful for treating ventricular arrhythmias. Reversal therapies for hyperkalemia include glucose with insulin or sodium polystyrene sulfonate, but this patient has only mildly elevated potassium. However, AH exhibits a life-threatening intoxication of digoxin that warrants the use of digoxin antibodies. She is bradycardic and not responding to atropine. The antibodies work by binding to digoxin, therefore rendering it unavailable for binding to cells in the body. Clinical improvement can be seen within 30 minutes of administration. Side effects including allergic reactions are rare. However, removing the pharmacologic effect of digoxin may precipitate exacerbation of CHF or atrial fibrillation.

Case 7

1. B This patient reports that he hasn't used this particular bottle of sublingual tablets for over a year. Because the SL tablets are volatile and lose potency when exposed to air, they must only be used for a maximum of 6 months after the original container is opened. Monitoring of the expiration date must be strict, and expired SL nitroglycerin should be replaced. This medication should be stored in a cool, dry place and should be closed tightly after each opening. In addition, the SL nitroglycerin must be protected from light and therefore be kept in the original amber bottle. Nitrate tolerance is not correct because tolerance occurs with continuous exposure to nitrates. Because short-acting nitrates have a rapid onset of action and short duration, it is unlikely to cause tolerance.

2. A Isosorbide dinitrate tablets. Adding atenolol or verapamil for angina is not uncommon. However, this patient's BP and HR are within normal range. Adding nitroglycerin ointment is messy and is not the best alternative for an active lifestyle. Sublingual isosorbide dinitrate has a slower onset of action but does not offer any advantage over SL nitroglycerin. Isosorbide dinitrate tablets are longer acting and can control symptoms throughout the day, especially for patients with active lifestyles. Isosorbide dinitrate should be given three times daily over a 10-hour period (e.g., at 7:00 A.M., 12:00 P.M., and 5:00 P.M.).

Case 8

1. B With long-term use of beta-blockers, there is an upregulation of the beta-receptors. When beta-blockers are abruptly stopped after chronic use, these agents can cause rebound HTN. Exacerba-

tion of angina, MI, arrhythmias, and death may occur. A gradual tapering of beta-blockers over 1 to 2 weeks may avoid the rebound. It is possible that the antihypertensive medications were not adequate; since he has not taken his medications for 5 days, this would be difficult to assess. Loratadine, asthma, or hyperglycemia are also unlikely to increase blood pressure.

2. C The patient has COPD and renal impairment; thus, the beta-blocker selected should be β_1 selective and hepatically cleared. Atenolol is renally cleared. Nadolol is nonselective and renally excreted. Both propranolol and labetolol are nonselective. Metoprolol is the best choice because it is β_1 selective and hepatically eliminated.

Case 9

1. C Diltiazem. Quinidine can be used to maintain normal sinus rhythm (NSR) after cardioversion of atrial fibrillation. Metoprolol is commonly used to control ventricular rate before conversion to NSR. However, this patient has two contraindications (COPD and diabetes) for beta-blocker use. Unlike diltiazem, amlodipine and nimodipine do not block AV nodal conduction; therefore, they would be ineffective at rate control.

2. D Verapamil. Verapamil has been the calcium channel blocker most studied for migraine prophylaxis. In addition, verapamil is the calcium channel blocker associated with inducing both constipation and gingival hyperplasia. Nifedipine and diltiazem should not be used since studies have shown that their efficacy is questionable for migraine prophylaxis. Bepridil is used only for chronic stable angina. Amlodipine may be used for migraine prophylaxis, but it is not as likely to produce the side effects that this patient is experiencing.

Case 10

1. B Unlike other diuretics, furosemide at high infusion rates is associated with ototoxicity. Ototoxicity may occur with all loop diuretics, but the frequency is less with bumetanide and it has not been reported with torsemide. In addition, hypocalcemia is a side effect also experienced with loop diuretics and not with thiazide diuretics. In contrast, hydrochlorothiazide decreases urinary excretion of calcium, which may result in an elevation of serum calcium levels. Thus, thiazide diuretics may potentially reduce the risk of osteoporosis and be beneficial in postmenopausal women.

2. B Diuretics that act on the distal tubule (thiazides and potassium-sparing diuretics) lose their effectiveness when CrCl decreases to less than 30 to 50 mL/min. The loop diuretics are more potent and retain their effectiveness at low CrCl ($>$ 5 mL/min).

Case 11

1. E One of the primary adverse effects of ACE inhibitors is hypotension. It may be manifested as dizziness, lightheadedness, presyncope, or syncope. It occurs most commonly with the first dose. Patients at risk for developing hypotension are those with hyponatremia (serum sodium < 130 mEq/L), recent increases in diuretic dose, and hypovolemia. Hypotension can be minimized by temporarily withholding or reducing the diuretic dose and/or starting the ACE-I at lower doses.

2. B ACE inhibitors such as captopril may cause angioedema. The incidence of angioedema is less than 1% and may occur any time during therapy. The swelling is usually confined to the face, lips, tongue, glottis, and larynx. Antihistamines may be used to relieve discomfort, but symptoms usually resolve without treatment. If the swelling obstructs the airway, then epinephrine should be administered immediately. Patients should not be rechallenged with an ACE inhibitor if they have a history of angioedema. The other adverse effects are not likely caused by captopril. The bradycardia is caused by metoprolol, flushing is caused by isosorbide dinitrate, and morphine may cause hallucinations, especially in the elderly.

Case 12

1. A Both ACE inhibitors and ARBs are contraindicated in patients with bilateral renal stenosis. Patients with bilateral renal stenosis have decreased blood flow to the glomerulus. When given ACE inhibitors or ARBs, the effects of angiotensin II are reduced, which leads to vasodilatation of the efferent arterioles. This will result in a decrease in pressure and glomerular filtration rate and a worsening of the renal function.

2. E ACE inhibitors and ARBs may induce or potentiate renal impairment and elevate serum potassium, especially in patients who have underlying renal dysfunction or are taking concurrent medications that can increase serum potassium. Upon initiation of ACE inhibitors and ARBs, baseline serum Cr, BUN, and serum potassium should be obtained and then monitored periodically. BP also should be monitored regularly to evaluate efficacy and risk of hypotension.

Case 13

1. D Amiodarone may decrease warfarin metabolism within a week of coadministration, or the effects of the interaction may be delayed for several weeks. Patients who develop hyperthyroidism secondary to amiodarone may have an additional increased anticoagulant effect, because the turnover of clotting factors is more rapid. If amiodarone is discontinued, effects of the decreased warfarin metabolism may last 1 to 3 months.

2. A Patient's INR is supratherapeutic. She is not having any major bleeding other than the slight nosebleed. Having a poor appetite may have decreased the amount of vitamin K that is absorbed. In addition, fevers also can increase the turnover of clotting factors. Because the patient has taken her morning dose of warfarin, her INR may continue to increase. Giving vitamin K orally at 2.5 mg would reverse the INR back toward the therapeutic range. Because it is given PO, effects are more predictable, compared to doses given SC. The IV route is not necessary in this patient, because she is not bleeding. Also, there may be a small percentage of anaphylaxis with the IV route.

Case 14

1. C Clopidogrel. Patients with preexisting asthma may develop hypersensitivity reactions to aspirin; therefore, a thienopyridine should be used. Clopidogrel should always be considered before ticlopidine because it is associated with fewer side effects. Ticlopidine has been associated with life-threatening neutropenia and other blood dyscrasias. Abciximab and eptifabitide are GpIIb/IIIa inhibitors that are only available IV.

2. E Discontinue abciximab, aspirin, and heparin and give a platelet transfusion. Because abciximab is associated with thrombocytopenia, platelet counts should be monitored carefully. The manufacturer recommends that a platelet count be obtained prior to initiation of abciximab, 2 to 4 hours following the bolus dose, and 24 hours after discontinuing abciximab or prior to patient discharge. If thrombocytopenia is verified, then the following should be employed (see Table A-14).

Table A-14

Platelet count	Action
< 100,000 cells/mm³	Discontinue abciximab
< 60,000 cells/mm³	Discontinue aspirin and heparin
< 50,000 cells/mm³	Give platelet transfusion

Case 15

1. B The sustained-release formulation of oxycodone would be inappropriate to administer via gastric tube since crushing the tablet would eliminate the sustained-release mechanism. The drug would then have to be administered more frequently to control pain, defeating the purpose of the long-acting formulation. IV opioids, liquid formulations, and immediate-release tablets that may be crushed are viable options.

2. E Oxycodone/acetaminophen would be the most appropriate drug to start for this patient's acute postsurgical pain. The onset of action is rapid, and it can be titrated to effect. Morphine and meperidine have active metabolites that can accumulate in this patient with renal dysfunction, increasing the risk for seizures, sedation, and respiratory depression. The fentanyl patch is primarily indicated in chronic pain. The onset is slow, and the patches cannot be titrated up rapidly to cover acute pain, nor titrated down as the patient recovers and requires less opioid.

Case 16

1. D Gabapentin, a membrane stabilizer, should be continued with incremental increases in dose until pain is relieved or adverse effects occur. Individual response to neuropathic pain treatment is highly variable, with effective doses of gabapentin ranging from 300 mg/day to greater than 3000 mg/day. If there is no response, other agents may be added, one at a time. Each agent should be given an adequate trial to assess effectiveness. Imipramine, a tri-

cyclic antidepressant, is a good option with fewer anticholinergic effects and may be used instead of, or added to, an existing pain regimen. Carbamazepine, a membrane stabilizer, is associated with many CYP450 enzyme drug interactions and side effects, and is usually reserved for refractory neuropathic pain. Lidocaine, a membrane stabilizer, is used locally as a nerve block in diagnostic studies. It does not provide long-term neuropathic pain relief.

2. B Sustained-release morphine should be dosed every 8 to 12 hours. The total dose of immediate-release morphine used during the day should be added up and converted to sustained-release morphine. Immediate-release morphine may be dosed around the clock, but this is labor intensive and does not provide long periods of pain control. Methadone has a longer T½ than other immediate-release opioids, but is still dosed at least twice daily for adequate pain control. Once daily, high doses of methadone are reserved for dependence treatments. The dose may be converted to another immediate-acting agent if the patient is not experiencing satisfactory pain relief from the current regimen. Otherwise, direct conversion from an immediate-release form that is effective to its sustained formulation is preferable.

Case 17

1. E Virtually all of the oral combination products available for migraine treatment have been associated with **analgesic overuse headaches.** This phenomenon also has been noted with ergotamine. Most analgesics are recommended to be used only twice weekly to minimize the risk of this syndrome. Serotonin agonists, although still susceptible to overuse, are less prone than other agents to cause this syndrome. In patients with frequent migraine headaches (more than three migraines per month), **migraine prophylaxis** also may be a consideration (in addition to trigger avoidance). A variety of treatments are effective for migraine prophylaxis, including beta-blockers (propranolol), calcium channel blockers (verapamil), anticonvulsants (divalproex sodium), and tricyclic antidepressants.

2. A Cluster headaches typically develop over 5 to 15 minutes and resolve within 90 minutes. Due to the short duration of the headache attacks, oral pharmacologic therapy is often ineffective. Narcotics are often not effective in treating cluster headaches. Oxygen therapy is very effective for aborting cluster headaches, but is limited by inconvenience. Ergotamine sublingual tablets are an inexpensive, quick option for treatment. Another alternative, if the patient is agreeable to giving himself or herself an injection, would be sumatriptan SC. It is an effective, rapid treatment for cluster headaches. Cluster headache prophylaxis may be a consideration for the future if abortive therapy is ineffective, or the patient continues to have frequent headaches (cluster headaches have been reported up to eight times per day in some patients).

Case 18

1. B In patients with low albumin, their phenytoin levels should be "corrected," because phenytoin is a highly protein bound drug. In this patient with an albumin of 2.8 g/dL, her phenytoin level of

5 μg/mL functions as a level of 7 to 8 μg/mL (still below the desired target), necessitating a dose adjustment. If a patient has the phenytoin level drawn a few hours after taking the dose, the level will appear falsely elevated. This patient's level was drawn appropriately, and her compliance was verified. The therapeutic level of an antiepileptic is only as effective as the control of a patient's seizures. Although 10 to 20 μg/mL is generally the target for phenytoin, based on patient presentation, the target may differ. In a patient such as this one, with no history of seizures, a target of at least 10 μg/mL is typically the goal. Her transaminases were normal and would not influence a decision to change her dosage at this time.

2. C Valproic acid can be given IV while the patient is NPO and then she can be converted back to her oral regimen as soon as possible. Valproic acid has no interactions with propoxyphene or doxycycline. Valproic acid troughs (not peak levels) should be monitored to ensure minimal effective concentrations.

Case 19

1. E Respiratory depression is seen with benzodiazepines (lorazepam, diazepam) and with barbiturates (phenobarbital, pentobarbital). Both classes are associated with sedation, somnolence, and respiratory depression. However, both phenytoin and fosphenytoin do not affect respiratory rate.

2. F Lorazepam is less lipid soluble than diazepam, and hence has a longer duration of activity in the CNS. Diazepam is quicker acting in the brain than lorazepam due to its high lipophilicity, but quickly exits out of the brain to fatty tissues (statement A). Phenytoin has a higher incidence of hypotension and cardiac arrhythmias than fosphenytoin (statement B). Once you achieve seizure control with a benzodiazepine, a longer-acting anticonvulsant is necessary to ensure adequate serum levels in the system. Phenytoin or fosphenytoin should be administered as well (statement C). After two failed trials of either phenytoin or fosphenytoin, the next preferred agent is phenobarbital (statement D). Status epilepticus is defined as more than **30** minutes of continuous seizure activity (statement E).

Case 20

1. A Benzodiazepines have long been used to treat social phobia, but RM is particularly afraid of the potential for physiologic and psychological dependence. Buspirone has not been found to be particularly effective for social phobia. Beta-blockers may be worth considering, particularly if his symptoms are more suggestive of stage fright, but issues around decreased exercise tolerance may discourage their use in a professional athlete such as RM. Because SSRIs are quite effective for this condition, sertraline and paroxetine are excellent options to consider, and because paroxetine appears to carry a greater propensity for weight gain, sertraline is the preferred treatment in this patient.

2. C The abrupt discontinuation of long-term benzodiazepines may precipitate a serious withdrawal syndrome consisting of anxiety, restlessness, insomnia, agitation, sensory disturbances, and diaphoresis. Seizures may result from the abrupt discontinuation of benzodiazepines, although this is much more common with the more potent short-/intermediate-acting agents (e.g., alprazolam, triazolam). The onset of withdrawal symptoms is usually 2 to 3 days for short-/intermediate-acting agents, and 5 to 6 days for longer-acting benzodiazepines (e.g., clonazepam).

Case 21

1. B Sexual dysfunction is generally believed to be a dose-dependent side effect with SSRIs and may be relieved or prevented with lower doses. Although RH may run the risk of relapse at a lower dose, many patients will achieve a therapeutic response at lower doses. If this approach is unsuccessful, bupropion is an excellent antidote and may also provide additional antidepressant effects (i.e., augmentation). Sildenafil has actually been found to reverse SSRI-induced sexual dysfunction but is an expensive alternative with potential cardiovascular complications that should only be considered after other measures fail.

2. C Although a more complete history and physical examination is recommended to confirm the diagnosis (including vitals, CK, LFT, BUN/CR, and complete medication history), the constellation of symptoms that this patient is reporting is strongly suggestive of SSRI withdrawal syndrome. It is now widely recognized that the abrupt discontinuation of certain antidepressants (most notably paroxetine and venlafaxine) will precipitate the sudden onset of symptoms 48 to 72 hours after drug discontinuation. Although this syndrome is ordinarily self-limiting, it can be quite uncomfortable for patients or incapacitating. Often, younger patients are reluctant to take psychotropic medications for a full course of therapy, and it is quite possible that she stopped the venlafaxine when she felt better or simply ran out. It may be necessary to remind her that antidepressants need to be continued for at least 4 to 9 months after remission is achieved. If the antidepressant is to be discontinued at a later date, it should be slowly tapered over a few weeks.

Case 22

1. C Risperidone. Although the incidence of adverse effects associated with hyperprolactinemia is rare with atypical antipsychotics, risperidone can increase prolactin levels in a dose-dependent manner. Blockade of the dopaminergic tone in the hypothalamus and 5HT-2 antagonism by risperidone may explain this effect. Other adverse effects associated with persistent prolactin elevation include sexual dysfunction, female menstrual disorders, and reduced bone mineral density.

2. B Diphenhydramine. Diphenhydramine would not be the optimal choice in this patient who is also taking haloperidol. Anticholinergic agents such as diphenhydramine have the potential to decrease the efficacy of antipsychotic agents due to their effects on the cholinergic-dopamine receptor balance. The other agents do not significantly interact with antipsychotic medications.

Case 23

1. B Triazolam. Triazolam has short onset of action and short duration of action. These properties increase the risk for withdrawal reactions. The other benzodiazepines have longer durations of action that decrease the potential for withdrawal reactions.

2. D Bupropion. Bupropion is the only agent that has the highest likelihood of causing jitteriness and insomnia at therapeutic doses. All of the other choices have significant sedative properties. Trazodone is commonly used as a hypnotic rather than as an antidepressant.

Case 24

1. A Methimazole has a longer $T\frac{1}{2}$ than PTU and can be dosed once daily; PTU requires three to four daily doses, which may affect compliance. PTU does not cause pretibial myxedema; rather Graves' hyperthyroidism leads to pretibial myxedema. Methimazole does not interact with amiodarone; however, amiodarone can affect thyroid function, leading to both hypo- and hyperthyroidism. PTU therapy may result in spontaneous remission, but patients typically require therapy for many years (1 to 15 years).

2. B Of the thioamides, PTU is less likely to cross the placenta compared with methimazole and is the preferred agent in pregnancy. PTU is also preferred over methimazole because it decreases the peripheral conversion of T_4 to T_3, whereas methimazole does so minimally. Both thioamides are used before surgery to decrease thyroid hormone stores and prevent intraoperative complications. PTU is routinely used during thyroid storm and not myxedema coma.

Case 25

1. D Levothyroxine is the drug of choice for hypothyroidism since it provides the necessary hormone without causing the increase peak effect of T_3 administration. Levothyroxine is converted to T_3 in the periphery. Liotrix contains T_4 and T_3 in a 4:1 ratio. This combination is not necessary since the T_4 is converted to T_3 and the short $T\frac{1}{2}$ of liotrix requires multiple daily doses. Desiccated thyroid is unreliable in potency since it is standardized to iodine content and not to T_4 or T_3 content. Triiodothyronine is also not preferred since rapid gastric absorption can lead to hyperthyroid symptoms and can lead to cardiac effects.

2. C Calcium carbonate can interfere with the absorption of levothyroxine in the GI tract and may lead to inadequate replacement. Digoxin requirements may be decreased during hypothyroidism due to a decrease in metabolic breakdown of digoxin. Rifampin and phenytoin are both CYP450 enzyme inducers that will increase levothyroxine breakdown in the liver, requiring higher levothyroxine doses. During hypothyroidism, an increase in warfarin dose may be necessary since hypothyroidism decreases turnover of clotting factors. Warfarin does not directly interfere with levothyroxine absorption.

Case 26

1. D She is currently experiencing hypoglycemic episodes in the mid-afternoon. This can be attributed to too much insulin lispro at lunchtime. It also would be a good idea to assess her food intake at each meal to see if she has consistent carbohydrate intake. While an A1C of 7.1% is close to goal, she is not in good glycemic control because she is experiencing hypoglycemia with her current insulin regimen.

2. E Absorption of SC insulin can be affected by a number of factors. In order to achieve the most predictable pattern absorption of insulin, it is important to minimize factors that can affect the absorption. In general, factors that increase blood flow to the site of injection will increase the insulin absorption rate. For example, patients should not take a shower immediately after injecting insulin as heat can cause the insulin to be absorbed more quickly. Lipohypertrophy can result when a person uses the same injection site repeatedly. Fat deposits can build up, which will cause a delay in insulin absorption.

Case 27

1. B AK has renal dysfunction and therefore metformin is contraindicated. Use of an alpha-glucosidase inhibitor would likely not achieve the target A1C, which requires a 1.5% lowering to attain the goal of less than 7%. He is not overweight (BMI is in normal range of 18.5 to 24.9). Therefore, a sulfonylurea would be an appropriate oral agent to select. It is important to select a sulfonylurea that is metabolized to inactive metabolites given his renal dysfunction. In renal dysfunction, metabolites can accumulate; thus, using a sulfonylurea with active metabolites would increase the risk of hypoglycemia. While not a choice in the answers, a thiazolidinedione would be a possibility. However, in a thin patient, where insulin resistance is likely playing a lesser role in hyperglycemia, a thiazolidinedione would not be the most appropriate choice. Thiazolidinediones also require frequent liver function monitoring (every month for the first year and periodically thereafter). Thiazolidindiones bind to the PPARγ (peroxisome proliferator activated receptor, gamma) nuclear receptors, which causes an upregulation of the glucose transporter, GLUT 4, resulting in enhanced insulin sensitivity.

2. A The blood pressure goal for a person with diabetes is less than 130/80 mm Hg. His blood pressure is well controlled on the ACE inhibitor benazepril. His A1C is above goal at 7.8% (goal is less than 7%). The LDL-C goal for a person with diabetes is less than 100 mg/dL (HDL cholesterol more than 45 mg/dL in men; TG less than 150 mg/dL); he is above goal with an LDL-C of 137 mg/dL. He should have a dilated retinal examination at least once yearly and a pneumococcal vaccination at least once. A one-time revaccination is recommended for people over 64 years of age if they were previously vaccinated at less than 65 years of age and it was administered more than 5 years ago. Finally, a microalbumiuria test is recommended annually, which requires a patient to bring a urine sample to the laboratory for assessment of protein in the urine (and thus renal function).

Case 28

1. E Response to a change in therapy should be evaluated at 6 weeks. Upon achieving goals, response to therapy and patient adherence should be evaluated every 4 to 6 months.

2. F Before initiating statin therapy, it is recommended to have baseline measurements of the lipoprotein profile and LFTs. If the LFTs are more than three times the upper limit of normal (ULN), statins should be avoided. If the LFTs are less than three times the ULN, statin therapy can be initiated, but the patient should be monitored closely. If LFTs become elevated, reversal of the transaminase elevation is common upon discontinuation of the statin. Some experts also recommend obtaining a baseline creatine kinase (CK) level. If the CK level is more than 10 times the ULN while on a statin, the statin should be discontinued. The combination of a statin with niacin or a fibrate should be used cautiously because of an increased risk of myopathy. Although most statins are taken at dinner or bedtime, atorvastatin can be taken at any time of the day due to its longer T½ (~14 hours). Lovastatin should be taken with food because this increases its bioavailabilty.

Case 29

1. A The preferred treatment for exercise-induced bronchospasm is pretreatment with a short-acting inhaled β₂-agonist (e.g., albuterol) just prior to exercise. Aerosolized albuterol induces bronchodilatation shortly after administration, and JC should be instructed to use his albuterol inhaler 5 to 15 minutes before engaging in physical activity. Oral β₂-agonists are not recommended due to the increased potential for systemic adverse effects (tremor, tachycardia) and slower onset of action. Similarly, nonselective β₂-agonists (epinephrine, metaproterenol) are not recommended due to the increased potential for excessive cardiac stimulation. Regular administration of short-acting inhaled β₂-agonists is not recommended in the management of intermittent asthma due to the increased risk of adverse effects without additional clinical benefit. Although daily administration of inhaled corticosteroids is effective in the management of EIB, given JC's mild intermittent asthma symptoms, the initiation of high-dose inhaled corticosteroid therapy is not appropriate at this time.

2. D This patient has symptoms consistent with oral candidiasis (thrush), a fungal infection caused by *Candida albicans.* Thrush presents as discrete white plaques or small red spots on the oral (especially the tongue) and pharyngeal mucosa. The lesions are generally painless, but some patients experience "burning" pain or pain on swallowing. Other symptoms of thrush include nausea and taste alterations. Oral candidiasis is one of the most common side effects associated with inhaled corticosteroids. Local corticosteroid deposition on the oral and pharyngeal mucosa facilitates fungal colonization and overgrowth. Thrush is more likely to occur with high doses of inhaled corticosteroids. Appropriate preventative measures include the use of a spacer device and rinsing of the oral cavity with water after inhalation to decrease oral and pharyngeal corticosteroid deposition. All inhaled corticosteroid formulations cause thrush, and the substitution of an alternative corticosteroid without instituting the above measures is unlikely to help. Oral corticosteroids are associated with more severe systemic side effects and should not be used in the management of asthma unless absolutely necessary.

Case 30

1. C PJ is exhibiting symptoms of COPD progression with increasing shortness of breath, cough, and sputum production. The patient is currently receiving a short-acting inhaled β_2-agonist as needed for shortness of breath with limited symptomatic relief. Inhaled corticosteroids should be reserved for patients with a documented spirometric response to corticosteroids or for those patients with moderate-severe COPD (FEV$_1$ < 50% predicted) and frequent exacerbations requiring treatment with antibiotics or systemic corticosteroids. Chronic use of systemic corticosteroids has not been shown to improve outcomes and should be avoided due to an increased risk of serious adverse effects. Combination therapy with bronchodilators with different mechanisms of action (e.g., β_2-agonists and anticholinergics) may enhance therapeutic response with a reduced incidence of adverse effects. Given PJ's worsening symptoms on albuterol monotherapy, the addition of ipratropium is a reasonable intervention at this time. Antimicrobial therapy, while effective in the treatment of COPD exacerbation in patients with purulent sputum, has no prophylactic role in the chronic management of COPD. Although patients with COPD often experience chronic cough, the regular use of antitussives is not recommended due to the protective role of cough in clearing respiratory secretions. Furthermore, narcotics such as codeine should be used with caution in patients with COPD due to the potential for respiratory depression.

2. E Adverse reactions associated with β_2-agonist therapy are primarily caused by stimulation of beta-receptors outside the respiratory tract. Hypotension can occur as a result of stimulation of β_2-receptors in the peripheral vasculature. Tachycardia is commonly observed and may be a reflex response to reduced peripheral vascular resistance or a direct effect resulting from stimulation of β_1-receptors in cardiac tissue because β_2-selectivity may be lost with high-dose therapy. Even with recommended dosing, skeletal muscle tremor and CNS tremor are common adverse effects. It is unlikely that albuterol would contribute to somnolence in this clinical setting. Stimulation of beta-receptors in hepatocytes and skeletal muscle promotes glycogenolysis and the intracellular movement of potassium, resulting in hyperglycemia and hypokalemia.

Case 31

1. B Diphenhydramine is effective at treating EPS or dystonic reactions associated with extended or high-dose antipsychotic or phenothiazine use. EPS or dystonic symptoms are due to dopamine antagonism and the subsequent central imbalance between dopamine and acetylcholine. These symptoms may be treated with anticholinergic agents, including antimuscarinic agents such as benztropine and trihexyphenidyl. Many providers prefer to use antihistamines because they are associated with less severe adverse reactions. Antihistamines, however, have different levels of anticholinergic activity. Diphenhydramine has a high anticholinergic profile, whereas tripelennamine, brompheniramine,

cyproheptadine, and cetirizine have moderate to low anticholinergic profiles and would not be as effective at treating these reactions.

2. E A transdermal scopolamine disc has an onset of action of 4 hours and provides 72 hours of continuous antiemetic coverage. This option would provide long-lasting antiemetic medication without the need for frequent dosing. Meclizine is an antihistamine that is very helpful in preventing vertigo, nausea, and vomiting associated with motion sickness, but it would require frequent dosing and its adverse effect profile may be augmented in this elderly patient. Chlorpheniramine also has undesirable side effects, and has a low level of anticholinergic activity so may not be as effective in the prevention and treatment of motion sickness. Loratadine and fexofenadine, second-generation antihistamines, are structurally more polar compounds, preventing penetration into the CNS. As a result of the lack of CNS penetration, these antihistamines tend to have less antiemetic or sedative effects and are primarily used for the treatment of seasonal allergies.

Case 32

1. E Due to her concomitant disease states, AK should avoid beta-blockers, adrenergic agents, and sulfa medications. Pilocarpine is not a good choice for AK due to its bothersome local side effects. Latanoprost is a good initial choice for AK due to its convenient once daily dosing and mild local and systemic side effects.

2. D JC is most likely suffering from brimonidine-induced conjunctivitis. Brimonidine, an α_2-agonist, concentrates locally in the conjunctiva upon instillation and may act as an α_1-agonist to cause conjunctivitis. Hence, other α_1-agonists such as epinephrine, dipivefrin, and tetrahydrozoline (Visine) should also be avoided. Brinzolamide is a carbonic anhydrase inhibitor which causes conjunctivitis in fewer than 1% of patients and would be a good alternative. JC should be encouraged to remain compliant since glaucoma is a progressive disease without a known cure.

Case 33

1. B Mannitol is the preferred hyperosmotic agent in treating glaucoma accompanied by hyperemia or uveitis because it does not penetrate the eye as well as the other agents. Agents that enter the eye readily produce a lower osmotic gradient and a shorter duration of action. Because inflammation greatly increases ocular permeability, agents such as glycerin and urea are not as favorable as mannitol.

2. E If the IOP is not reduced prior to surgery, surgical manipulation may induce the ciliary process to increase production of aqueous humor, therefore raising the IOP even further. Hence, the IOP needs to be lowered before surgery can be performed. Strong miotic agents, such as pilocarpine 10%, are contraindicated because they may potentiate angle closure. TK's initial treatment should include pilocarpine 2% to 4%, timolol, acetazolamide, and a hyperosmotic agent that is not contraindicated in a diabetic patient with poor renal function. Apraclonidine may also be considered presurgically to further reduce/stabilize the IOP.

Case 34

1. E Antiplatelet and anticoagulant medications such as aspirin and warfarin would increase the risk of bleeding during surgery. Heparin and anticoagulant therapy will likely be required, however, immediately postoperatively because this surgery involves the lower extremity and will require prolonged immobilization. COC use should be discontinued at least 4 weeks prior to surgery to avoid increasing the risk of blood clots postsurgically. COC use should be reinitiated only after the patient is ambulating.

2. B A mean delay of 10 months is observed after the discontinuation of Depo-Provera injections. All of the other formulations listed are associated with minimal delay in return to fertility (typically 1 month or less).

Case 35

1. C Oral administration of estrogen may increase the synthesis of triglycerides due to first-pass metabolism. Transdermal estrogen will alleviate a majority of her menopausal symptoms, while avoiding first-pass metabolism. Because MJ has an intact uterus, she should receive progesterone in combination with an estrogen to prevent endometrial hyperplasia. Topical progesterone is insufficient in avoiding endometrial hyperplasia caused by transdermal estrogen. Vaginal estrogen/progesterone may improve vaginal atrophy, but is unlikely to affect her hot flashes.

2. E The addition of testosterone to HRT regimens can promote new bone formation, improve libido and sex drive, and improve moodiness, anxiety, and irritability (psychological symptoms). Negative effects, however, can include hirsutism, virilization, an increase in acne, and a reduction in HDL-C.

Case 36

1. A Postpartum hemorrhage (PPH) is still one of the leading causes of maternal mortality worldwide. Because it is often due to uterine atony, it can generally be well controlled pharmacologically with uterotonic agents such as oxytocin and prostaglandins. PGE_{1M} and $PGF_{2\alpha}$ are the commonly used prostaglandins for PPH, since PGE_2 causes more adverse reactions when given systemically. Methergine (methylergonovine), an ergot alkaloid is also used for PPH, but because of its contractile effect on vascular smooth muscle, it is relatively contraindicated in patients with uncontrolled HTN. Heparin is an anticoagulant used to treat thrombotic events, and would be contraindicated in any case of excessive bleeding. IV estrogen stabilizes the endometrial lining and is used to treat bleeding in menorrhagia. It has not been used in the setting of PPH.

2. E Patients with prior vaginal deliveries generally have more successful inductions. In this patient who has a favorable cervix, already dilated to 3 cm, there is no reason to undergo cervical

ripening so prostaglandins are unnecessary. Similarly, laminaria tents and the use of a Foley bulb to dilate the cervix further would be unnecessary. In addition to oxytocin, the other way to induce her labor is via artificial rupture of the membranes.

Case 37

1. A In this patient with well-documented CAD who is s/p CABG, either terbutaline or nifedipine would be contraindicated. It is not entirely clear which would be the safest, but based on studies, the use of nifedipine in patients with documented CAD can lead to an increase in mortality. Of the other three, the next most dangerous medication is likely to be $MgSO_4$, which can lead to cardiopulmonary arrest at toxic levels. The safest choice between indomethacin and the oxytocin antagonist is difficult to sort out. Indomethacin has a higher risk characterization at baseline than the oxytocin antagonist, and in a patient with CAD, there should be concerns about renal function which is an issue with NSAIDs.

2. C There are a subgroup of patients who will have frequent uterine contractions with minimal cervical change for long periods of time in the third trimester. Although PO agents, nifedipine and terbutaline have not been shown to improve the outcome preterm delivery, they have been shown to decrease contractions and with that, patient anxiety. IV $MgSO_4$ is not commonly used long-term and can be associated with bone loss and hypocalcemia if it is. SC terbutaline and IV ritodrine are also not commonly used long term. There are several studies looking at SC terbutaline used at home on pumps, and not only has efficacy not been shown, it has been associated with adverse events. The oxytocin antagonists are not used other than in IV form at this point.

Case 38

1. B Methylprednisolone. Given the patient's electrolyte abnormalities, all of the other corticosteroid options would be ruled out since they have mineralocorticoid effects that may make this patient's electrolyte abnormalities worse. Methylprednisolone has anti-inflammatory properties and no mineralocorticoid activity. For patients who are hospitalized and present with electrolyte abnormalities, corticosteroids with high anti-inflammatory properties and minimal mineralocorticoid activity are preferred.

2. D Hydrocortisone. Hydrocortisone is the only corticosteroid that is available as suppositories, enemas, and foams for rectal use. It is the best choice for this patient since the rectal route may have the potential to minimize systemic toxicities (i.e., behavioral disturbances, insomnia) that the patient previously experienced with the IV and PO corticosteroids. This patient's exacerbation is mild and his disease is localized to the rectum and distal colon. Therefore, per rectum corticosteroids will be able to target these areas successfully.

Case 39

1. D Indomethacin is a drug of choice for an acute gout attack. Because he has no history of ulcer disease, there is no evidence that this patient would not tolerate this NSAID. Indomethacin has a short T½ that will result in a fast onset of action to relieve the pain. Prednisone and colchicine are not first-line agents for treatment of acute gout. Allopurinol and probenecid are agents used to prevent acute gout attacks and as treatment in patients with symptomatic hyperuricemia.

2. C This patient is a candidate for allopurinol. Allopurinol is the drug of choice for patients with renal impairment. Probenecid is not recommended for patients with a CrCl rate of less than 50 mL/min. Indomethacin, ibuprofen, and colchicine are agents to treat acute gouty attacks.

Case 40

1. E Naproxen would be the reasonable choice because of the relatively infrequent (twice to three times daily) dosing regimen and more tolerable side effect profile compared with aspirin and indomethacin. Celecoxib and rofecoxib would be alternatives if the patient could not tolerate naproxen. These agents should be reserved for patients with known GI bleeding disorders or intolerance to the other nonspecific NSAIDs. COX-2 inhibitors are still second-line therapy due to high cost and not well studied for the treatment of OA.

2. A Acetaminophen would be the drug of choice to try in this patient. If an adequate response were not achieved, due to the patient's age and medical history, it would be reasonable to begin a COX-2 inhibitor such as celecoxib. Aspirin, ibuprofen, and indomethacin should be avoided in this patient with a history of GI bleeding.

Case 41

1. E Naproxen would be the best choice for this patient. Although aspirin is less expensive than naproxen and equally efficacious, the convenient dosing regimen and improved side effect profile makes naproxen a better choice. Celecoxib and rofecoxib (COX-2 inhibitors) should be reserved for patients who are intolerant of the other NSAIDs due to their increased cost and similar efficacy. Sulfasalazine is a second-line agent for RA.

2. C Hydroxychloroquine would be a reasonable choice for this patient. It is hard to predict how a specific DMARD will work in an individual patient. SSZ is not an option since the patient has a sulfa allergy. MTX could be another alternative, but it has more side effects than HCQ. It can be reserved for use at a later time if an adequate response is not achieved with HCQ. Injectable gold is quite toxic, and patients must be willing to give themselves injections.

Case 42

1. A Famotidine, as well as some of the other antisecretory agents, can lead to headaches, dizziness, and other CNS side effects. This is particularly true in older patients or in those with compromised renal elimination.

2. C Of the agents listed, only tetracycline has activity against *H. pylori* when used in combination with other antimicrobials. Although doxycycline belongs to the tetracycline family, it has not been shown to have activity against *H. pylori.* Miconazole is an antifungal agent and has no activity against *H. pylori.* Amoxicillin but not ampicillin has activity against *H. pylori.*

Case 43

1. A PPIs are most effective when given 30 minutes before a meal or breakfast (and not with food). This ensures that large amounts of inactive H^+/K^+-ATPase pumps are present. PPIs should not be coadministered with H_2 antagonists. PPIs work best if taken routinely to promote healing rather than on an as-needed basis.

2. E Cardiac arrhythmias have been observed when cisapride has been used at greater than recommended doses or in those patients taking drugs that are CYP450 inhibitors. Cisapride can help to relieve constipation and nausea because it has prokinetic effects, facilitating the emptying of gastric contents. Cough and anemia also may resolve because cisapride will help to reduce the frequency of reflux episodes and allow time for healing of the esophageal erosions.

Case 44

1. E Lorazepam is most effective for anticipatory nausea and vomiting, or emesis that occurs prior to chemotherapy administration. The antiemetic effects may be related to the sedative and anxiolytic properties of lorazepam. $5-HT_3$ antagonists and dopamine antagonists are poor choices because efficacy has not been shown in anticipatory nausea and vomiting.

2. C Metoclopramide with dexamethasone has been shown to be effective in delayed nausea and vomiting, which occurs more than 24 hours after chemotherapy administration and may last as long as 7 days. Cisplatin is a classic agent that causes significant delayed nausea and vomiting. 5-HT3 antagonists, even in combination with dexamethasone, have not been shown to be effective for delayed nausea and vomiting. Metoclopramide may be given in high doses, but dystonic and EPS reactions often associated with such high doses makes this an undesirable choice (even with coadministration of diphenhydramine).

Case 45

1. C Calcium and iron supplementation are common causes of constipation. Polycarbophil, a bulk-forming laxative, exerts its therapeutic effect by increasing the mass and water content of stool and by speeding transit time in the colon. Cascara sagrada and sennosides are cathartics, which speed colonic transit time and alter water and electrolyte transport across the colonic mucosa. Sodium biphosphonate is a saline cathartic, which increases intestinal peristalsis by osmotic properties. Docusate sodium is a stool softener that allows penetration of the stool by fat and water, facilitating its transport through the intestines.

2. D When diarrhea or frequent bowel movements are experienced with the use of laxatives, the laxatives should be held until resolution of diarrhea. Lactulose can be used routinely, especially in patients who have failed stool softeners or bulk-forming laxatives. Lactulose can be titrated to number of stools per day by increasing or decreasing the dose and frequency. Cathartics and mineral oil should not be used on a daily or regular basis.

Case 46

1. D The patient has signs and symptoms consistent with cellulitis. Because the patient does not have any drug allergies and requires an oral outpatient regimen, cephalexin is the best choice. Cephalexin provides adequate empiric coverage against the most likely pathogens that cause cellulitis, *Streptococcus pyogenes* and *Staphylococcus aureus*.

2. D Because the patient is exhibiting signs of an IgE-mediated reaction to nafcillin, the best choice is a non–beta-lactam antibiotic with good gram-positive activity such as clindamycin. While rare, IgE-mediated reactions or type 1 reactions to penicillin are the most worrisome adverse effects. IgE-mediated reactions usually occur within 72 hours of starting penicillin and are characterized by laryngeal edema, wheezing, and urticaria. Anaphylaxis usually occurrs within the first hour of administration. In this patient, it would be prudent to avoid the use of cephalosporins as well since the risk for cross-reactivity between penicillins and cephalosporins is 3% to 7%.

Case 47

1. B The potential for antagonism exists when two beta-lactam antibiotics are used in combination. Carbapenems are unsuitable in combination with another beta-lactam because they are potent inducers of beta-lactamases. Although both agents have similar adverse event profiles, overlapping spectrums of activity, and are both renally excreted, these are not contraindications to use the two agents together. Also, imipenem is not inactivated by tazobactam.

2. F Meropenem is the best choice. Ertapenem and ampicillin/sulbactam do not adequately cover *Acinetobacter baumannii*. Also, with her history of renal insufficiency and seizures, imipenem would not be appropriate because the patient would be at increased risk for seizures.

Case 48

1. E Because JK has experienced anaphylaxis to amoxicillin, prescription of any type of penicillin or cephalosporin should be avoided. Cross-reactivity between penicillins and cephalosporins is incomplete, but with a history of anaphylaxis to penicillins, cephalosporins should not be prescribed. Clindamycin would be an appropriate alternative to use to treat the cellulitis.

2. C Cephalosporins do not have clinically significant drug interactions. However, drugs containing a methylthiotetrazole group such as cefotetan can cause disulfiram-like reactions when taken with ethanol. While MN is receiving cefotetan he will have to refrain from drinking alcohol.

Case 49

1. A Although pneumococcus remains the most common cause of acute otitis media, CT's otitis media is due to *Haemophilus influenzae*, a gram-negative coccobacilli. Although amoxicillin is active against *H. influenzae*, approximately 30% of *H. influenzae* strains in the United States are beta-lactamase producing; thus, CT may be infected with a beta-lactamase-producing strain. The addition of clavulanic acid to amoxicillin prevents the degradation of the amoxicillin beta-lactam ring. Levofloxacin is not indicated due to early reports of tendonitis in young animals given fluoroquinolones. Similarly, tetracyclines are not indicated in children under 8 years of age due to their deposition in bone and tooth, and propensity to cause tooth discoloration. Erythromycin does not have activity against *H. influenzae*, unlike clarithromycin and azithromycin.

2. C Metoclopramide is the best choice. Erythromycin and cisapride can cause QTc prolongation, particularly in patients with pre-existing cardiac disease or receiving antiarrhythmics. Although azithromycin is less likely to cause QTc prolongation compared to erythromycin, it is also not as effective at stimulating GI motility as erythromycin.

Case 50

1. B Nongonococcal urethritis is primarily caused by *C. trachomatis*. Infections caused *by C. trachomatis* can be treated with tetracyclines, azithromycin, or macrolides. Doxycyline is contraindicated in pregnant women because of the effects on fetal teeth and bone growth. In the setting of pregnancy, erythromycin is the recommended regimen; however, preliminary data suggest that azithromycin is also safe and effective.

2. C The tetracyclines interact with multivalent cations such as Ca^{+2}, Mg^{+2}, Fe^{+2}, or Al^{+3}. The major mechanism of these drug interactions is the formation of iron-drug complexes (chelation or binding of iron by the involved drug).

Case 51

1. C Ciprofloxacin is the best choice due to its good penetration into the prostate. Although TMP-SMX also has good penetration into the prostate, it should be avoided due to his allergy to sulfa medications. Beta-lactams and nitrofurantoin are not used for prostatitis because they do not adequately penetrate into the prostate.

2. D Trimethoprim is the best option since it can be taken by patients with sulfa allergies and has not been shown to increase

QTc interval. Gatifloxacin and moxifloxacin should be avoided in this situation due to her cardiac history and increased risk of QTc prolongation with the quinolones. Also, due to the minimal excretion of moxifloxacin into the urine, it is not a preferred agent for UTIs. TMP-SMX should be avoided due to her history of anaphylaxis to sulfa medications.

Case 52

1. H Risk factors for ototoxicity include preexisting renal dysfunction, prolonged therapy, and concomitant receipt of other ototoxic drugs such as furosemide. Because KC is only 45 years old, age is not a risk factor. Beta-lactam antibiotics and ACE inhibitors are not typically ototoxic and would not contribute to KC's otoxoticity.

2. C Of the aminoglycosides, tobramycin has the best activity against *P. aeruginosa*. Streptomycin is typically reserved for infections due to *mycobacterium* tuberculosis. Amikacin is typically reserved for resistant gram-negative infections or infections due to atypical mycobacteria. Neomycin is an oral agent that is poorly absorbed in the GI tract and is used for GI decontamination only.

Case 53

1. C Treatment for catheter-related infections is often initiated empirically, with definitive therapy based on culture results and susceptibility. Dialysis catheters are usually permanently inserted lines, and patients on chronic hemodialysis are at higher risk for developing catheter-related infections secondary to staphylococcal species, particularly coagulase-negative staphylococci. Oral vancomycin is not appropriate because it does not achieve adequate blood levels to treat systemic infections.

2. F "Red man" syndrome is an infusion-related reaction that is mediated by release of histamine and is not considered a hypersensitivity or allergic reaction. Thus, treatment with epinephrine is not warranted. In patients who experience red man syndrome, prolonging the duration of infusion or premedication with diphenhydramine will prevent further reactions.

Case 54

1. B Antibiotic-associated diarrhea due to *C. difficile* can occur with any antibiotic, but particularly with clindamycin. With the administration of antibiotics, normal GI flora is inhibited, which allows *C. difficile* to overgrow. Metronidazole is the treatment of choice for *C. difficile* infections. Although oral vancomycin also has activity against *C. difficile*, it is typically used as second-line treatment.

2. C Alcohol ingestion should be avoided when taking metronidazole. The coadministration of alcohol with metronidazole can result in an uncomfortable disulfiram-like reaction in patients due to inhibition of aldehyde dehydrogenase, leading to an accumulation of acetaldehyde. A disulfiram reaction manifests as flushing, nausea, vomiting, throbbing headache, sweating, and HTN. The effect may last 30 minutes in mild cases to several hours in severe cases.

Case 55

1. D The most appropriate therapy would be a neuraminidase inhibitor such as oseltamivir since amantadine and rimantadine do not cover influenza B. Treatment of influenza must be initiated within 48 hours of symptoms for maximum efficacy. Influenza vaccination is only effective for the prevention of influenza and not for symptomatic therapy. If this were influenza A and amantadine was chosen to treat this patient, dose adjustments would be necessary due to her renal insufficiency. She would also be at increased risk of CNS toxicity due to her age and possible accumulation of the drug due to her renal insufficiency.

2. A Because CD is currently receiving amantadine for Parkinson's disease, he does not require additional prophylaxis with rimantadine because both medications are equally effective for the treatment and prophylaxis of influenza A. Zanamivir is unnecessary because he does not need additional prophylaxis for influenza B. In addition, zanamivir may cause bronchospasms in patients with asthma or chronic obstructive pulmonary disease. If CD requires zanamivir in the future, he should be instructed to use his beta-agonist inhaler prior to zanamivir.

Case 56

1. E The dose of ganciclovir should be decreased due to his worsening renal function, which is a risk factor for increased bone marrow suppression. His neutropenia can be managed by administering filgrastim (granulocyte colony-stimulating factor) in an attempt to increase his WBC count. Cidofovir and foscarnet can both exacerbate SL's renal insufficiency so would be contraindicated at this time.

2. F Because foscarnet is an inorganic pyrophospate analogue, foscarnet can cause electrolyte disturbances, particularly hypocalcemia, and hyper- or hypophosphatemia. Thrombophlebitis with foscarnet can be severe, requiring a central line for administration. The main adverse effect of foscarnet is renal insufficiency, including acute tubular necrosis and interstitial nephritis.

Case 57

1. G Infusion-related toxicities secondary to amphotericin are common and may be prevented with premedication with diphenhydramine and acetaminophen. Meperidine is effective in halting rigors and muscle spasms. Thus, it is typically given in response to rigors, and not as premedication. Sodium loading with normal saline may prevent some of the renal toxicities, particularly prerenal azotemia, associated with amphotericin and is administered prior to amphotericin.

2. B GM is at risk for vulvovaginal candidiasis due to her poorly controlled insulin-dependent diabetes. Vulvovaginal candidiasis can be effectively treated with any of the topical azole antifungals such as clotrimazole. Because this is not a systemic infection, amphotericin is not warranted. Ketoconazole, itraconazole, and voriconazole may be alternatives in patients with refractory disease. However, ketoconazole and itraconazole require an acidic environment for adequate oral absorption. PPIs, such as omeprazole, and H_2-receptor blockers can increase the gastric pH and thus inhibit absorption. If GM required systemic therapy for treatment of her vulvovaginal candidiasis, fluconazole would be the preferred agent because it is not dependent on gastric pH for absorption.

Case 58

1. D Rifampin significantly reduces the plasma concentrations of the calcium channel blockers verapamil, diltiazem, and nifedipine. Diltiazem is a substrate of CYP3A4 and rifampin is an inducer of CYP3A4. Rifampin does not interact with metoprolol, aspirin, pravastatin, or nitroglycerin. However, if the patient had been on another HMG-CoA reductase inhibitor such as atorvastatin, lovastatin, or simvastatin instead of pravastatin, rifampin would have reduced the plasma concentrations of these agents since they are also metabolized via CYP3A4.

2. C This patient appears to be experiencing isoniazid-induced neuropathy and is at increased risk for isoniazid-induced neuropathy due to his diabetes and history of alcoholism. The treatment of choice is to add pyridoxine to his regimen. Ethambutol and rifampin are not usually associated with peripheral neuropathy. Discontinuing isoniazid is not the best option since isoniazid is a first-line agent for MTB.

Case 59

1. B Zidovudine and TMP-SMX are both known to suppress bone marrow and cause anemia. Nelfinavir, lamivudine, and fluconazole are not usually known to cause anemia.

2. E Simvastatin is metabolized by CYP3A4. Nevirapine is an inducer of CYP3A4, whereas lopinavir and ritonavir are inhibitors of CYP3A4. Thus, the effect of these two drugs on simvastatin levels is unpredictable. Lamivudine is not metabolized by the CYP450 system and will not affect simvastatin levels.

Case 60

1. F CW has decompensated liver disease (based on the findings of hepatic encephalopathy [asterexis] and presence of ascites [abdominal fluid wave and recent weight gain]). Treatment with interferon (interferon-α or pegylated interferon-α) or the combination of interferon plus ribavirin is contraindicated. Patients with decompensated liver disease do not respond well to therapy and may be at risk for further hepatic decompensation when therapy is initiated. In addition, the side effects such as bone marrow suppression, flulike symptoms, fatigue, and depression are poorly tolerated in this patient population. Ribavirin by itself is ineffective in the treatment of HCV infection.

2. D Ribavirin causes dose-related hemolytic anemia. Metabolites of ribavirin accumulate within the RBCs, which cause cell damage. Although interferon can cause anemia, it is usually the result of bone marrow suppression. Hemolytic anemia tends to occur within 1 to 2 weeks after initiation of therapy. It is recommended that a baseline hematocrit and hemoglobin be checked prior to therapy and then regularly during therapy.

Case 61

1. D Dexrazoxane. Dexrazoxane has been found to provide some protection against anthracycline-induced cardiotoxicity without compromising antitumor effectiveness. The mechanism of protection is thought to be related to intracellular iron chelation, which lessens formation of toxic oxygen free radicals. It has been most studied with doxorubicin and is indicated for patients who have received cumulative doses of doxorubicin > 300 mg/m^2 who would benefit from continued anthracycline therapy. The other agents listed do not clinically reduce cardiotoxicity from anthracyclines. Leucovorin has been used to rescue normal cells from high-dose methotrexate toxicity. Mesna binds toxic acrolein metabolites of ifosfamide and cyclophosphamide and reduces hemorrhagic cystitis. Amifostine is used to reduce renal toxicity from cisplatin. Although N-acetylcysteine has been postulated to reduce anthracycline-induced cardiotoxicity via sulfhydryl repletion and antioxidant effects, it has not been found to provide effective cardioprotection.

2. E Bilirubin. Cholestasis may dramatically impair clearance of anthracyclines (including doxorubicin), and dose reductions are recommended for elevated bilirubin levels. Diabetes and asthma are unlikely to affect doxorubicin clearance or toxicity. Although the baseline platelet count is somewhat low in this patient, the myelosuppression from anthracyclines is primarily seen as leukopenia, and thrombocytopenia is rarely severe. Because anthracyclines are primarily eliminated in the bile, renal impairment (often present in patients with multiple myeloma) does not affect routine dosing.

Case 62

1. D Cisplatin has been associated with severe hypomagnesemia. Replacement with both PO and IV supplementation has been shown to be of benefit. Cisplatin is also the most emetogenic chemotherapy agent. Blocking serotonin receptors with **serotonin type III antagonists** (ondansetron, granisetron, or dolasetron) has led to complete prevention of nausea and vomiting in approximately 50% of patients. Dacarbazine is not known to cause pulmonary toxicity, but other alkylating agents (carmustine and busulfan) have been associated with delayed **pulmonary fibrosis.** Pulmonary effects usually present as shortness of breath, nonproductive cough, and hypoxia. Steroids are often used for symptomatic treatment.

2. E Adequate hydration is absolutely necessary for the safe administration of high-dose cyclophosphamide. Often NS is used as hydration, since cyclophosphamide can be associated with the development of SIADH. The sodium will help minimize the incidence of hyponatremia. Mesna is often used with high-dose cyclophosphamide. As with ifosfamide, cyclophosphamide forms the acrolein metabolite that can be directly toxic to the bladder, leading to hemorrhagic cystitis. The incidence of hemorrhagic cystitis is much lower with cyclophosphamide than ifosfamide, so usually only higher doses (> 2000 mg) will require mesna, whereas all doses of ifosfamide should be given with mesna. High doses of cyclophosphamide can be very emetogenic. It causes both acute and delayed nausea and vomiting. Acute chemotherapy-induced nausea and vomiting (occurring within 24 hours of chemotherapy administration) is mediated by the stimulation of serotonin type III receptors which then stimulate the vomiting center. Blocking the receptors with serotonin antagonists will help minimize acute nausea and vomiting. On the other hand, delayed chemotherapy-induced nausea and vomiting (nausea and vomiting occurring more than 24 hours after chemotherapy administration) is not serotonin mediated, so the use of serotonin antagonists is of minimal benefit. Only the use of steroids, such as dexamethasone, has been shown to offer significant benefit for delayed nausea and vomiting.

Case 63

1. E All of the above conditions should be evaluated in patients receiving high-dose cytarabine. Although cytarabine is hepatically metabolized, one of the major active metabolites, Ara-U, is renally eliminated. Ara-U accumulation may lead to feedback inhibition of cytidine deaminase, which will lead to accumulation of ara-CTP, which is a neurotoxin. In the presence of renal impairment (which may be common in the elderly population), the accumulation of Ara-U may cause cerebellar toxicity. Often cerebellar toxicity is manifested as nystagmus, dysarthria, ataxia, and slurred speech. The cerebellar toxicity may be slowly reversible or it may be permanent in some cases. Cytarabine is extensively excreted through the lacrimal ducts, causing chemical conjunctivitis. The use of steroid eye drops during treatment and for at least 48 hours after the end of high-dose cytarabine may significantly minimize conjunctivitis. Rashes, characteristically starting on the soles and palms, are common with cytarabine administration. Diphenhydramine, topical steroids, and hydroxyzine are often used for pruritis associated with these rashes. Narcotic analgesics may be necessary for pain. Fevers are also a common side effect. In many situations, drug-induced fevers must be distinguished from fevers due to infections.

2. B Fluorouracil is a prodrug that is metabolized to FdUMP and a triphosphate metabolite. FdUMP binds and interferes with thymidylate synthase, whereas the triphosphate metabolite interferes with RNA function. Leucovorin is a reduced form of folic acid. Leucovorin provides folate cofactors that stabilize the binding of FdUMP and thymidylate synthase, thus enhancing the cytotoxic effects of fluorouracil.

Case 64

1. E All of the above. Vinblastine is hepatically eliminated and must be dose adjusted for hepatic dysfunction. Because vinca alkaloids may cause neurotoxicity (including paralytic ileus), it is important

to evaluate the patient's bowel status prior to administration. Of the vinca alkaloids, vinblastine is the most likely to cause severe myelosuppression (may be dose limiting), and baseline WBC counts should be obtained. Vinblastine is a vesicant. It can only be given as an IV infusion via a central line. It also may be given as a slow IV push if there is no central line and good peripheral access.

2. B Administer via a central line. The risk of extravasation is too high if a vesicant is administered via peripheral venous access. If vesicants are to be administered as a continuous infusion, a central line is mandatory. Applying warm compresses to the affected area or administration of hyaluronidase are often used as measures to treat extravasations should they occur.

Case 65

1. C It is recommended that all patients receiving paclitaxel receive pretreatment to reduce the risk and severity of hypersensitivity reactions. The preferred regimen includes a combination of a corticosteroid (such as dexamethasone), an antihistamine (diphenhydramine or equivalent), and an H_2 antagonist (such as cimetidine or ranitidine). Omeprazole and other PPIs will not block H_2-receptor sites and do not provide protection against hypersensitivity reactions.

2. E It is recommended that all of the above laboratory parameters be evaluated prior to each course of docetaxel. Myelosuppression (especially neutropenia) is dose limiting with docetaxel, and patients with absolute neutrophil counts of less than 1500/mm^3 should not receive this drug. Patients with baseline abnormalities in LFTs are at higher risk for severe side effects (including myelosuppression and death). Docetaxel should not be administered to patients with bilirubin levels above the ULN. Additionally, patients with AST or ALT levels greater than 1.5 times the ULN with concomitant alkaline phosphatase greater than 2.5 times the ULN should generally not receive docetaxel.

Case 66

1. A Irinotecan use is commonly associated with both early (within 24 hours) and late diarrhea complications. The mechanisms underlying the diarrhea may differ. The early diarrhea may be preceded by diaphoresis or abdominal cramping and is thought to be cholinergic in nature. IV atropine may be useful for patients experiencing early diarrhea. There is some thought that the cholinergic syndrome is partly mediated by serotonin receptors, and premedication with a serotonin antagonist (such as ondansetron) may be useful (in addition to preventing nausea and vomiting associated with irinotecan). However, these agents are unlikely to produce significant relief once the diarrhea starts. Loperamide is very useful in management of *late* diarrhea associated with irinotecan. Stool softeners and promotility agents should be avoided in patients receiving irinotecan.

2. E Myelosuppression (primarily neutropenia) is the dose-limiting side effect of topotecan. The median nadir occurs at about 11 days, with a duration of 7 days. Total alopecia may occur with topotecan but is not considered dose limiting. Nausea and vomiting are usually mild to moderate and can be reduced with appropriate antiemetics. Other side effects of topotecan include mild paresthesia and diarrhea.

Case 67

1. C Tamoxifen. This patient is premenopausal with a breast cancer expressing hormone receptors (ER and PR positive). She may benefit from interventions aimed at decreasing estrogenic stimulus to the cancer tissue. Because she expressed an interest in having children, oophorectomy may not be an acceptable option for her. Tamoxifen acts by inhibiting estrogen effects and may be useful in treating this type of breast cancer. Ethinyl estradiol is an estrogenic compound and should be avoided in this patient because it may stimulate the growth of her breast cancer. Letrozole acts as an aromatase inhibitor to decrease conversion of androgens to estrogens, but it is only indicated for use in women with breast cancer who are postmenopausal. Flutamide and nilutamide are antiandrogenic compounds used in the treatment of metastatic prostate cancer.

2. B Hot flashes. Anastrozole is an aromatase inhibitor used to treat metastatic breast cancer in postmenopausal women. It is generally well tolerated, although patients may experience hot flashes and other mild side effects such as diarrhea, headache, and nausea. Severe myelosuppression is unlikely. Elevated transaminases can occur infrequently in patients with liver metastases, but it is unclear whether these changes resulted from progression of liver metastases or from drug effects. Anastrozole (compared with aminoglutethimide) is a specific inhibitor of aromatase enzymes and does not prevent production of endogenous cortisol, so adrenal insufficiency would not be expected.

Case 68

1. H All of the above. Alemtuzumab is targeted against the CD52 antigen, which is expressed on many different cell types (including normal and malignant cells). As a result, this agent has been associated with profound immunosuppression, and patients are at high risk for developing opportunistic infections. Use of alemtuzumab is absolutely contraindicated in patients with active infections. In addition, it is strongly recommended that all patients undergoing treatment with this agent be given prophylactic antibiotics to prevent PCP (i.e., TMP-SMX) and herpes virus infections (i.e., acyclovir). Because alemtuzumab (like all MoAbs) can cause infusion-related reactions, including severe hypersensitivity, patients should receive acetaminophen, antihistamines, and possibly corticosteroids prior to each infusion to minimize these reactions.

2. D Gemtuzumab ozogamicin. Gemtuzumab ozogamicin contains an MoAb directed against CD33 antigens, which are expressed on immature myeloid cells and leukemic cells. The MoAb is linked to a toxin (calicheamicin), which is released inside the cells once the complex is internalized. Gemtuzumab ozogamicin is approved for treatment of adults with CD33-positive AML who are greater than 60 years of age who are not considered candidates for standard AML therapy. Rituximab is directed against CD20 antigens and is used for B-cell NHL. Trastuzumab is indicated for metastatic breast cancer in patients who overexpress Her2/neu, and alemtuzumab is used for refractory chronic lymphocytic leukemia. Daclizumab is an MoAb directed against the IL-2 receptor and is used to prevent rejection in solid organ transplantation.

Case 69

1. E All of the above. Although imatinib is relatively well tolerated compared with other antineoplastic agents, it does have a number of significant toxicities. It may cause fluid retention and edema so patients should be weighed and monitored regularly for signs of fluid retention. Fluid retention is more common in elderly patients (over 65 years) and in those patients receiving higher doses. Imatinib also may be associated with cytopenias such as neutropenia and thrombocytopenia, especially in patients in accelerated phase or blast crisis. It is recommended that complete blood counts be monitored weekly for the first month, biweekly for the second month, and periodically thereafter. Baseline LFTs are important for two reasons. First, imatinib is metabolized by the liver, and impaired liver function may lead to increased imatinib exposure. Second, hepatotoxicity has been reported in patients treated with imatinib. If patients experience elevated LFTs while on imatinib, dose reduction or treatment interruption may be considered.

2. E Itraconazole. Imatinib is primarily metabolized by the CYP3A4 hepatic enzyme system. Drugs that may inhibit this enzyme (such as ketoconazole, itraconazole, erythromycin, clarithromycin, etc.) may impair clearance of imatinib and result in increased toxicity. Imatinib itself is also a fairly potent inhibitor of the CYP3A4 enzyme and may result in toxicity due to other drugs that are substrates for this enzyme (such as simvastatin, warfarin, benzodiazepines, etc.). The other medications listed are unlikely to affect the function of CYP3A4 or interact adversely with imatinib.

Case 70

1. B Mycophenolate mofetil and other antiproliferative agents frequently cause **leukopenia** and **thrombocytopenia**. Mycophenolic acid (active form of mycophenolate mofetil) inhibits the enzyme inosine monophosphate dehydrogenase, the key enzyme in the de novo pathway for purine biosynthesis. Activated T-lymphocytes cannot use the salvage pathway for purine biosynthesis, and therefore are sensitive to the effects of mycophenolic acid. The calcineurin inhibitors, IL-2 receptor antagonists, and corticosteroids do not cause bone marrow suppression.

2. E Antithymocyte globulin can be used in the treatment of acute rejection. Antithymocyte globulin is a polyclonal antibody that is directed against T-lymphocytes that express cell surface markers such as CD2, CD3, CD4, CD8, CD25, etc. Once bound to the receptor, antithymocyte globulin inactivates the T-lymphocyte and removes it from circulation. Muromonab CD3, a monoclonal antibody, also can be used for the treatment of rejection. High-dose corticosteroids such as methylprednisolone are usually first-line therapy. If ineffective, then an antilymphocyte antibody will be used. The calcineurin inhibitors, antiproliferative agents, and IL-2 receptor antagonists are used to prevent acute rejection, not treat it.

Index